Unlocking the Potential of Patients With ADHD

Unlocking the Potential of Patients With ADHD

A MODEL FOR CLINICAL PRACTICE

VINCENT J. MONASTRA

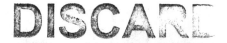
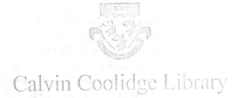
AMERICAN PSYCHOLOGICAL ASSOCIATION
WASHINGTON, DC

Published by
American Psychological Association
750 First Street, NE
Washington, DC 20002
www.apa.org

To order
APA Order Department
P.O. Box 92984
Washington, DC 20090-2984
Tel: (800) 374-2721; Direct: (202) 336-5510
Fax: (202) 336-5502; TDD/TTY: (202) 336-6123
Online: www.apa.org/books/
E-mail: order@apa.org

In the U.K., Europe, Africa, and the Middle East, copies may be ordered from
American Psychological Association
3 Henrietta Street
Covent Garden, London
WC2E 8LU England

Typeset in Goudy by Stephen McDougal, Mechanicsville, MD

Printer: Book-mart Press, Inc., North Bergen, NJ
Cover Designer: Berg Design, Albany, NY
Technical/Production Editor: Devon Bourexis

The opinions and statements published are the responsibility of the authors, and such opinions and statements do not necessarily represent the policies of the American Psychological Association.

Library of Congress Cataloging-in-Publication Data

Monastra, Vincent J.
   Unlocking the potential of patients with ADHD : a model for clinical practice / Vincent J. Monastra. — 1st ed.
      p. ; cm.
   Includes bibliographical references.
   ISBN-13: 978-1-4338-0238-6
   ISBN-10: 1-4338-0238-4
   1. Attention-deficit disorder in adolescence. 2. Attention-deficit hyperactivity disorder.
I. American Psychological Association. II. Title.
   [DNLM: 1. Attention Deficit Disorder with Hyperactivity. 2. Adolescent. 3. Child.
WS 350.8.A8 M736u 2008]
   RJ506.H9M654 2008
   618.928589—dc22
                                                                    2007017474

British Library Cataloguing-in-Publication Data
A CIP record is available from the British Library.

Printed in the United States of America
First Edition

This book is dedicated to my wife, Donna,
whose faith and wisdom inspire me, and
whose love sustains me.
To my father, James, who taught me how
to be focused and calm in the face of adversity.
To my mother, Mary, who showed me
the value of common sense.
To my big kids, Reuben and Bridget, who helped
me realize the importance of honest communication.
To my little kids, Julian and Diego, who helped me realize
that with love and perseverance, anything is possible.
To my brothers, Sam and Andrew, and my sister, Mary, who
shared so much of life's journey with me.
And to all the children, teens, and adults who
I have treated, whose pain, integrity, determination,
intelligence, humor, and noble spirit
will remain etched in my heart forever.

CONTENTS

PREFACE

When I began my professional career nearly 30 years ago, I never intended to become a specialist. During my graduate and postgraduate years of study, I believed that it was my responsibility to learn effective treatments for every condition listed in the diagnostic manual for mental health providers. I read great volumes of books and journal articles, sought supervision from highly skilled doctors, and attempted to apply the knowledge that I acquired in my daily clinical work. With a background rooted in behavioral therapy, family therapy, neuropsychology, biochemistry, and neurophysiology, I found that I was able to effectively treat a wide range of psychiatric disorders. However, there was one group of patients who appeared largely unresponsive to the strategies that I had learned during my graduate and postgraduate studies: patients presenting with attention deficits and hyperactivity.

In my early clinical work, I sought to apply principles of behavioral and systems-based therapies in the treatment of these patients but found little success. Children and teenagers diagnosed with an attention-deficit disorder (with or without hyperactivity) did not demonstrate sustained positive response to a variety of reward, response cost, or punishment paradigms, no matter how consistently applied. On a similar note, interventions designed to reduce conflict, promote parenting skills, and enhance the family relationships of these individuals yielded little sustained improvement in the patient's core attention-deficit disorder symptoms. After applying behaviorally and family-systems–based treatments for nearly a decade, I became convinced that factors other than trauma, impaired family relations, and unsystematically applied reinforcement contingencies were responsible for the onset and maintenance of attention-deficit and hyperactivity disorders.

For the next 2 decades, I concentrated on conducting studies that could contribute to an understanding of the causes of attention-deficit and hyperactivity disorders and the development of valid assessment and clinically effective treatment protocols. During this time period, I collaborated with a team of clinical researchers, who systematically collected data from patients in eight diverse regions of the United States and engaged in dialogue with some of the most highly respected clinical researchers of our time. As a result of this research and dialogue, neurophysiologically based assessment and treatment procedures were developed and examined in a series of studies, involving over 10,000 individuals who presented with impairment of attention and/ or behavioral control.

The setting for my research has been a private, outpatient clinic dedicated to the care of patients with attention deficits and/or problems of behavioral control (i.e., hyperactivity and impulsivity). The clinic is located in an upstate New York community, with a population of approximately 500,000 within a 50-mile catchment area. This region is racially and ethnically diverse and provides a wide range of employment possibilities for residents, including teaching hospitals, multiple colleges and universities, and a variety of manufacturing plants (primarily computer hardware and software). The socioeconomic status of our patients ranges widely, as we care for individuals whose finances are below the poverty level, as well as those in the lower through upper middle classes.

The purpose of this book is to provide clinicians with a practical, empirically supported model for the assessment and care of patients who present with symptoms of inattention, impulsivity, and hyperactivity. Although rooted in the clinical research conducted at our center, the model presented in this book integrates existent neurological and neurobehavioral findings reported by numerous clinical researchers into an intervention program that can be systematically and sequentially applied and investigated in a wide range of clinical settings. Throughout this book, emphasis is placed on the application of assessment techniques that can clarify the specific causes of attention-deficit/hyperactivity disorder (ADHD) symptoms in a specific patient. To facilitate the application of our evaluation procedures in other settings, samples of our assessment instruments are presented in this book for use in clinical practice. Similarly, because of the multiple types of functional impairments found in patients with ADHD, the book provides detailed descriptions for providing comprehensive care in school and outpatient clinical settings, including models for academic support programs; individual, parent, and marital counseling; as well as social skills and attention training programs.

Although the integrative, neurobehavioral model for assessment and treatment presented in this book is founded on a substantial body of scientific literature, it is important to recognize that the process of translating neuroscientific findings into clinical practice is in the early stage of development. Advances in molecular genetics, neuroimaging, and quantitative electroencephalography seem likely to lead to the development of more accurate diagnostic procedures. Such enhanced diagnostic accuracy, and the identification of specific neural pathways that are causing ADHD symptoms in a specific individual, also seems likely to result in improved medication selection and, as a result, improved treatment response.

On a similar note, as increased awareness of the neurological foundations of ADHD is established among health care providers and as a shift from trauma, behavioral, and family-systems models for ADHD occurs, increased effort can be placed on developing skill training programs to improve attention, behavioral control, and a wide range of functional impairments that persist despite pharmacological treatment. Although several training models are presented in detail in this book, I anticipate that future research efforts will lead to the development of protocols that achieve more enduring results in a more rapid and efficient manner.

Despite these limitations, my hope is that clinicians will find the model for clinical practice presented in this book to be helpful in their daily clinical work. Unlike other comprehensive texts, this book is not intended to be archived on a bookshelf. Instead, this book seeks to translate existing research into a workable base of knowledge that can enhance patient care on a daily basis, stimulate the development of applied clinical research programs at the community level, and serve as a guide for the formulation of the more effective treatments that will emerge in the years to come.

ACKNOWLEDGMENTS

To complete a book like this requires thousands of hours of work, not only by the author but also by family, colleagues, and support staff. First, I want to express my heartfelt gratitude to my wife, Donna, for finding the strength and energy to assume so many of the daily responsibilities at home and at our clinic so that I could complete this book. I also want to thank her for helping me remain focused as I worked on this highly complex and multifaceted task and for her review of drafts of this text. I also express my appreciation to the members of my research team, T. Nick Fenger, George Green, Michael Linden, Joel Lubar, Arthur Phillips, Peter Van Deusen, and William Wing, who devoted countless hours, without financial compensation, to explore the neurophysiological realities of attention-deficit/hyperactivity disorder (ADHD) with me.

In particular, I want to express my appreciation to Joel Lubar, for his willingness to teach me the value of quantitative electroencephalography as a tool for understanding brain functions. As a graduate student at the University of Southern Mississippi, I had learned from Douglas Lowe that the brain generated electricity. It was only after my discussions with Joel Lubar and Barry Sterman that I began to understand the dynamics of brain activity and how to translate the meaning of these electrical signals in ways that could benefit patients with ADHD. I am indebted to both of these highly esteemed colleagues for their willingness to share their incredible foundation of knowledge with me.

I also express my appreciation to the Association for Applied Psychophysiology & Biofeedback (AAPB) and the International Society for Neurotherapy & Research (ISNR). In particular, I thank Tom Brownback, Jay Gunkelman, Lynda Kirk, Ted LaVaque, Michael Linden, Judith Lubar, Alan Strohmayer, Paul Swingle, Hershel Toomim, and the other members of AAPB and ISNR for their enthusiasm and willingness to engage in the kinds of thought-provoking discussions that inspire the development of new approaches to long-standing problems.

Likewise, I consider it important to recognize the impact of my early training in systems theory and structural family therapy on the Parenting and Life Skills Programs developed by me and taught at our clinic. Although I am convinced that ADHD is founded on neurological rather than psychosocial factors, I have been impressed by the important role performed by parents in teaching essential life skills and the value of systemic interventions in promoting the health and well-being of individuals. The lessons taught by my mentors in family therapy at the Philadelphia Child Guidance Clinic (Jorge Colapinto, Ken Covelman, Barbara Forbes-Bryant, Salvador Minuchin, Jamshed Morenas, and Carl Whitaker) guide me still.

I also wish to acknowledge the contribution of my research staff, particularly my assistant, Gary Truax, for his efforts in conducting numerous literature searches and collecting the scientific articles reviewed in this text. I am also thankful for the contributions of my interns from Binghamton University—Frank Hoppie, Flora Poleshchuk, and Erin Street—who facilitated data collection and statistical analyses needed for the completion of scientific studies conducted at our clinic. The illustrations for this book were created by my talented daughter Bridget. As a typical proud Poppi, I was pleased that she was able to spare the time to help me with this project.

Recognition is also due to Susan Reynolds, Susan Herman, Ron Teeter, and the members of the editorial staff in the Books department at the American Psychological Association. Although an author may spend thousands of hours in the preparation of a manuscript, the members of the editorial staff devote an inordinate amount of time reviewing and helping to guide text revisions while ensuring the scientific accuracy of the information presented. For this, they receive little recognition. Yet without their efforts, the quality of a text like this can be compromised. I have always appreciated the efforts of my publisher and the in-house and external reviewers and hope that the reader will realize that the final version of this text truly represents a team effort.

Finally, I thank God for giving me the health and stamina to complete this task. Throughout the years of my clinical practice, I have operated from the premise that although God is the source of all wisdom, knowledge is derived from countless hours of work and the willingness of human beings to share their observations with each other. I have truly been blessed by the generosity of scientists, clinicians, parents, teachers, and patients with ADHD who shared their perspectives with me, so that the model of patient care described in this book could emerge. My hope is that the assessment and treatment strategies described in this book will help to improve the lives of the patients we serve.

Unlocking the Potential of Patients With ADHD

INTRODUCTION

Scientific studies conducted throughout the world indicate that between 2% and 29% of children and adolescents present with symptoms of inattention alone or in combination with symptoms of hyperactivity and impulsivity that are sufficiently severe to meet criteria for a diagnosis of attention-deficit/hyperactivity disorder (ADHD; American Psychiatric Association, 2000; Barkley, 2006; Bhatia, Nigam, Bohra, & Malik, 1991; Costello, Costello, & Edelbrock, 1988; Simonoff et al., 1995). The condition appears to be chronic in nature and there is substantial evidence that the majority of children with disorders of attention and behavioral inhibition will continue to exhibit such symptoms into adulthood (e.g., Barkley, 2002; Spencer, Biederman, Wilens, & Faraone, 1998; G. Weiss, Hechtman, Milroy, & Perlman, 1985; Wilens & Dodson, 2004). As extensively reviewed by Barkley (2006), without accurate diagnosis and effective treatment, such patients are at significantly greater risk to have a history of academic underachievement, failure and withdrawal, substance abuse, accidental injury, involvement in criminal activities, and a variety of comorbid psychiatric conditions (e.g., anxiety, mood disorders).

Because multiple medical and psychiatric disorders other than ADHD can cause symptoms of inattention, impulsivity, and hyperactivity, a significant task for clinicians is to clarify which disorder(s) or condition(s) are responsible for the impairment of attention and behavioral control evident in a specific patient. For some patients, the cause is ADHD. For other patients, the cause is traumatic brain injury; anemia; hypoglycemia; hypothyroidism; diabetes; allergies; sleep disorders; visual impairment; auditory processing disorder; deficiencies of iron, vitamin B-12, zinc, or magnesium; mood disorder; anxiety disorder; or other conditions. Consistent with the fundamental principles of medicine (Beeson, McDermott, & Wyngaarden, 1979), the effective treatment of persistent, enduring symptoms of inattention and/or impulsivity and hyperactivity in an individual depends on the clinician's ability to identify the specific cause(s) of such symptoms in a specific patient and to initiate a treatment plan that addresses the underlying causes on a case-by-case basis.

Clinicians of our era now have the benefit of an array of assessment procedures, including interview, patient observation, standardized behavioral rating scales, neuropsychological tests of executive functions (e.g., attention, working memory, motor organization and regulation), quantitative electroencephalography (qEEG), functional magnetic resonance imagery (fMRI), positron emission tomography (PET), and single photon emission computed tomography (SPECT). Owing to significant advances in genetics, chromosomal studies are also available for research and clinical purposes. The addition of these technologies to previously available biochemical assays of blood, urine, and tissue samples creates a context in which the specific underlying causes of impairments of attention and behavioral regulation can begin to be accurately understood on an individual basis.

Despite the availability of such assessment procedures, there is considerable scientific debate regarding the validity and clinical use of behavioral, neuroimaging, neuropsychological, and neurophysiological measures (Barkley, 2006; Loo & Barkley, 2005). As is extensively presented in this book, a review of the scientific literature supports several conclusions at this time.

First, although the diagnosis of ADHD cannot be made on the basis of a behavioral rating scale or on the outcome of a specific neuroimaging, neuropsychological, or neurophysiological measure in isolation, each of these procedures provides information that can contribute to the evaluation process. Behavioral rating scales and observational measures provide a description of the kinds of symptomatic behaviors that require intervention. Neuropsychological tests of attention (e.g., continuous performance tests) provide a standardized context for evaluating attention and behavioral control that is not confounded by rater bias, contextual variations, or specific learning disabilities. The use of qEEG and fMRI techniques can provide an initial indicator that medical factors are contributing to the presence of symptoms in a given patient.

Second, parents of children with impairments of attention and behavioral control are generally uncomfortable with a diagnostic process limited to interview, conversations with teachers, and the use of rating scales (Angold,

Erkanli, Egger, & Costello, 2000; Costello et al., 1996; Monastra, 2005b). Such parents tend to decline or discontinue treatment within 6 months of the diagnosis following such assessment practices (Angold et al., 2000; Costello et al., 1996; P. S. Jensen, 2000; Monastra, 2005b). When an assessment process that includes behavioral, neuropsychological, and neurophysiological evaluations, as well as medical evaluation, is conducted, marked increase in treatment initiation and retention rates has been reported (Monastra, 2005b).

Third, chronic impairments of attention and behavioral control can be caused by a number of divergent medical conditions (including anemia, hypoglycemia, thyroid disorders, sleep disorders, dietary insufficiencies, visual impairments, etc.), as well as other psychiatric disorders (e.g., mood, anxiety, and conduct disorders). Because of the prevalence rates of such disorders in the general population, it seems unlikely that any of the currently available neurological or neurophysiological measures will be proven to be specific for ADHD, as the rates for these other disorders constitutes a substantial error factor. However, the identification of abnormal physical findings during qEEG or fMRI alerts the clinician that medical conditions are contributing to the manifestation of symptoms in a specific patient. Such a condition may prove to be ADHD or one of the other medical conditions associated with enduring symptoms of inattention, impulsivity, and hyperactivity.

As is reviewed in this book, the existent scientific literature suggests a genetic foundation of ADHD, which is expressed in various neurological, neurochemical, neurophysiological, and behavioral characteristics and a wide range of functional impairments. Patients who undergo a thorough and comprehensive evaluation and are treated with a targeted, carefully monitored combination of medical and psychosocial treatments have demonstrated enhanced clinical response compared with those treated from a behavioral perspective or from a standard community-care model of drug therapy alone (Arnold et al., 2004; P. S. Jensen, Hinshaw, Swanson, et al., 2001; Monastra, 2005b; Multimodal Treatment Study of Children With ADHD [MTA] Cooperative Group, 2004). The purpose of this book, therefore, is to provide clinicians with a practical, empirically supported, integrative model for the assessment and care of patients who present with symptoms of inattention, impulsivity, and hyperactivity that can be applied in a wide range of clinical settings. Throughout this book, emphasis is placed on using a combination of assessment procedures that can clarify the specific causes of these symptoms in a specific patient. Emphasis is placed on an individualized, multidimensional assessment process and a matching between etiology and treatment selection to optimize clinical outcome for each patient who seeks assistance.

In chapter 1, a review of the core symptoms of ADHD, comorbid psychiatric disorders, and areas of functional impairment is provided. This chapter is intended to provide an overview of the multiple types of psychiatric symptoms, strategies for differentiating ADHD from other psychiatric disorders, and an indication of the types of functional problems that will require systematic assessment and treatment in clinical practice. In chapter 2, the causes of ADHD are examined from a neuroscience perspective. As noted previously, the existing neuroanatomical, neurophysiological, neurochemical, and genetic evidence appears to support the theory that ADHD is an inherited condition, characterized by structural and functional abnormalities of both the central nervous system and, in all likelihood, the autonomic nervous system as well. Recent neurophysiological studies, using qEEG techniques (summarized by Chabot, di Michele, & Prichep, 2005; Clarke, Barry, McCarthy, & Selikowitz, 2001b; Clarke, Barry, McCarthy, Selikowitz, & Croft, 2002; Hermens, 2006; Monastra, 2005a, 2005b) have suggested that there are two primary neurophysiological subtypes of patients with ADHD. These studies point to the possibility of patient matching to type of pharmacological treatment to maximize clinical response and minimize adverse effects and treatment discontinuation. Early studies that test such a hypothesis are also reviewed in this chapter.

In chapter 3, an overview of common medical conditions that can cause symptoms of inattention, impulsivity, and hyperactivity is provided. This overview is intended to alert practitioners to the need for a thorough medical evaluation when a child, adolescent, or adult presents with a symptom profile that meets *Diagnostic and Statistical Manual of Mental Disorders* (4th ed., text rev.; American Psychiatric Association, 2000) criteria for a diagnosis of ADHD. Such disorders have been responsible for the ADHD-like symptoms presented by approximately 5% of patients examined at our clinic (Monastra, 2005b; Monastra, Monastra, & George, 2002)

Chapter 4 describes a neurobehavioral assessment process. This multidimensional evaluation procedure includes the behavioral assessment of a patient (incorporating clinical interview, rating scales, and other observational techniques), as well as neuropsychological and neurophysiological strategies. Specific assessment protocols used in our clinical research are highlighted in this chapter, and samples of the semistructured interview, checklists, and other patient monitoring procedures used at our clinic are provided.

Treatments for patients with ADHD are then reviewed, beginning with the foundation of attention in any individual: nutrition, adequate sleep, and exercise. Although such factors are not considered causative of ADHD, a substantial body of research supports the functional importance of nutrition, sleep, and exercise. Because of the general lack of emphasis on dietary, sleep, and exercise in the clinical research literature on ADHD, clinicians may find chapter 5 to be particularly helpful in enhancing clinical response. To facilitate patient education, self-monitoring, and progress, sample checklists and forms used in clinical practice are provided.

Following this presentation of healthy dietary, sleep, and exercise habits is a review of pharmacological treatments for ADHD. Strategies for assessing and revising medical treatments are also included in chapter 6. Because areas of functional impairment commonly persist even after effective pharmacological treatments are introduced, a process for evaluating such skill deficits is essential in clinical practice. Chapter 7 provides a framework for conducting such functional assessments

The content of the book then shifts to a series of chapters presenting nonpharmacological treatments for ADHD. In chapter 8, a thorough review of electroencephalographic (EEG) biofeedback (neurotherapy) is provided, as this type of treatment has been examined in multiple, controlled group studies and been reported to be effective in at least 75% of the cases studied (Monastra, 2005a). Although not widely incorporated into clinical practice at present, given the substantial minority of patients who do not respond to stimulant therapy (30%; Swanson, McBurnett, Christian, & Wigal, 1995), the high rate of patients with ADHD who either decline medication or discontinue pharmacotherapy within a year (at least 40%–50%; Angold et al., 2000; Costello et al.,1996; P. S. Jensen, 2000), and the effectiveness of EEG biofeedback (Hirshberg, Chiu, & Frazier, 2005; Monastra, 2005a), a detailed review of this type of treatment is included.

Once effective treatment of the core symptoms of ADHD has been established, interventions directed at improving the educational, social and occupational functioning of patients can be initiated. In chapter 9, the process for developing comprehensive plans of academic support and accommodation in school settings is presented. Included in that chapter is a review of current educational laws specifying the educational rights of patients with ADHD as well as assessment strategies for determining areas of functional impairment caused by ADHD. Chapter 9 also provides an overview of classroom interventions, modifications, and motivational strategies that appear helpful in promoting the success of students.

Chapters 10 and 11 describe how practitioners can incorporate structured parenting and social skills classes in their practice. On the basis of the findings reported by members of the MTA Cooperative Group (e.g., Arnold et al., 2004; Hinshaw et al., 2000; Pelham & Hoza, 1996), as well as research conducted at our clinic (Monastra, 2005c; Monastra et al., 2002), incorporating such programs in outpatient clinical settings appears beneficial in the care of patients. These chapters provide detailed instructions for conducting such classes to facilitate use in a wide range of clinical settings.

Because ADHD does not simply fade away, chapter 12 highlights diagnostic and treatment issues in adults with ADHD. The chapter provides a review of research on pharmacological, marital, and family interventions, as well as cognitive behavior therapy and adult coaching. Finally, chapter 13 provides case illustrations and discusses common problems encountered in clinical practice.

Until persons with ADHD encounter health care providers who can accurately diagnose and initiate effective, comprehensive care for the specific causes of their symptoms, they will continue to experience the daily frustration, embarrassment, disappointment, and functional failures that are a by-product of this disorder. However, by understanding the neuroscience of ADHD and initiating neurologically founded, medical, nutritional, social, educational, and rehabilitative interventions, health care providers can address the multiple sources of distractibility, impaired concentration, impulsivity, and restlessness, thereby unlocking the potential of patients with ADHD.

1

ADHD: CORE SYMPTOMS, DIFFERENTIAL DIAGNOSIS, AND AREAS OF FUNCTIONAL IMPAIRMENT

In clinical practice, health care professionals are routinely asked to evaluate and treat patients who are struggling to succeed at home, work, and in their social relationships because of a lack of attention, a persistent sense of restlessness, and an inability to control impulsive actions. Although the specific criteria for diagnosing an attention-deficit/hyperactivity disorder (ADHD) vary between the guidelines adopted in the United States (*Diagnostic and Statistical Manual of Mental Disorders, Fourth Edition, Text Revision* [*DSM–IV–TR*]; American Psychiatric Association, 2000) and those used in Europe and in other international communities (*International Classification of Diseases, Tenth Edition*; ICD-10; World Health Organization, 1994), it is clear that a significant minority of individuals throughout the world experience significant functional impairments that are caused by impaired attention and lack of behavioral control. Central to the diagnosis of ADHD in either system is the presence of symptoms of inattention, impulsivity, and hyperactivity that are present to a degree that is atypical on the basis of age.

The primary difference between the two systems is that the ICD-10 requires that the patient demonstrate a sufficient number of symptoms of both inattention and hyperactivity–impulsivity in order to meet diagnostic criteria. In the *DSM–IV–TR*, the diagnosis can be made on the basis of the presence of a sufficient number of symptoms of inattention (i.e., ADHD, Predominately Inattentive Type) or hyperactivity–impulsivity (i.e., ADHD, Predominately Hyperactive–Impulsive Type) or both (i.e, ADHD, Combined Type). Throughout this book, the term *ADHD* is used to refer to individuals who meet the criteria established by the American Psychiatric Association (2000). Because of the different diagnostic criteria, estimated prevalence rates based on the ICD-10 system tend to be lower than when *DSM–IV–TR* criteria are used (see reviews by Barkley, 2006; Bird, 2002).

In this chapter, the core symptoms of ADHD are presented, together with a review of symptoms of other psychiatric disorders that are often evident in patients diagnosed with this disorder. In addition, areas of functional impairment are examined. Such a review appears essential for several reasons. First, because effective treatment of any psychiatric disorder is dependent on accurate diagnosis, the ability to differentiate among various disorders with shared symptoms is essential in clinical practice. Second, because patients with ADHD commonly have multiple psychiatric disorders, each requiring treatment, an understanding of common patterns of comorbidity can alert practitioners to the need for combined treatments in a specific patient. Third, although the core symptoms of ADHD are the primary initial targets of clinical interventions, the eventual impact that ADHD treatments exert on the broad spectrum of functional impairments is perhaps the most significant measure of the efficacy of any treatment program.

Although many practitioners are familiar with the core symptoms of ADHD, the range and degree of comorbid psychiatric disorders and functional impairments is extensive. As is emphasized in this book, effective treatment for patients with ADHD begins with assessment and intervention not only for inattention, impulsivity, and hyperactivity but also for the defiance, depression, anxiety, social skill deficits, health problems, and occupational and educational problems that are commonly noted in these patients.

CORE SYMPTOMS AND PREVALENCE OF ADHD

According to the *DSM–IV–TR*[1], the diagnostic criteria for ADHD are as follows:

Criterion A: Either (1) or (2):
   (1) six (or more) of the following symptoms of inattention have persisted for at least 6 months to a degree that is maladaptive and inconsistent with developmental level:

---

[1]Reprinted with permission from the *Diagnostic and Statistical Manual of Mental Disorders, Fourth Edition, Text Revision* (Copyright 2000). American Psychiatric Association.

Inattention

   (a) often fails to give close attention to details or makes careless mistakes in schoolwork, work, or other activities
   (b) often has difficulty sustaining attention in tasks or play activities
   (c) often does not seem to listen when spoken to directly
   (d) often does not follow through on instructions and fails to finish schoolwork, chores, or duties in the workplace (not due to oppositional behavior or failure to understand instructions)
   (e) often has difficulty organizing tasks and activities
   (f) often avoids, dislikes, or is reluctant to engage in tasks that require sustained mental effort (such as schoolwork or homework)
   (g) often loses things necessary for tasks or activities (e.g., toys, school assignments, pencils, books, or tools)
   (h) is often easily distracted by extraneous stimuli
   (i) is often forgetful in daily activities

(2) six (or more) of the following symptoms of hyperactivity–impulsivity persisted for at least 6 months to a degree that is maladaptive and inconsistent with developmental level:

Hyperactivity

   (a) often fidgets with hands or feet or squirms in seat
   (b) often leaves seat in classroom or in other situations in which remaining seated is expected
   (c) often runs about or climbs excessively in situations in which it is inappropriate (in adolescents or adults, may be limited to subjective feelings of restlessness)
   (d) often has difficulty playing or engaging in leisure activities quietly
   (e) is often "on the go" or often acts as if "driven by a motor"
   (g) often talks excessively

Impulsivity

   (a) often blurts out answers before questions have been completed
   (b) often has difficulty awaiting turn
   (c) often interrupts or intrudes on others (butts into conversations or games)

Criterion B: Some hyperactive–impulsive or inattentive symptoms that caused impairment were present before age 7 years.

Criterion C: Some impairment from the symptoms is present in two or more settings (e.g., at school [or work] and at home).

Criterion D: There must be clear evidence of clinically significant impairment in social, academic, or occupational functioning.

Criterion E: The symptoms do not occur exclusively during the course of a Pervasive Developmental Disorder, Schizophrenia, or other Psychotic Disorders and are not better accounted for by another mental disorder (e.g., Mood Disorder, Anxiety Disorder, Dissociative Disorder, or a Personality Disorder).

Depending on the number of symptoms of inattention and hyperactivity–impulsivity, the following diagnostic subtypes have been established:

Attention-Deficit/Hyperactivity Disorder, Combined Type: If both Criteria A1 and A2 are met for the past 6 months;

Attention-Deficit/Hyperactivity Disorder, Predominately Inattentive Type: If Criterion A1 is met but Criterion A2 is not met for the past 6 months;

Attention-Deficit/Hyperactivity Disorder, Predominately Hyperactive–Impulsive Type: If Criterion A2 is met but Criterion A1 is not met for the past 6 months.

As noted in the *DSM–IV–TR*, the prevalence of ADHD is estimated to be approximately 3% to 7% of school-age children, although rates as low as 2% (August, Realmuto, MacDonald, Nugent, & Crosby, 1996; Costello, Costello, & Edelbrock, 1988) and as high as 29% (Bhatia, Nigam, Bohra, & Malik, 1991) have been reported (see reviews by Barkley, 2006; Bird, 2002). This condition is not limited to the United States, as comparable prevalence rates are reported in Canada (Breton et al., 1999; Offord et al., 1987; Romano, Tremblay, Vitaro, Zoccolillo, & Pagini, 2001; Szatmari, Offord, & Boyle, 1989a, 1989b), Brazil (Rohde et al., 1999), Australia (Graetz, Sawyer, Hazell, Arney, & Baghurst, 2001), New Zealand (Anderson, Williams, McGee, & Silva, 1987; Fergusson, Horwood, & Lynskey, 1993; McGee et al., 1990), Germany (Baumgaertel, Wolraich, & Dietrich, 1995; Esser, Schmidt, & Woerner, 1990), The Netherlands (Kroes et al., 2001; Verhulst, van der Ende, Ferdinand, & Kasius, 1997), Italy (Gallucci et al., 1993), India (Bhatia et al., 1991), China (Leung et al., 1996), and Japan (Kanbayashi, Nakata, Fujii, Kita, & Wada, 1994). There is substantial evidence that this disorder has a strong genetic foundation, as the heritability of ADHD is approximately .75 (Swanson & Castellanos, 2002).

Investigations of the effect of age and gender on prevalence have revealed that ADHD continues to be evident in approximately 4% of the adult samples studied in the United States (Barkley, 2006; Murphy & Barkley, 1996). The ratio of ADHD in males to females ranges from 2:1 to 10:1 in published studies (see review by Ross & Ross, 1982). Barkley (2006) averaged the prevalence rates in the United States and in international studies and estimated a 3.4:1.0 ratio of males to females. Further examination of symptom retention rates reveals that 30% to 80% of children diagnosed with ADHD continue to display a significant number of core ADHD symptoms into adolescence and adulthood (August, Stewart, & Holmes, 1983;

Biederman et al., 1996; Cantwell & Baker, 1989; Claude & Firestone, 1995; Mannuzza, Klein, & Addalli, 1991).

LIMITATIONS OF THE CURRENT DIAGNOSTIC CRITERIA

Examination of the *DSM–IV–TR* criteria reveals that the diagnosis is to be made on the basis of observation, interview with multiple informants, and review of clinical history. The *DSM–IV–TR* advises practitioners to rule out conditions such as Pervasive Developmental Disorder (PDD), Schizophrenia, or other Psychotic Disorder, Mood Disorder, Anxiety Disorder, Dissociative Disorder, or Personality Disorder. However, no specific recommendations are given with respect to the evaluation of medical conditions that can cause symptoms of inattention or restlessness (e.g., anemia, hypoglycemia, allergies). Instead, the *DSM–IV–TR* notes that there are no laboratory tests that have been established as diagnostic and no specific physical features have been associated with ADHD.

Unfortunately, such statements minimize the reality that there are a number of medical conditions that can cause symptoms of inattention, hyperactivity, and impulsivity. Although the diagnosis of ADHD requires that other medical conditions be ruled out, the types and prevalence of medical conditions that excluded individuals from participation in studies of ADHD are not routinely reported in published scientific articles. However, several published reports that did conduct a comprehensive medical evaluation (including blood assays) as part of the assessment process have indicated that approximately 5% of patients who met *DSM–IV–TR* criteria for ADHD were subsequently diagnosed with another medical condition that was the cause of their symptoms (Monastra, 2005a, 2005b; Monastra, Lubar, & Linden, 2001; Monastra et al., 1999; Monastra, Monastra, & George, 2002). A detailed presentation of a comprehensive assessment process that is useful in ruling out other relevant medical conditions is provided in chapter 4.

Beyond minimizing the need for evaluation of other medical conditions when a patient presents with chronic symptoms of inattention, impulsivity, or hyperactivity, the *DSM–IV–TR* provides little guidance with respect to the process for determining symptom severity. It is left to the individual practitioner to determine what constitutes "often" and how to define "inconsistent with developmental level." Guidelines presented by the American Academy of Child & Adolescent Psychiatry (1997) and the American Academy of Pediatrics (2000) recommend an evaluation process that emphasizes parent and/or caregiver and teacher report, as well as an examination of the individual's behavior in a variety of situations. However, the inconsistency of such reports in clinical practice is problematic, and the research literature has consistently revealed low correlation rates between informants, particularly parent versus teacher reports (e.g., Achenbach,

McConaughy, & Howell, 1987; Derks, Hudziak, Dolan, Ferdinand, & Boomsma, 2006; Hewitt et al., 1997; Simonoff et al., 1995). Additionally, low correlation is found between diagnoses based on unstructured clinical interview and those based on a standardized process, such as the Diagnostic Interview Schedule for Children (A. Jensen & Weisz, 2002; Lewczyk, Garland, Hurlburt, Gearity, & Hough, 2003).

Although not directly addressed in the *DSM–IV–TR*, this lack of interrater reliability is a serious impediment to behaviorally based assessment and treatment protocols. Hewitt et al. (1997; the Virginia Twin Study of Adolescent Behavioral Development) reported interrater correlations ranging from .05 to .35 across informants in their study of 1,412 pairs of twins. Such findings are quite consistent with those noted by Achenbach et al. (1987), Simonoff et al. (1995), and Verhulst and Koot (1992). Despite the face validity of rating scales, the frequent divergence of opinion between mother, father, teacher, and patient confounds diagnostic efforts that rely on this type of information, leading to a recommendation that "evidence-based diagnosis," incorporating the results of standardized assessment measures, is needed to enhance the accuracy of the diagnostic process (Jensen-Doss, 2005; Lewczyk et al., 2003). As is reviewed in chapter 4 (this volume), neuropsychological and neurophysiological measures, developed to directly assess attentional processes, have demonstrated test reliability, sensitivity, and specificity, and can be helpful in determining the degree of "deviation" of an individual from age peers with respect to attention and capacity for behavioral regulation.

COMORBID PSYCHIATRIC DISORDERS

In clinical practice, the majority of patients diagnosed with ADHD will also meet diagnostic criteria for another psychiatric disorder (Barkley, 2002, 2006; Klein & Mannuzza, 1991; Pliszka, 2000; Pliszka, Carlson, & Swanson, 1999; Spencer, Biederman, & Wilens, 1999; Waxmonsky, 2003). Among the numerous studies cited in these reviews, the research conducted by Barkley, Fischer, Edelbrock, and Smallish (1990); Biederman et al. (1996, 1997); Claude and Firestone (1995); M. Fischer, Barkley, Smallish, and Fletcher (2002); Mannuzza and his colleagues (Mannuzza, Klein, & Addalli, 1991; Mannuzza, Klein, Bessler, Malloy, & LaPadula, 1993; Mannuzza, Klein, Bonagura, et al., 1991); the Multimodal Treatment Study of Children With ADHD (MTA) Cooperative Group (1999; P. S. Jensen, Hinshaw, Kraemer, et al., 2001); Szatmari et al. (1989a, 1989b); M. Weiss and Hechtman (1993); and Wilens et al. (2002) are particularly noteworthy.

To promote a better appreciation of the rate of comorbidity between ADHD and other psychiatric disorders, Table 1.1 may prove useful to clinicians. A more detailed examination of comorbidity rates and strategies for differential diagnosis follows.

TABLE 1.1
Comorbidity Rates of Attention-Deficit/Hyperactivity Disorder (ADHD)
and Other Psychiatric Disorders

DSM–IV–TR disorder	General population (%)	Patients with ADHD (%)
Conduct Disorder	1–10	15–56
Oppositional Defiant Disorder	2–16	23–63
Anxiety Disorders	5–15	20–50
Mood Disorders	10–25	15–75
Learning Disorders	2–10	40–60
Substance Use Disorders	20–25	40–50
Tic Disorders	4–18	4–18
Eating Disorders	1–3	11–17
Autistic Spectrum Disorders	<1	<1

Note. Data from Barkley, Fischer, Edelbrock, and Smallish (1990); Biederman et al. (1996, 1997); Claude and Firestone (1995); M. Fischer, Barkley, Smallish, and Fletcher (2002); P. S. Jensen, Hinshaw, Kraemer, et al. (2001); Manuzza, Klein, and Addalli (1991); Mannuzza, Klein, Bessler, Malloy, and LaPadula (1993); Mannuzza, Klein, Bonagura, et al. (1991); Multimodal Treatment Study of Children With ADHD Cooperative Group (1999); Szatmari, Offord, and Boyle (1989a, 1989b); M. Weiss and Hechtman (1993); and Wilens et al. (2002). *DSM–IV–TR = Diagnostic and Statistical Manual of Mental Disorders* (4th ed., text rev.; American Psychiatric Association, 2000).

Conduct Disorder

According to the *DSM–IV–TR*, patients with Conduct Disorder (CD) present with symptoms of aggression to people and animals, destruction of property, deceitfulness or theft, and serious violations of rules (e.g., failure to comply with parental rules regarding curfew, running away, truancy). Age of onset is prior to 13. Duration of symptoms is at least 6 months. Prevalence in the population is estimated to be between 1% and 10%. The male-to-female ratio is approximately 2:1, and children with CD tend to have family backgrounds that include lower socioeconomic status, greater incidence of family conflict and/or violence, and a higher prevalence of psychiatric and substance abuse disorders (see review by Maughan, Rowe, Messer, Goodman, & Meltzer, 2004). Comparison with the diagnostic criteria for ADHD indicates no common symptoms. Hence, the behavioral characteristics of CD are easily distinguishable from ADHD.

Examination of the cited literature indicates that 15% to 56% of children with ADHD will also meet diagnostic criteria for a diagnosis of CD. Subtype analysis has indicated that children with ADHD, Combined or Predominately Hyperactive–Impulsive types, are approximately 3 times more likely to also have CD than children diagnosed with ADHD, Predominately Inattentive Type (Lalonde, Turgay, & Hudson, 1998). When present in a patient with ADHD, CD typically occurs in combination with Oppositional Defiant Disorder (ODD; Lalonde et al., 1998). From a prognostic perspective, the presence of a comorbid CD in a child with ADHD significantly decreases the likelihood of successful adolescent and adult outcomes. Children diagnosed with either ADHD or ODD and CD are at increased risk for substance abuse, criminal behavior, and academic failure. Although there is scientific debate whether ADHD in combination with CD represents a unique subtype of ADHD, there is little question that the presence of this type of comorbidity creates serious long-term risks for a child.

Oppositional Defiant Disorder

The *DSM–IV–TR* describes ODD as a disorder characterized by disruptive behaviors that "are of a less severe nature than those of individuals with CDs and typically do not include aggression toward people or animals, destruction of property or a pattern of theft or deceit" (American Psychiatric Association, 2000, pp. 101–102). Instead, this disorder is determined by a "pattern of negativistic, hostile, and defiant behavior," characterized by loss of temper, argumentativeness, defiance, refusal to comply with parental requests, deliberate annoyance of others, spitefulness, and a tendency to blame others for mistakes (p. 101).

As with ADHD, the process for assessing developmental deviance is determined by the individual practitioner, as the criteria for defining "often" are not provided. Duration of symptoms must be at least 6 months, and significant impairment of social, academic, or occupational functioning must be noted. Prevalence of ODD is noted in 2% to 16% of the population (according to the *DSM–IV–TR*), tending to occur more often in families where there is serious marital discord and maternal depression. The male-to-female ratio is similar to that for CD (1:1–2:1).

Unlike CD, the differentiation of ADHD from ODD is not easily established. Whereas CD is characterized by chronic patterns of aggression and serious violations of rules, and most often appears during later childhood and adolescence, both ADHD and ODD are evident during early childhood. In addition, common symptoms of ADHD, such as impairment of attention while listening to instructions or directions, loss of concentration, impaired mental stamina, and avoidance of tasks requiring sustained mental effort, can be expressed in a variety of ways. For example, children with ADHD or ODD may become argumentative, irritable, and verbally and/or physically aggressive when asked to do homework or complete a household chore such as cleaning their room. They may also display a variety of hyperactive and impulsive behaviors that annoy others. These emotional reactions could be interpreted as a manifestation of the loss of mental stamina and impaired behavioral or emotional control, which are the defining characteristics of ADHD, rather than an indication of ODD.

In addition, a child with ADHD who is being treated with either an immediate or sustained release type of stimulant or a nonstimulant ADHD medication (e.g., atomoxetine) is also more likely than age peers to display symptoms of irritability and defiance, particularly during the morning (prior to initiating stimulant medication) and during the late afternoon and early evening (as stimulant effects dissipate). In these instances, such symptoms appear to be more consistent with the known side effects of medication rather than to represent an indication of an additional psychiatric diagnosis such as ODD. As is discussed in later chapters on the assessment and treatment of ADHD and comorbid features, the essential differentiation between ADHD and ODD is the presence of significant impairment of attention. There are several neuropsychological tests that can help clinicians directly examine attentional abilities, which are reviewed in chapter 4.

Perhaps owing to the similarity in functional problems evident in both ADHD and ODD (e.g., failure to follow instructions, rules, and directions; task avoidance) and the difficulty in differentiating the causes of these behaviors (e.g., neurological impairment of attention and behavioral inhibition vs. psychosocial factors such as maternal depression, inadequate parenting style, and marital discord), a substantial percentage of patients with ADHD are also diagnosed with ODD. The degree of comorbidity between these two disorders is quite high, ranging from 23% to 63%. Unlike CD, the functional problems associated with ODD during adolescence and adulthood are not as great, prompting certain researchers to postulate that perhaps ADHD plus ODD is an "intermediate subgroup between those who have ADHD alone and those with ADHD plus CD" (Spencer et al., 1999, p. 917).

Although those diagnosed with ADHD in combination with ODD or CD have a higher rate of school dysfunction than children with ADHD alone, the children with ODD or ADHD plus ODD do not have as severe a problem as those with CD. In addition, the risk for criminal behavior and substance abuse, although increased, is not as great for patients with ODD or ADHD plus ODD than for patients with CD. As summarized by Spencer et al. (1999), "in the absence of CD, ODD does not necessarily progress to CD and does not share the poor outcome of CD" (p. 917). However, the high degree of functional similarity between ODD and ADHD can contribute to inadequate treatment of a child with ADHD who is exhibiting characteristics of both disorders. As with the differentiation of ADHD from CD, the direct evaluation of attentional abilities can assist clinicians in the assessment process as significant impairment of attention is not a symptom of ODD.

Anxiety Disorders

The *DSM–IV–TR* lists 11 different types of anxiety disorders, ranging from Agoraphobia to Substance-Induced Anxiety Disorder. Common among the various disorders is the experience of a subjective state of sudden panic or more persistent panic-like states in which symptoms such as accelerated heart rate, sweating, shortness of breath, nausea, dizziness, paresthesias (numbness or tingling), and chills or hot flashes are evident

Depending on the specific subtype of anxiety disorder, the patient may become psychologically paralyzed (e.g., Panic Disorder); avoid the anxiety provoking context (e.g., Agoraphobia, Simple Phobia, Social Phobia); experience persistent, intrusive ideas, thoughts, impulses, or images (obsessions); or engage in repetitive, compulsive behaviors (e.g., handwashing, ordering, checking). In children, avoidance may also be combined with symptoms of aggression and tantrums. Age of onset is not a defining criterion of anxiety disorders, as symptoms can emerge at any age. As with other *DSM–IV–TR* disorders, the duration of symptoms is at least 6 months and evidence of significant functional impairment is required.

The prevalence of anxiety disorders reported in clinical studies is approximately 5% to 15% of the general population. Both males and females develop anxiety disorders. Certain types of disorders are diagnosed twice as frequently in females than males (e.g., Specific Phobias, Panic Disorder with or without Agoraphobia). In other types of anxiety disorders, the rate is equivalent (e.g., Obsessive–Compulsive Disorder). Among children diagnosed with a childhood-onset Obsessive–Compulsive Disorder, more boys than girls are identified. Anxiety disorders have a high degree of heritability, occurring up to 20 times more frequently among first-degree biological relatives of patients with this disorder than in the general population.

Like with disruptive behavioral disorders, there is a high degree of comorbidity between ADHD and anxiety disorders, with 20% to 50% of patients diagnosed with ADHD also meeting *DSM–IV–TR* criteria for an anxiety disorder. Subtype analysis indicates that these disorders occur more often in patients with ADHD, Predominately Inattentive Subtype (Lahey et al., 1988), than in Hyperactive/Impulsive or Combined Types. As noted by Rutter (1989), the presence of an anxiety disorder in childhood or adolescence is a poor prognostic sign for later adult functioning. Consequently, as concluded by Spencer, Biederman, and Wilens (1999), "having both ADHD and anxiety disorders may substantially worsen the outcome of children with both disorders" (p. 921).

Differentiation of anxiety disorders from ADHD alone or in combination with an anxiety disorder hinges on the degree of deviation of the patient from age peers on measures of both attention and anxiety. Whereas ADHD is not characterized by symptoms of anxiety, patients with an anxiety disorder can exhibit impaired attention and concentration. Hence, it is important to assess the patient's attention under low-anxiety contexts or in standardized testing contexts after anxiety is being medically treated, as the pharmacological interventions for an anxiety disorder diagnosed in combination with ADHD will be markedly different than for anxiety disorders alone.

As is reviewed in chapter 6 (this volume), there is little indication that the antidepressants commonly prescribed for anxiety disorders (e.g., the selective serotonin reuptake inhibitors [SSRIs]) have any significant effect on the core symptoms of ADHD. Instead, as noted in a study of over 1,500 patients (Monastra, 2005a, 2005b), a combination of SSRI-type medications (or antihypertensive medications such as guanfacine or clonidine) and stimulants seems more effective in treating patients who have ADHD and a comorbid anxiety or mood disorder. The findings of the MTA Study (P. S. Jensen, Hinshaw, Swanson, et al., 2001) likewise indicate positive response to stimulant therapy in patients diagnosed with ADHD in combination with an anxiety disorder, thereby supporting the use of stimulants as a first-line treatment where both conditions are present.

Mood Disorders

The *DSM–IV–TR* lists 10 different types of mood disorders; however, clinical research has centered on an examination of Major Depressive Disorder, Dysthymia, and Bipolar Disorder alone and in combination with ADHD. The primary symptoms consist of indicators of either depression or mania (or both). As presented in detail in the *DSM–IV–TR*, depression is characterized by feelings of sadness or emptiness that persist most of the day, nearly every day. In children and teenagers, mood disorders can also be associated with irritability. There is typically a loss of interest or pleasure in daily activities, significant weight loss or gain, insomnia or hypersomnia, agitation, fatigue, feelings of worthlessness, guilt, diminished ability to think, and thoughts of death or suicide. Mania is characterized by symptoms such as inflated self-esteem, decreased need for sleep, talkativeness, pressured speech, flight of ideas, distractibility, increase in goal-directed activity, and involvement in pleasurable activities with high risk for adverse consequences.

As with other psychiatric disorders, the diagnosis requires that symptoms cause significant distress or impairment in social, occupational, or other important areas of functioning. For a diagnosis of a major depressive episode, five symptoms of depression must be noted for at least 2 weeks and represent a change from previous functioning, and one of the symptoms must be depressed mood or loss of interest or pleasure. For a diagnosis of a Dysthymic Disorder, the depressed mood must persist most of the day for at least 2 years. For a diagnosis of a bipolar disorder, three symptoms of mania must be noted for the diagnosis of a manic episode. For a mixed episode, the criteria for both a manic and a depressive episode must be met.

Examination of age of onset and distribution by gender indicates that mood disorders can occur during childhood, adolescence, or adulthood. However, the prevalence of mood disorders varies depending on age. According to the *DSM–IV–TR*, Major Depressive Disorder is estimated to occur in fewer than 1% of preschoolers, 1% to 2% of children in the elementary grades, and 5% of adolescents. Lifetime prevalence rates for Major Depressive Disorder range from 10% to 25% of women, to 5% to 12% of men. Dysthymia will develop in at least 6% of the adult population; Bipolar Disorder, in approximately 1% to 2% of the adult population, with 15% to 30% of patients diagnosed with Bipolar Disorder exhibiting at least one manic episode by the age of 19. Overall, mood disorders tend to occur 2 to 3 times as frequently in females than males, and are identified more often among first-degree biological relatives of persons diagnosed with mood disorders than in the general population.

The percentage of patients diagnosed with Mood Disorders who also meet *DSM–IV–TR* criteria for a diagnosis of ADHD is also quite high, ranging from 15% to 75%, with the majority of studies reporting a comorbidity rate between 9% and 32% (Pliszka, 2000; Waxmonsky, 2003). As with other psychiatric disorders that occur in combination with ADHD, the presence of a mood disorder with ADHD worsens the prognosis for recovery. Because patients diagnosed with a combination of these disorders tend to respond positively to pharmacological treatments for mood disorders and ADHD, antidepressant medications, as well as lithium and anticonvulsant medications (e.g., carbamazepine, valproic acid, gabapentin) are often introduced first for the treatment of moderate to severe depression, followed as needed with stimulant medications for residual symptoms of inattention and impaired concentration. When depressive symptoms are mild, relative to core ADHD symptoms, pharmacological treatment for ADHD alone may prove beneficial in reducing both the ADHD symptoms and depression (Spencer, Biederman, Wilens, & Faraone, 2002; Waxmonsky, 2003).

Review of the symptoms of ADHD and Mood Disorders reveals multiple overlapping characteristics that can impede accurate diagnosis, including diminished ability to think or concentrate and psychomotor agitation. In addition, several of the core symptoms of depression (e.g., poor appetite, insomnia, low self-esteem) are commonly reported by patients being treated for ADHD. For example, in Food and Drug Administration clinical trials, appetite suppression was noted in 22% of patients treated with mixed amphetamine salts, 14% of patients treated with atomoxetine, and 4% of those treated with extended release types of methylphenidate. Insomnia likewise was present in patients that were being pharmacologically treated for ADHD, occurring in 17% of those treated with mixed amphetamine salts, 16% of those treated with atomoxetine, and 4% of those being treated with methylphenidate (*Physicians' Desk Reference*, 2007).

In clinical practice, the differential diagnosis currently hinges on an examination of the age of onset of the patient's depression, the persistence of symptoms of depression, and the severity of depressive symptoms. Both Pliszka (2000) and Waxmonsky (2003) recommended that the diagnosis of a mood disorder should be made only when the depressed mood is present nearly every day for several hours and vegetative symptoms are prominent. Quantitative electroencephalographic (qEEG) procedures have also been developed to assist in the process of differential diagnosis among various psychiatric disorders, including depression, anxiety, and ADHD (see reviews by Chabot, di Michele, & Prichep, 2005; Monastra, 2004). In particular, the research of Davidson and Hugdahl (1995) has revealed specific qEEG characteristics in patients diagnosed with mood disorders. These electrophysiological indicators (i.e., cerebral asymmetry in the production of certain brain frequencies in the frontal lobe) are not prominent in patients diagnosed with ADHD. The use of such strategies in the assessment process are reviewed in detail in chapter 4.

Learning Disorders

The *DSM–IV–TR* lists three types of learning disorders: Reading Disorder, Mathematics Disorder, and a Disorder of Written Expression. The diagnostic criteria for the learning disorders are similar, requiring achievement that is substantially below that expected on the basis of an individual's age, measured intelligence, and level of education. In addition, the individual's skill level must significantly interfere with academic achievement or activities that require reading, mathematics, or written expression, respectively. The *DSM–IV–TR* criteria exclude skill deficits caused by a sensory impairment (e.g., vision, hearing, motor coordination). Typically, a level of performance 1.5 to 2.0 *SD* below age peers and/or below level of intelligence as measured by standardized tests of academic achievement and intellectual functions is considered sufficient to meet the first criterion for a diagnosis of a learning disorder. Onset of symptoms of each of these disorders is commonly noted in kindergarten; however, a diagnosis of a learning disorder is rarely made prior to the end of the first grade.

Estimates of the prevalence of learning disorders range from 2% to 10%, with the U.S. Department of Health and Human Services Centers for Disease Control and Prevention (CDCP) reporting approximately 4% of children aged 6 to 11 had been identified with a learning disorder (Pastor & Reuben, 2002). The CDCP report, prepared by Pastor and Reuben (2002), indicated that reading disorders occur in approximately 4% of the school-age population in the United States. Mathematics Disorder is estimated to occur in 1% of the population; the rate of Disorders of Written Expression is estimated to be less than 1%. Reading disorders occur more frequently in males than females (4:1), although referral bias is noted in the *DSM–IV–TR*. No gender features were cited for Mathematics Disorder or Disorder of Written Expression. In approximately 80% of diagnosed cases, multiple learning disorders are noted. As with ADHD, a high degree of heritability is reported, as learning disorders are more prevalent among first-degree biological relatives of individuals with learning disorders, according to the CDCP report.

In contrast with the low rate of occurrence of learning disorders in the general population, patients diagnosed with ADHD are commonly diagnosed with a learning disorder. Comorbidity rates ranging from 10% to 92% are reported, with most studies reporting that 40% to 60% of students diagnosed with ADHD will also meet diagnostic criteria for at least one learning disorder. Because several of the diagnostic criteria for ADHD involve impairment in the performance of academic tasks (e.g., makes careless mistakes in schoolwork, has difficulty sustaining attention on tasks, does not follow through on instructions, fails to finish schoolwork, avoids tasks that require sustained mental effort such as schoolwork or homework), it is often difficult to differentiate ADHD from a specific Learning Disorder without direct assessment of attention and core academic skills. Where evidence of both disorders is noted, the use of stimulant therapy has been suggested by several clinical researchers (Plizka, 2000; Waxmonsky, 2003), as improvements in both types of disorders have been reported following such treatment.

Substance Use Disorders

The *DSM–IV–TR* lists 12 specific types of disorders characterized by a maladaptive pattern of substance use that leads to clinically significant functional impairment or distress. The substances listed with the potential for dependence or abuse include alcohol, amphetamines, caffeine, cannabis, cocaine, hallucinogens, inhalants, nicotine, opioids, phencyclidine, sedatives, hypnotics or anxiolytics, and polysubstance use. The specific criteria for a diagnosis of Substance Dependence are described in the *DSM–IV–TR* and include evidence of increased tolerance; withdrawal syndrome; failure of efforts to reduce or control substance use; excessive expenditure of time to obtain the substance; discontinuation of involvement in social, occupational, or recreational activities; and continuation of use despite knowledge that the substance is causing physical or psychological problems. The diagnosis of Substance Abuse is characterized by recurrent substance use that causes a failure to fulfill major role obligations; use of the substance in situations in which it is hazardous; and repeated legal, social, or interpersonal problems related to substance use. Both Substance Dependence and Abuse require the persistence of symptoms for a consecutive 12-month period.

Onset of intoxication varies with substance; however, the first episode of alcohol, cannabis, and nicotine usage typically occurs by the midteen years. Although an estimated 20% to 25% of the general population has at least one substance use disorder (SUD), the rate nearly doubles in individuals diagnosed with ADHD (Biederman, Wilens, Mick, Faraone, & Spencer, 1998; Biederman, Wilens, et al., 1995; Molina & Pelham, 2003). Males and females are equally likely to develop at least one SUD. There is a high degree of heritability of SUD, with rates approximately 3 times greater in first-degree relatives of an individual with an SUD than the general population. Although at one time it was hypothesized that early exposure to stimulant medications was responsible for the increased risk for SUD, more recent studies have indicated that the use of pharmacotherapy for ADHD actually reduces the risk for SUD (Barkley, Fischer, Smallish, & Fletcher, 2003; Biederman, Wilens, Mick, Spencer, & Faraone, 1999). Because patients with ADHD and SUD can have loss of attention, concentration, and memory, it is essential that adolescent and adult patients presenting with ADHD symptoms be screened for psychoactive use. On the basis of the high prevalence rate in the general public and increased risk among patients with ADHD, laboratory testing for illegal psychoactives merits consideration in the assessment of patients older than 11 years of age.

Tic Disorders

The *DSM–IV–TR* lists four types of tic disorders: Tourette's Disorder, Chronic Motor or Vocal Tic Disorder, Transient Tic Disorder, and Tic Disorder Not Otherwise Specified. A *tic* is defined as "a sudden, rapid, recurrent, nonrhythmic, stereotyped motor movement or vocalization" (American Psychiatric Association, 2000, p. 108). Examples of simple motor tics include eye blinking, facial grimacing, nose wrinkling, neck jerking, and shoulder shrugging. Complex motor tics can include nonfunctional hand gestures, jumping, repetitive touching, stomping, retracing steps, twirling while walking, and assuming and holding unusual postures. More dramatic symptoms such as copropraxia (i.e., sudden vulgar, sexual, or obscene gesture) and echopraxia (i.e, mirroring of another's movements), are also examples of complex motor tics.

A variety of vocal tics are also listed in the *DSM–IV–TR*. Examples of simple vocal tics are throat clearing, grunting, sniffing, snorting, and chirping. Complex vocal tics include the sudden expression of single words or phrases; speech blocking; sudden and nonfunctional changes in the pitch, emphasis, or volume of speech; palilalia (i.e., repeating one's own speech), echolalia (i.e., repeating the last-heard sound, word, or phrase); and coprolalia (i.e., the sudden, inappropriate expression of a socially unacceptable word or phrase). Onset of a tic disorder can occur as early as the age of 2 years, with a median age of onset of motor tics of 6 to 7 years of age. Motor and vocal tics occur in a relatively large percentage of children and adolescents, with an estimated prevalence between 4% and 18% reported (Peterson, Pine, Cohen, & Brook, 2001; Spencer et al., 1999). Tourette's Disorder is far less common, occurring in fewer than 50 individuals in 10,000. Tourette's Disorder appears more common among males than females, with ratios ranging from 2:1 to 5:1. Like ADHD, there is a greater risk for Tourette's Disorder among first-degree blood relatives of individuals diagnosed with this disorder.

Although the risk for Tourette's Disorder does not significantly increase in patients with ADHD, the development of simple and complex tics can be precipitated by treatment with psychostimulants. When present, such symptoms typically require a reduction in the dosage of stimulant, a change of medication to a nonstimulant (e.g., atomoxetine, buproprion), or the initiation of treatment with an antihypertensive medication (e.g., clonidine, guanfacine). Individuals diagnosed with Tourette's Disorder are at greater risk for ADHD (25%–85%; Comings, 2000), necessitating the need for treating both disorders concurrently in clinical practice.

Examination of shared symptoms reveals that both ADHD and tic disorders are characterized by the presence of nonfunctional motor and verbal behaviors. In ADHD, the symptoms include excessive, intrusive speech, running, jumping, climbing, fidgeting, and squirming, in the absence of sudden involuntary simple or complex behaviors called *tics*. In tic disorders, excessive running, stomping, and intrusive speech can also occur; however, the defining characteristic of this disorder is the presence of sudden, involuntary vocal or motor behaviors. Differential diagnosis is typically determined by review of parent and teacher reports and direct observation of the child.

Eating Disorders

Two specific types of eating disorders (EDs) are described in *DSM–IV–TR*, Anorexia Nervosa and Bulimia Nervosa. Although the *DSM–IV–TR* notes an association between EDs and mood and anxiety disorders, the effect of dietary insufficiency on attention and concentration is also well documented (and is reviewed in chap. 5). Studies directly examining the degree of comorbidity between ADHD and EDs indicates that approximately 11% to 17% of patients diagnosed with ADHD will also meet diagnostic criteria for an ED (Surman, Randall, & Biederman, 2006; Wentz et al., 2005). Consequently, because of the impact of dietary deficiencies on attention and concentration, the comorbidity of these disorders among patients seen at our clinic, and the impact of this dual diagnosis on treatment, EDs are included among the conditions that require consideration in the evaluation and treatment of patients with ADHD.

According to the *DSM–IV–TR*, Anorexia Nervosa is a disorder that affects approximately 0.5% of the population, with a mid- to late-adolescent onset. It occurs more frequently in females than males (10:1) and is more prevalent among first-degree blood relatives of individuals diagnosed with this disorder. Symptoms include refusal to maintain body weight within 85% of expectations for age and height, fear of gaining weight, disturbance in body image, and amenorrhea.

Bulimia Nervosa, likewise, is a disorder with an onset in late adolescence that affects approximately 1% to 3% of the population at some point in their lives. It also occurs more frequently in females than males (10:1) and is more commonly found among first-degree biological relatives of diagnosed individuals than in the general population. According to the *DSM–IV–TR*, Bulimia Nervosa is characterized by recurrent episodes of eating an amount of food (within a discrete period of time) that is definitely larger than expected for most people, a sense of loss of control over eating during the episode, and the use of inappropriate behaviors to prevent weight gain (e.g., self-induced vomiting; use of laxatives, diuretics, or other medications). The frequency of such episodes is at least twice per week for 3 months.

Although there are no similarities between the core symptoms of either type of ED and ADHD, symptoms of inattention can result from this disorder. Because of the earlier age of onset of ADHD versus ED, review of school records for an indication of the onset of impairment of attention, as well as interviews with the patient and family members regarding early childhood history, can facilitate the process of differential diagnosis.

Childhood Developmental Disorders

Several other developmental disorders emerging during early childhood have also been associated with impairment of attention and executive functioning, in addition to their defining core symptoms: Autistic Disorder (AD), Asperger's Disorder (ASP), Central Auditory Processing Disorder (CAPD), and Sensory Integration (or Modulation) Disorder (SIMD). As described by Barkley (1997), B. F. Pennington and Ozonoff (1996), and Russell (1997), patients with ADHD exhibit deficits in a variety of skills, including attention, response inhibition, working memory, cognitive flexibility, planning, and fluency. However, investigations of the capacity for attention and executive functions in children with AD, ASP, CAPD, and SIMD reveal that children with these disorders also display impairment of attentional and executive functions (e.g., Chermak, Hall, & Musiek, 1999; Geurts, Verte, Oosterlaan, Roeyers, & Sergeant, 2004; Holtmann, Bolte, & Poustka, 2005; Mangeot et al., 2001; Noterdaeme, Amorosa, Mildenberger, Sitter, & Minow, 2001; Riccio, Hynd, Cohen, Hall, & Molt, 1994). A brief review of the comorbidity of each of these disorders with ADHD is provided in the following sections.

Autistic Disorder

As described in the *DSM–IV–TR*, the defining symptoms of AD include a delay in (or lack of) the development of spoken language, markedly abnormal social and communication skills, and a highly restricted range of activities and interests. Prevalence of AD is estimated to be approximately 5 cases per 10,000 individuals, occurring 4 to 5 times more often in males than females and an increased risk for emergence of AD is reported among family members. According to the CDCP (2007), prevalence of autistic spectrum disorders (ASD; including AD, ASP, and PDDs) is approximately 1 in 150. Onset of symptoms occurs prior to the age of 3 years.

There is no overlap between the specific diagnostic criteria for ADHD and AD; however, children with ADHD have numerous social skills and communication deficits and children with AD often have executive functioning deficits. As reviewed by Barkley (2006) and Hinshaw (2002), children with ADHD have difficulty tracking and engaging in mutually enjoyable conversations, struggling with the challenges of word retrieval. Like children with AD, they can become highly fixated on particular areas of interest. Conversely, children whose core symptoms are defined in social or relational terms (i.e., AD) demonstrate difficulty in cognitive flexibility, planning, and working memory (Ozonoff & Strayer, 1997; Russell, 1997). Hyperactivity and impulsivity are also commonly observed in children diagnosed with AD (Goldstein & Schwebach, 2004; D. O. Lee & Ousley, 2006).

Asperger's Disorder

Like those diagnosed with AD, individuals diagnosed with ASP exhibit significant impairment in the development of social and communication skills and demonstrate a markedly restricted range of interests and activities. Unlike patients with AD, children with ASP do not demonstrate a significant delay in language development. Definitive prevalence rates have not been established to date, although there appears to be an increased rate of occurrence among family members. There are no shared symptoms with ADHD, according to *DSM–IV–TR* criteria; however, as noted with AD, patients with ADHD show significant impairment of social functioning and patients with ASP display evidence of impairment of attention and executive functions.

Studies of attention and executive functions among patients diagnosed with ASP have revealed a high rate of attentional problems (Holtmann et al., 2005), as well as comorbid ADHD (Ehlers & Gillberg, 1993; Ghaziuddin, Weidmer-Mikhail, & Ghaziuddin, 1998). Holtmann et al. (2005) reported that 65% of 104 patients with ASP were rated as having clinically significant levels of "attention problems" on the Child Behavior Checklist. Ghaziuddin et al. (1998) noted that approximately 33% (10 of 36) of their ASP patients also met criteria for a diagnosis of ADHD. A higher percentage of comorbid ADHD (80%; 4 of 5 patients) was noted in the study of patients with ASP reported by Ehlers and Gillberg (1993).

Because of the high degree of comorbid ADHD among patients with ASP, Fitzgerald and Kewley (2005) and Holtmann et al. (2005) recommended that the current *DSM–IV–TR* criteria be revised to improve the care of patients presenting with characteristics of both disorders. Currently, the presence of a PDD (like ASP) precludes the diagnosis of ADHD. In clinical practice, Fitzgerald and Kewley (2005) and Holtmann et al. (2005) asserted that when ADHD and ASP are present, initial treatment for ADHD merits consideration. Once effective treatment for core ADHD symptoms has been initiated, then residual social and communication skill deficits can be addressed. A study using such an approach (Monastra, 2005a, 2005b) reported that patients presenting with ADHD with comorbid ASP or AD responded positively to treatment with antihypertensive medication (e.g., guanfacine, clonidine) or SSRIs (e.g., paroxetine) in combination with low doses of methylphenidate or mixed amphetamine salts).

Central Auditory Processing Disorder

CAPD is defined by the American Speech–Language–Hearing Association Task Force on Central Auditory Processing Consensus Development (1996) as a deficiency in one or more of the following abilities: sound localization–lateralization, auditory discrimination or pattern recognition; temporal resolution, masking, integration, or ordering; or auditory performance decrements with competing or degraded acoustic stimuli. It is not specifically listed among the disorders included in *DSM–IV–TR*. Comparison between the characteristics of CAPD and ADHD reveal multiple overlapping symptoms, particularly inattention while listening, distractibility, and the associated functional symptoms related to such lack of attention (e.g., does not follow through on instructions, does not attend to or fails to remember verbal instructions).

This high degree of similarity between CAPD and ADHD has prompted researchers to examine patterns of comorbidity between the two disorders. Riccio et al. (1994) reported that 15 of 30 children diagnosed with CAPD also met criteria for a diagnosis of ADHD. Jerome (2000) likewise noted a high level of ADHD among children diagnosed with CAPD, reporting that 72% of his sample (*n* = 62) met criteria for a diagnosis of ADHD, as well as CAPD. Such comorbidity rates have prompted certain researchers (e.g., Keller, 1992) to suggest that the diagnosis of CAPD versus ADHD is a function of the professional training of the evaluator, asserting that the child with attentional and language disorders will be diagnosed with CAPD by an audiologist and ADHD by a psychologist.

To address the question of whether ADHD and CAPD were distinct disorders, several research teams have examined response to stimulant medication. A review of the literature revealed five studies examining stimulant effects in children diagnosed with either ADHD or CAPD or both (Cook et al., 1993; Gascon, Johnson, & Burd, 1986; Jerome, 2000; Keith & Engineer, 1991; Tillery, Katz, & Keller, 2000). In each of the studies, significant improvement in performance on tests of central auditory processing was reported in patients from both of the groups, although Tillery et al. (2000) reported significant improvement in only one of four CAP measures (an auditory continuous performance test).

As noted by Riccio et al. (1994), it remains premature to conclude whether CAPD and ADHD represent two distinct clinical entities. However, in clinical practice, use of stimulant medications in the treatment of children diagnosed with CAPD appears to merit consideration. On a similar note, close collaboration between speech–language pathologists and mental health providers is recommended (e.g., Riccio et al., 1994), as is the provision of speech–language therapy for patients with ADHD who manifest language and communication deficits. Such treatment appears particularly imperative if impairment of language functions persisted despite effective pharmacological treatment of the core symptoms of ADHD.

Sensory Integration (or Modulation) Disorder

Another type of developmental disorder that is not specifically listed in the *DSM–IV–TR* is SIMD. Research dating to the early 1990s indicates that children with ADHD exhibit a variety of motor and sensory abnormalities, in addition to core ADHD symptoms (Cermak, 1991; A. Fisher, Murray, & Bundy, 1991; Lane, Miller, & Hanft, 2000; D. N. McIntosh, Miller, Shyu, & Dunn, 1999). These include symptoms of impaired sensory integration (i.e., poor balance, impaired motor coordination, poor visuomotor skills, and motor planning deficits), which have been postulated to be related to inadequate or inefficient sensory processing of the vestibular, somatosensory, and other sensory systems (Ayres, 1979), as well as symptoms of impaired sensory modulation (i.e., "the ability to regulate and organize the degree, intensity, and nature of responses to sensory input in a graded and adaptive manner, so that an optimal range of performance and adaptation to challenges can be maintained"; Mangeot et al., 2001, p. 399).

As described by Mangeot et al. (2001), the behavioral expressions of SIMD in children include both sensation seeking (e.g., touches too hard, invades others' "personal space," is overly active, craves jumping or "bump-and-crash"–type activities) and sensation avoidance (e.g., aggressive response to touch, withdrawing from unexpected touch or from situations where unexpected touch might occur, fearful reaction with movement or when feet leave the ground, overreaction to touch such as holding hands, feelings of discomfort when jumping or running). Children with SIMD often appear poorly coordinated and lack motor planning, balance, and visuomotor skills (e.g., tying shoes, writing).

Estimates of the degree of comorbidity between ADHD and SIMD have not been definitively established. However, several studies provide some indication of the presence of characteristics of SIMD in children diagnosed with ADHD. Mangeot et al. (2001) examined 26 children diagnosed with ADHD and 30 "typically developing" control children, using a battery of tests designed to assess SIMD symptoms (Sensory Challenge Protocol; D. N. McIntosh, Miller, Shyu, & Hagerman, 1999), as well as electrodermal response. Results indicated that 20 of the 26 children with ADHD (77%) had scores >1.0 standard deviations below the mean. Conversely, within the control group, only 1 of 30 children (3%) performed below the "normal" range. Such findings are consistent with the results of a more recently published study by Pitcher, Piek, and Hay (2003), who reported motor dysfunction in 58% of their sample diagnosed with ADHD, Predominately Inattentive Type; 49% of those diagnosed with ADHD, Predominately Hyperactive–Impulsive Type; and 47% of those diagnosed with ADHD, Combined Type.

A larger, retrospective examination of the performance of 5,680 children on the Sensory Integration and Praxis Test (SIPT; Ayres, 1989) was reported by Mulligan (1996). In her study, Mulligan compared the performance of children diagnosed with ADHD (*n* = 309) with that of matched peers who had been referred for evaluation because of concerns about motor delays (*n* = 5,371). In both groups, evidence of significant impairment was noted on the SIPT. In both the ADHD patients and the non-ADHD participants with motor delays, significantly poorer performance was noted on the following subtests: standing and walking balance, design copy, postural praxis, praxis on verbal command, sequencing praxis, oral praxis, kinesthesia, and graphesthesia. It is surprising to note that patients diagnosed with ADHD demonstrated a greater degree of overall impairment on the SIPT than individuals who were initially referred because of concerns about motor development.

In subsequent analyses, Mulligan (1996) investigated whether certain of the deficits found on the SIPT could be related to impairment of vestibular processing and found significant differences between 309 patients diagnosed with ADHD and 309 matched control participants. Because the semicircular canals within the inner ear and the otolithic utricles–saccules of the vestibular system activate the autonomic nervous system (Yates, 1992) and stimulate attentional processes, other researchers examined whether vestibular stimulation (through the use of swings, hammocks, swivel chairs, and other rhythmic motion devices) could reduce ADHD symptoms (Arnold, Clark, Sachs, Jakim, & Smithies, 1985; Bhatara, Clark, Arnold, Gunsett, & Smeltzer, 1981). Although the initial results of these studies have been positive, the degree of improvement that can result from this type of intervention remains an empirical question. However, as reviewed by Arnold (2002), there appears to be support for considering such stimulation as part of the overall treatment for children with ADHD.

In summary, research examining the extent of comorbidity between ADHD and certain developmental disorders (e.g., AD, ASP, CAPD, SIMD) indicates that at least 50% of patients with ADHD will manifest significant impairment of sensorimotor, auditory processing, language, communication, or social functions that will further impede the successful adjustment of these individuals. Because of the degree of impairment and the high percentage of affected individuals, consultation with both speech–language pathologists and therapists and occupational therapists seems likely to enhance the prognosis of patients with ADHD.

AREAS OF FUNCTIONAL IMPAIRMENT

Beyond the core symptoms of ADHD and comorbid psychiatric, learning, and developmental disorders, patients diagnosed with ADHD also exhibit evidence of significant functional impairment at home, school, work, and in their social relationships. As thoroughly reviewed by Barkley (2006) and Hinshaw (2002), the vast majority of patients with ADHD experience a high degree of peer and parental rejection, underachieve in educational settings, are unemployed or underemployed, are more frequently arrested and convicted of criminal actions, and are at higher risk for accidental injury.

Barkley (2006) provides a detailed examination of the specific social impairments exhibited by children with ADHD. These children live in families where there is a greater degree of intrafamilial conflict, particularly in the parent–child dyad. Their parents tend to fluctuate between so-called lax and overreactive disciplinary styles, using more coercive management strategies than the parents of children without ADHD. Perhaps owing to the physical and psychological demands of supervising these children or the increased rate of ADHD among the first-degree biological relatives of children with ADHD, parents tend to be less responsive in social interactions and more critical and less rewarding of the behavior of children with ADHD.

Children and teens with ADHD tend to have difficulty engaging in mutually enjoyable conversations at home. Although the majority of children with ADHD are overly talkative, others struggle to produce language in social contexts. Both types of children are less likely to respond to questions or statements made by peers. The children with ADHD are also more likely to be viewed as defiant, noncompliant, and less able to engage in work and play activities than age peers. They are also more likely to be viewed as detached or aggressive in play contexts.

The impact of such behavioral tendencies is evident in peer acceptance as well. A detailed examination of the peer relationships of children with ADHD was conducted by Hoza et al. (2005) and summarized by Hoza (2007). In their comparison of 165 children diagnosed with ADHD and 1,298 classmates, Hoza et al. examined social preference and "likability." They found that children with ADHD were less well-liked, had fewer dyadic friends, and were commonly placed in the "rejected" social status category by their peers. Within the social context of the school, they were not selected for friendship by the children of higher social preference and likability.

The combination of a high frequency of learning disorders and low peer acceptance seems likely to contribute to the pattern of retention, suspensions, and school drop-out rates. As reviewed by Barkley (2006), over 50% of children with ADHD require tutoring, approximately 33% require the assistance of special education teachers, and between 30% and 40% are retained in at least one grade. Suspensions occur in approximately 50% of patients; between 10% and 33% of children with ADHD drop out of school prior to completion of their high school diploma requirements.

Consistent with these reports of academic problems, Mannuzza et al. (1993) reported that approximately 25% of their ADHD sample did not graduate from high school or attain an equivalency diploma (vs. 2% of the comparison group). Adults without ADHD were approximately 4 times more likely to attain a bachelor's degree (34% vs. 9%) and pursue postgraduate degrees (7% vs. 2%) than adults with ADHD. Using the Hollingshead and Redlich (1958) Occupational Scale, a significant difference in the level of occupational status was also reported by these authors.

With such high rates of academic and social problems, increased risks for legal problems would be anticipated. An investigation of a nationally representative sample of over 6,000 adult inmates from 431 jails in the United States revealed that approximately 10% of inmates had dyslexia or ADHD (Harlow, 1998). Similarly, Mannuzza et al. (1993), Murphy and Barkley (1996), and M. Weiss and Hechtman (1993) reported increased risk for criminal behavior in adults with ADHD. Among adolescents diagnosed with ADHD, the rate of incarceration is substantially higher, with approximately 50% of "delinquent" youths being diagnosed with ADHD (Foley, Carlton, & Howell, 1996; Zagar, Arbit, Hughes, Busell, & Busch, 1989).

A final area of functional impairment centers on the increased risk for accidental injury or poisoning in patients with ADHD. Multiple studies have indicated that patients with ADHD are 2 to 3 times more likely to experience an accidental injury sufficient to require sutures or hospitalization. Hartsough and Lambert (1985) reported that approximately 16% of children with ADHD in their sample had at least four or more serious accidental injuries (e.g., bone fractures, lacerations requiring sutures, head injury). Only 5% of their comparison group had a similar history of injury. P. S. Jensen, Shervette, Xenakis, and Bain (1988) noted a twofold increase in incidence of any physical trauma sufficient to require sutures or hospitalization in their study (68.4% vs. 39.5%).

Increased risk for multiple automobile accidents has also been consistently reported in the literature (Barkley, Guevremont, Anastopoulos, DuPaul, & Shelton, 1993; Barkley, Murphy, & Kwasnik, 1996a; Woodward, Fergusson, & Horwood, 2000). These studies indicated that although there is no significant difference between ADHD patients and age peers in the occurrence of a single automobile accident, the rate of such accidents (1.5 vs. 0.4), as well as the percentage of multiple accidents (40.0% vs. 5.6%) is significantly greater in the ADHD group (Barkley et al., 1993), with the percentage of individuals involved in more severe crashes (involving injury) also being significantly greater in individuals diagnosed with ADHD (60% vs. 17%; Barkley et al., 1996a).

In addition to increased risk for accidental injuries at play or while driving, patients with ADHD are also more likely to have suffered from an accidental poisoning. Although the percentage of individuals with ADHD experiencing accidental poisoning has varied from 7.3% to 21.0% (compared with 2.6%–7.7% of individuals without ADHD), published research has consistently indicated that children with ADHD are 2 to 3 times more likely to have been poisoned (P. S. Jensen et al., 1988; Stewart, Thach, & Friedin,

1970; Szatmari et al., 1989a, 1989b). Such findings provide further impetus for the need for early intervention in the diagnosis and treatment of ADHD.

IMPLICATIONS FOR CLINICAL PRACTICE

In clinical practice, health care providers are asked to intervene to help promote the health, well-being, and social development of patients presenting with symptoms of inattention, impulsivity, and hyperactivity. These patients commonly present with at least one comorbid psychiatric disorder; are likely to be struggling to function effectively at home, school, occupational, and recreational settings; and are at heightened risk for injury and the development of patterns of psychoactive substance abuse and/or dependence. Despite the multiplicity of clinical problems and degree of functional impairments presented in this chapter, several lessons can be gleaned from the research literature.

First, ADHD presents as the only psychiatric disorder in a minority of cases seen in clinical practice. Comorbid learning and psychiatric disorders are likely to be present in nearly 75% of patients diagnosed with ADHD. Because of the wide range of psychiatric and functional problems found in patients with ADHD, it is unlikely that a treatment program consisting of stimulant medication alone will yield optimal results. Pharmacological and psychological treatment of each of the presenting psychiatric disorders is likely to be required to achieve alleviation of core clinical features, with initial emphasis typically placed on the introduction and maintenance of effective treatment for the core symptoms of ADHD.

Second, because developmental disorders of language and communication, auditory processing, and/or sensorimotor functions occur in at least 50% of patients diagnosed with ADHD, consultation with audiologists, speech–language therapists, and occupational therapists seems advisable in order to develop a care program that integrates multiple modalities of treatment to enhance the development and functioning of cortical regions involved in attention and other executive functions (e.g., motor planning, fluency).

Third, the presence of a high degree of comorbidity with learning, developmental, and other psychiatric disorders requires practitioners to use a combination of assessment strategies in determining a diagnostic formulation. An assessment protocol that includes direct assessment of attention and capacity for behavioral regulation, as well as auditory processing, and sensorimotor integration can help clarify diagnostic issues and promote a higher rate of treatment initiation, a reduction in frequency of adverse effects, and an increase in the likelihood of treatment maintenance.

Fourth, although interview and behavioral rating scales are commonly used in clinical practice in combination with clinical interview to determine a diagnosis of ADHD, the similarity between the behavioral characteristics of ADHD and other medical and psychiatric disorders—as well as the low interrater reliability among parent, teacher, and patient ratings—creates a context in which there is uncertainty regarding the validity of the diagnosis of ADHD when such a determination is made on the basis of history and behavioral symptoms alone. Recent estimates indicate that only 25% to 56% of diagnosed patients are receiving even minimal treatment (i.e., fewer than 12 prescriptions per year), primarily because of parental distrust of a diagnosis based on interview and rating scales alone (P. S. Jensen, 2000; Monastra, 2005a, 2005b). Consequently, more comprehensive assessment strategies that incorporate direct assessment of attention and capacity for behavioral regulation seem required to promote the sustained treatment of patients with ADHD.

Fifth, because of the range of functional problems exhibited by patients with ADHD, comprehensive care needs to proceed from an assessment of areas of functional impairment and the development of a treatment plan that systematically addresses such impairments at home, school, occupational, and other social settings. Recommendations for conducting such a functional assessment are provided in chapter 4.

2

THE ETIOLOGY OF ADHD:
A NEUROLOGICAL PERSPECTIVE

For decades, clinicians have been aware of the increased incidence of attention-deficit/hyperactivity disorder (ADHD) among family members. However, the process by which such family patterns were inherited, and the nature of the resultant neuroanatomical, biochemical, and neurophsysiological characteristics of ADHD remained largely unknown throughout much of the 20th century. By the conclusion of the century, techniques for genetic mapping became available in clinical research, and positron emission tomography (PET), single photon emission computed tomography (SPECT), functional magnetic resonance imaging (fMRI), and quantitative electroencephalography (qEEG) imaging techniques began to provide the view of ADHD from within.

No longer restricted to investigations of the behavioral expressions of ADHD, neuroscientists have been able to develop and test models of the cortical systems responsible for alerting, preparation for response, phasic cognitive and motoric responding to stimuli, and sustained concentration, through direct examination of the brain. As theoretical models were presented and critically evaluated, an understanding of the nature of specific cortical and subcortical regions responsible for attention and behavioral regulation began to emerge. Paralleling such developments was an examination of structural, biochemical, and electrophysiological anomalies in patients diagnosed with ADHD, and the development of brain-based formulations of the causes of ADHD. An understanding of the relationship between genetics, neuroanatomy, neurochemistry, neurophysiology, and the behavioral expressions of ADHD is essential to comprehend the nature of this disorder and those treatments that are effective.

The purpose of this chapter is to provide a review of the neuroscience research as related to ADHD. As concluded by recent examinations of this literature (Barkley, 2006; Bobb, Castellanos, Addington, & Rapoport, 2005; Giedd, Blumenthal, Molloy, & Castellanos, 2001; Monastra, 2005a), it is becoming clear that ADHD is associated with specific abnormalities of at least four genes and that such abnormalities appear to be expressed in anatomical differences in the frontal lobes, basal ganglia, corpus callosum, and cerebellum, as well as in neurochemical and neurophysiological anomalies of the brains of individuals diagnosed with ADHD. On the basis of this research, several models for understanding attention and behavioral regulation have been presented, with emphasis placed on understanding how neurological anomalies contribute to the disruption of these functions in patients diagnosed with ADHD (e.g., Barkley, 1997; Chabot, di Michele, & Prichep, 2005; F. Levy, 1991; Niedermeyer & Naidu, 1998; Nigg, 2000; Posner & Petersen, 1990; Sergeant, 2005).

As expressed by Chabot et al. (2005), the emerging consensus is that "ADHD cannot be conceptualized as a single disease entity with a narrow phenotype and distinct cause" (p. 42). Rather, as is illustrated in this review, ADHD appears to be associated with a dysregulation of the activation and interaction of multiple cortical and subcortical regions involved in various attentional functions, as well as the organization, regulation, and expression of behavioral response to situational demands. The implications of such research findings for patient assessment, as well as the selection and implementation of pharmacological and neurophsyiological treatments for ADHD, are discussed in this chapter as well.

GENETIC STUDIES OF ADHD

As reported in the *Diagnostic and Statistical Manual of Mental Disorders* (4th ed., text rev.; *DSM–IV–TR*; American Psychiatric Association, 2000), ADHD is a psychiatric disorder with a significantly greater incidence of occurrence among first- and second-degree relatives of identified patients. The risk for concordant ADHD among twins ranges from approximately 75% among monozygotic twins (R. Levy, Hay, McStephen, Wood, & Waldman, 1997; Silberg et al., 1996; Willcutt, Pennington, & DeFries, 2000) to approximately 30% to 35% among dizygotic twins (Bradley & Golden, 2001). In familial studies, siblings of children diagnosed with ADHD are at substantially greater risk for the development of this disorder. Estimates of the degree of risk place the likelihood for ADHD among siblings of children with ADHD to be 3 to 7 times greater than the prevalence rate in the general population (Biederman, Keenan, & Faraone, 1990; Biederman et al., 1992; Welner, Welner, Stewart, Palkes, & Wish, 1977). In summation, this research indicates that between 10% and 35% of the siblings of children with ADHD will also have this disorder. It is striking that both Biederman, Faraone, et al. (1995) and Smalley et al. (2000) noted that the likelihood of ADHD in a child dramatically increases in families containing a parent diagnosed with ADHD. Biederman, Faraone, et al. reported a risk rate of approximately 57%. Smalley et al. indicated that in families containing at least two children with ADHD, the likelihood that at least one parent had been diagnosed with ADHD at one point in their lives was 55%.

This clustering of ADHD within families supported the hypothesis that ADHD was an inherited disorder and stimulated extensive research to uncover the genetic foundation of this disorder. The review article by Bobb et al. (2005) as well as the chapter by Swanson and Castellanos (2002) provide a comprehensive perspective on the status of genetic research at this time. Bobb et al. reviewed the molecular genetic studies of ADHD that were published between 1991 and 2004. Their examination of the research encompassed 94 polymorphisms in 33 candidate genes. Neurotransmitter systems that were investigated included dopamine (DA), serotonin (5-HT), and noradrenalin, as well as other candidate genes selected because of their role in mediating the action of neurotransmitter systems (e.g., monoamine oxidase–A, –B), their role in addiction processes (e.g., nicotinic acetylcholine receptor, alpha-4 and alpha-7 subunits; cannabinoid receptor), or their neural function (e.g., glutamate receptor; ionotropic; N-methyl-D-aspartate–2A, a receptor involved in short-term and working memory). Genome-wide scans (i.e., studies examining the entire spectrum of the human genome) were also incorporated in their review.

Bobb et al. (2005) concluded that there was evidence of an association for four genes and ADHD: DA D4 and D5 receptors, the DA transporter DAT1, and the 5-HT transporter (5-HTT). Other candidate genes (e.g., the norepinephrine [NE] transporter gene [NET1]; the DA D2 and 5-HT 2A receptors) have also been implicated in a number of studies investigating their association with ADHD (e.g., Comings, 2001; Comings et al., 2000a, 2000b; Levitan et al., 2002; Li, Wang, Qian, Wang, & Zhou, 2002). The discovery of genetic anomalies on these specific candidate genes would be expected, given our understanding of the pharmacokinetics of certain medications commonly prescribed to treat core ADHD symptoms.

For example, methylphenidate, which inhibits DAT1 (thereby increasing the amount and duration of action of DA in the synapse; see Amara & Kuhar, 1993; Volkow et al., 1995) has been demonstrated to be an effective treatment for ADHD. Therefore, the association of anomalies of the genetic region responsible for the development of DAT1 and ADHD would be anticipated. Atomoxetine, an NET inhibitor, has also been shown to effectively reduce ADHD symptoms (Michelson et al., 2001). This medication inhibits the activity of noradrenergic reuptake transporters (such as NET1), increasing the amount and prolonging the synaptic availability of noradrenalin. The development of an effective pharmacological treatment that targets NET1 is again consistent with certain of the genetic findings.

Although the identification of specific genetic anomalies seems likely to continue to support the development of medications targeting DA, NE, and 5-HT receptors and transporters, a review of the genetic research does not lead to a conclusion that ADHD is a neuropsychiatric disorder that is inherited from a single polymorphism or specific combination of polymorphisms. Genome-wide scans, such as those conducted by Arcos-Burgos et al. (2003), Bakker et al. (2003), S. E. Fisher et al. (2002), and Ogdie et al. (2003), are less prone to selection bias and have provided additional support for examining genetic regions responsible for the development of DA receptors (D2, D1), as well as other structures (e.g., glutamate receptor, GRIN2A; nicotinic acetylcholine receptor, CHRNA7). However, at present, interpretation of the genetic research is greatly limited by the inconsistency in the definition of ADHD (categorical vs. dimensional). Review of the literature indicates that selection criteria exert a significant moderating effect on the outcome of genetic studies.

The impact of patient selection criteria on genetic research is clearly reflected in the analysis conducted by Bobb et al. (2005). For example, when a dimensional definition is used (in which severity of symptoms is measured and incorporated in the selection criteria), 60% of the genetic studies identify polymorphisms that are significantly associated with ADHD (25% yield negative findings; 15% yield positive trends). In contrast, when a categorical definition of ADHD is used (in which selection criteria are based on a diagnosis of ADHD made by a health care provider), only 33% of the studies identify polymorphisms that are positively associated with ADHD (50% yield negative findings).

Further impeding research efforts to clarify the specific genetic factors that are contributing to ADHD in a specific patient is the lack of control for comorbid psychiatric and medical disorders. The vast majority of patients diagnosed with ADHD meet *DSM–IV–TR* criteria for at least one other psychiatric disorder. In addition, as noted by Barkley (2006) and reflected in our study of 1,514 families with at least one member diagnosed with ADHD (Monastra, 2005b), a small but clinically significant percentage of patients (approximately 5%) demonstrate symptoms of inattention, impulsivity, and/ or hyperactivity due to other medical conditions. Such conditions include prenatal exposure to alcohol and tobacco smoke (in utero), lead poisoning, anemia, hypoglycemia, thyroid disorders, allergies, and other metabolic and nutritional disorders. Despite the significance of medical and psychiatric comorbidities in clinical practice, much of the genetic research conducted to date has not directly assessed or controlled for such factors.

Because of such methodological problems, genetic research has not provided a clear picture of the factors that are responsible for the high degree of concordance in twin studies and the increased incidence of ADHD among blood relatives. However, with the use of genome-wide scanning (to reduce selection bias), inclusion of a dimensional definition of ADHD, and improved screening for comorbid psychiatric and medical conditions, it seems quite likely that advances in molecular genetics will greatly contribute to an understanding of the underlying etiology of ADHD and the nature of effective treatments in the coming years. At this time, geneticists have identified several candidate genes that are associated with ADHD. Medications targeting the neuroanatomical expressions of these polymorphisms have been developed and are effective in the treatment of certain of the symptoms exhibited by patients diagnosed with ADHD.

Implications of Genetic Research for Clinical Practice

Given the variability of symptom presentation in clinical practice, it seems highly unlikely that any one polymorphism will be responsible for the range of symptoms manifested by patients with ADHD. Within the population of patients with ADHD, some exhibit evidence of impaired behavioral regulation, others do not. Some patients display significant impairment of mood regulation, exhibiting marked depression of mood or heightened anxiety; other patients do not. Some patients demonstrate marked difficulty in producing spontaneous language and avoiding eye contact and social interactions. Others are quite engaging. As examination of such differences is incorporated into genetic research, it seems likely that the delineation of multiple, genetically based, neuropsychiatric disorders that share symptoms of inattention and/or impaired behavioral regulation will be achieved.

Until such time, the current genetic research provides support for the investigation and application of pharmacological interventions that target DA, noradrenalin, and 5-HT receptors and transporters. In addition, the high rate of concordance found in twin studies and the increased prevalence of ADHD among blood relatives support the rationale for examining family psychiatric history in the assessment of patients for ADHD. Although the presence of ADHD in a blood relative does not indicate a diagnosis of ADHD in a specific patient, such a finding does significantly increase the likelihood of such a diagnosis.

Neuroimaging Studies of ADHD

Although genetic studies of patients with ADHD have provided evidence that neural systems that use DA, noradrenalin, and 5-HT may play a critical role in the development and maintenance of the core symptoms of ADHD, neuroimaging studies using magnetic resonance imaging (MRI), fMRI, PET, and SPECT have illustrated how such genetic anomalies may be expressed anatomically. Collectively, neuroimaging studies using MRI, fMRI, PET and SPECT have revealed abnormalities in regions of the brain involved in the regulation of attention, behavioral control, and judgment (particularly, the frontal lobes, basal ganglia, corpus callosum, and cerebellum; see Figure 2.1).

The arousal and activation of these regions have also been clarified in numerous studies examining the neurophysiology of those brain regions involved in alerting and executive functions (e.g., response inhibition, working memory, cognitive flexibility, planning, internalization of speech and reconstitution of language). Such neuronal activity is expressed in dynamic electrophysiological discharges, which are recorded on electroencephalographs (EEGs) and quantified via computerized power spectral analyses that define modern qEEG. In this section, MRI, fMRI, PET, SPECT, and qEEG findings are summarized, with an emphasis placed on clarifying the neurological foundation of ADHD at a cellular and regional level.

MRI and fMRI Studies

As extensively reviewed by Durston (2003), Giedd et al. (2001), and Swanson and Castellanos (2002), volumetric studies of total brain and regional brain volume have consistently revealed significant differences between groups of individuals diagnosed with ADHD and matched control participants. The brains of patients with ADHD are approximately 5% smaller than age- and gender-matched control participants in total volume. MRI examination of the volume of specific anatomic structures associated with the control of movement (basal ganglia and cerebellum), executive control functions (anterior cingulate gyrus), alerting functions (right frontal region), and the left dorsolateral region of the frontal lobe (verbal working memory and fluency) has revealed that each of these regions is approximately 10% to 12% smaller in patients diagnosed with ADHD.

In addition to overall and regional reduction in volume, evidence of asymmetry has been found in certain MRI studies. Asymmetry of one of the basal ganglia (caudate nucleus) has also been identified, with a tendency for the right caudate to be smaller than the left noted. Finally, reduced size in the rostral (anterior) region of the corpus callosum has been reported, although evidence of reduced size of the splenium area was reported in a study of stimulant nonresponders (Semrud-Clikeman, Filipek, Biederman, & Steingard, 1994). Also, fMRI studies (in which regional blood flow is monitored) have revealed lower blood flow into the striatum, a brain region that connects the frontal region and limbic system and includes the caudate nucleus. This pathway (the right inferior frontal lobe and its projections to the caudate nucleus) appears to be integral for response inhibition. Consis-

GROSS ANATOMY OF THE BRAIN

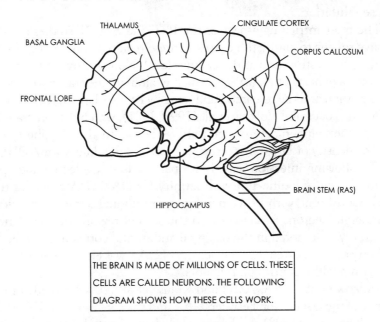

THE BRAIN IS MADE OF MILLIONS OF CELLS. THESE CELLS ARE CALLED NEURONS. THE FOLLOWING DIAGRAM SHOWS HOW THESE CELLS WORK.

CELLULAR LEVEL ACTIVITY OF A NEURON

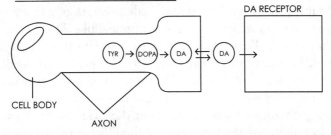

Figure 2.1. Brain regions responsible for attention and behavioral inhibition. DA = dopamine; DOPA = dihydroxyphenylaline; RAS = reticular activating system; TYR = tyrosine. Illustrated by Bridget Monastra.

tent with the results of genetic studies, the regions in which atypical findings were reported are also known to contain a high concentration of dopaminergic and noradrenergic brain cells.

PET and SPECT Studies

Similar to MRI and fMRI studies, abnormalities in the right lateral prefrontal cortex, the right middle temporal cortex, and the orbital and cerebellar cortices (bilaterally) have been noted on SPECT scans, with decreased blood flow emerging as the most consistent finding in patients diagnosed with ADHD. PET studies have likewise noted reduced glucose metabolism in the prefrontal cortex and basal ganglia in both adult and adolescent samples.

Again, as noted with fMRI and MRI studies, these regions are essential for response inhibition.

The most intriguing aspect of the PET and SPECT studies are those that have sought to clarify the causes of these regional abnormalities by examining specific structures at the cellular level. Noteworthy are the investigations of Dougherty et al. (1999), which examined DA transporter density in the striatum, and the research conducted by Krause, Dresel, Krause, Kung, and Tatsch (2000) and Volkow et al. (1998, 2001), which demonstrated the impact of methylphenidate on striatal DA levels. In the Dougherty et al. study, the density of DA transporters was assessed in adults with ADHD via SPECT, following injection with I-altropane, a highly selective radiopharmaceutical type of iodine-123 with affinity for DAT (DA reuptake transporter). Consistent with other neuroimaging findings, the distribution of dopaminergic neurons was greatest in the striatal region, with evidence of DA pathways also noted in the occipital and frontal cortex and cerebellum. Dougherty et al. reported that the density of DAT was elevated by 70% compared with healthy control participants.

Volkow et al. (1998, 2001) and Krause et al. (2000) provided further evidence of the association between DAT and the core symptoms of ADHD. Both Volkow et al. (1998) and Krause et al. demonstrated that methylphenidate blocks the activity of over 50% of the DAT in the striatum. Volkow et al. (2001) subsequently reported that the administration of methylphenidate caused significant increases in levels of extracellular DA in the striatum. Such findings led Volkow et al. (2001) to postulate that the symptoms of ADHD could be related to the excessive activity of DAT, in essence causing underarousal in the striatal region (and associated cortical regions). Such reduction in activity was effectively treated by the use of a pharmacological agent (methylphenidate) which increased the availability of extracellular DA, thereby enhancing the activation of the DA neural system.

qEEG Studies

MRI, fMRI, SPECT, and PET studies have sought to clarify specific abnormalities of brain structure at the cellular and regional level. Researchers using qEEG techniques have investigated electrophysiological abnormalities in the patterns of electrophysiological activation of specific brain regions. As reviewed by Chabot et al. (2005), Clarke and Barry (2004), and Loo and Barkley (2005), the electrical signals produced by the brain reflect the activity of multiple cortical and subcortical regions, including the brain stem and associated thalamic and cortical projections. The activity of the brain (as measured by surface electrodes) is similar to the beating of the heart. During resting phases, the beat (or frequency) is slower; during arousal phases, the frequency of the "beating" increases.

As described by Monastra (2005a, behavioral manifestations of various states of alertness are reflected in the beat or frequency of electrical activity recorded via qEEG. The frequency of electrical activity is measured in cycles per second, or hertz (Hz). Like the pulse of the heart, brain frequency is measured in the number of pulses per unit of time. Instead of beats per minute, brain electrical pulses are measured in frequency per second. During inattentive or "unfocused" states, slow EEG frequencies (3.5–8.0 Hz, called *theta*) are predominant over the prefrontal and frontal cortex and at certain midline locations (e.g., the vertex, situated over the middle of the Rolandic cortex). In relaxed, wakeful states, *alpha* rhythms (9.0–11.0 Hz) begin to be dominant over these same regions. As an individual transitions into a state of increased awareness and is preparing to engage in purposeful or planned action, further increase in the EEG frequency is noted and increased amplitude of the sensorimotor rhythm (12.0–15.0 Hz) is evident over the Rolandic (motor) cortex. Finally, during the performance of executive functions such as response inhibition, working memory, set shifting, planning, and fluency (Barkley, 1997; Welsh & Pennington, 1998), sustained bursts of more rapid EEG frequencies (*beta*; 16.0–20.0+ Hz) are evident over prefrontal, frontal, and central midline regions.

As reviewed by Barry, Clarke, and Johnstone (2003); Chabot et al. (2005); Clarke and Barry (2004); Hermens, Cooper, Kohn, Clarke, and Gordon (2005); and Loo and Barkley (2005), there is considerable scientific evidence that the structural abnormalities identified via MRI, PET, and SPECT scans are reflected in atypical patterns of electrophysiological activation as recorded during qEEG examination. Consistent with the findings of other neuroimaging studies, the qEEG research has detected dysregulation of cortical arousal over the same brain regions that appear to be atypical in their development from a structural perspective.

Examination of qEEG abnormalities has revealed two primary types of dysregulation in patients diagnosed with ADHD. The vast majority of patients (approximately 84%–94%) demonstrate excessive slow cortical activity, as evidenced by indicators such as high ratios of electrophysiological power in theta versus beta frequencies and excessive relative theta power over frontal regions of the brain. A secondary pattern, characterized by excessive beta over frontal and posterior regions, has also been consistently identified in approximately 5% to 15% of patients diagnosed with ADHD. As concluded by Loo and Barkley (2005), "current research findings show that most children with ADHD display fairly consistent EEG differences in brain electrical activity when compared to normal children, particularly regarding frontal and central theta activity" (p. 65).

The application of qEEG techniques in clinical settings has also been explored in numerous studies. Beginning with the early work of J. F. Lubar, Bianchini, and Calhoun (1985) and continuing in published reports by Bresnahan and Barry (2002); Chabot, Merkin, Wood, Davenport, and Serfontein (1996); Clarke, Barry, McCarthy, and Selikowitz (2001a); Mann, Lubar, Zimmerman, Miller, and Muenchen (1992); Monastra, Lubar, and

Linden (2001); and Monastra et al. (1999), researchers have reported test sensitivity and specificity rates of 80% to 95% when qEEG findings were used to differentiate patients with ADHD from healthy peers. Additional studies examining the use of qEEG findings to differentiate stimulant responders versus nonresponders (e.g., Clarke, Barry, McCarthy, & Selikowitz, 2001b; Satterfield, Schell, Backs, & Hidaka, 1984) have reported significant qEEG differentiation of the two groups, with responders tending to exhibit excessive slow-wave activity (hypoaroused type) and nonresponders tending to exhibit excessive fast activity. Consistent with such a neurophysiological subtyping of patients with ADHD, Chabot, di Michele, Prichep, and John (2001); Chabot et al. (1996); Prichep and John (1992); and Suffin and Emory (1995) have reported that approximately 70% to 80% of patients with ADHD will exhibit cortical slowing on qEEG and respond positively to stimulants. Such findings are quite consistent with the reported efficacy rates of stimulant medication (Barkley, 2006). Furthermore, "normalization" of qEEG profiles has been reported in multiple studies following administration of stimulant medication (Jonkman et al., 1997; Verbaten et al., 1994; Winsberg, Javitt, & Silipo, 1997).

ADHD: A DISORDER OF CORTICAL AROUSAL AND MODULATION

On the basis of the existent neuroscience literature, several researchers have postulated that the impairment of alerting and behavioral inhibition, as well as the multiple neurocognitive deficits found in patients with ADHD, is due to a dysfunction in cortical arousal and modulation (Hermens, 2006; Nigg, 2000; Pliszka, 2005; Sergeant, 2005). In contrast to earlier models of ADHD (e.g., Castellanos et al., 1996; F. Levy, 1991) that were primarily based on the role of dopaminergic pathways, the dysregulation of cortical arousal/modulation model (DCAM), considers the interaction among multiple cortical regions and the role of multiple neurotransmitters in conceptualizing the neurological foundations of ADHD. As such, the DCAM appears to be more consistent with emerging neuroscience findings, which implicate multiple neurotransmitters (DA, noradrenalin, 5-HT) and cortical regions (cerebellum, basal ganglia, corpus callosum, frontal lobes) in symptom onset and maintenance.

The DCAM perspective is that arousal and cortical activation involves an interplay of multiple regions of the brain, beginning with the ascending reticular activating system (ARAS), which involves noradrenergic, serotonergic, and dopaminergic pathways. In this model, external stimuli trigger the activation of noradrenergic pathways originating in the brain stem, priming the posterior attention system of the brain, and activating the release of adrenaline. The locus coeruleus (LC; a brain region that uses noradrenergic in neural transmission) appears to be particularly integral in this process, stimulating multiple brain regions that are responsible for arousal, attention, and orienting. The release of adrenaline further helps to prepare the body to react and simultaneously activates frontal regions (controlling executive functions), which are mediated by dopaminergic neurons. On qEEG examination, this process is reflected by a shift from slow (delta, theta) waves to faster (alpha, beta) frequencies appearing over frontal regions.

As the frontal regions of the brain are activated, a secondary process of arousal control can be initiated. As the degree of frontal cortical excitation becomes excessive, the frontal lobes provide feedback to the ARAS, triggering the slowing or "braking" of the system via serotonergic pathways. Hence from the DCAM perspective, both ascending and descending pathways are essential for the regulation of arousal and attention. The DCAM proposes that the core symptoms of ADHD can occur from excessive or deficient activation of neural systems involved in cortical arousal and activation. Such patterns of both excessive (hyperarousal) and deficient activation (hypoarousal) have been consistently reported in qEEG studies of patients with ADHD.

From this perspective, the selection of treatments based on evidence of level of cortical arousal over the frontal lobes and the motor cortex may lead to improved matching of patient to treatment and enhanced treatment response. The DCAM would predict that patients exhibiting cortical hypoarousal (i.e., excessive slow-wave activity) on qEEG examination would respond to stimulants; whereas those exhibiting hyperarousal (i.e., excessive beta activity) would be expected to respond to medications that inhibit the ARAS (e.g., antihypertensives). Initial qEEG studies exploring such patient matching (Monastra, 2005b) have reported positive results using such a technique.

The diversity of the psychiatric profiles presented by patients with ADHD makes it unlikely that any one model of ADHD will be sufficient to account for the multiplicity of clinical problems presented by patients. Until clinical researchers begin to use a multidimensional framework for the classification of patients with ADHD (i.e., one that incorporates the functional domains noted in chap. 1), it also seems unlikely that we will achieve clarification of the underlying genetic and neurological causes of the multiple, neuropsychiatric disorders currently defined as the three subtypes of ADHD.

IMPLICATIONS OF NEUROIMAGING STUDIES FOR CLINICAL PRACTICE

Collectively, the results of MRI, fMRI, PET, SPECT, and qEEG studies support the perspective that patients diagnosed with ADHD experience the effects of atypical development of brain regions that are responsible for alerting, sustained attention, and various executive functions, including response inhibition and planning, working memory, cognitive flexibility (set shifting), and fluency. These regions include the frontal lobes, the corpus callosum, the basal ganglia, and the cerebellar vermis. Neuroanatomical studies have consistently revealed reduction in the size of these structures, which is reflected in abnormal rates of blood flow and glucose metabolism, and abnormal patterns of electrophysiological activation.

On the basis of such neuroimaging studies, it appears to be highly unlikely that ADHD is caused by an abnormality of a single brain region or reflects the impact of a single genetic polymorphism. Instead, the identification of multiple, specific polymorphisms by genetic researchers, combined with neuroimaging findings of atypical development of multiple brain regions, suggests that the relationship between neural pathways emanating from the brain stem, incorporating posterior regions, as well as thalamic and frontal regions, is involved in the development and maintenance of the wide range of symptoms exhibited by patients with ADHD.

In contrast with earlier formulations of ADHD as a disorder of attention and/or impaired behavioral regulation, it is quite evident that patients with ADHD can exhibit atypical development across at least nine domains: alerting, concentration, behavioral inhibition, affective control, socialization, memory, language processing, word retrieval, and fine and/or gross motor development. Although patients with ADHD will not typically exhibit significant impairment in all of these domains, nearly all will display marked functional impairment in at least three areas. From an assessment standpoint, the recognition that patients diagnosed with ADHD will commonly exhibit multiple functional impairments supports an evaluation process that incorporates specific assessment techniques to evaluate the patient in each of these multiple, relevant domains.

The consistent finding of atypical neurological development in specific brain regions of patients with ADHD also supports the need to consider neurological and/or neurophysiological evaluation of patients with ADHD, particularly in those instances where the diagnostic formulation is confounded by the presence of multiple, comorbid psychiatric disorders. Although fMRI, PET, and SPECT studies have provided information that is essential in understanding the neurological foundations of ADHD, PET and SPECT scans are quite intrusive (involving injections of radioactive isotopes), and fMRI is highly sensitive and easily confounded by movement artifact. In contrast, qEEG techniques have been shown to have a high degree of test sensitivity and specificity for ADHD, are well tolerated by patients, and can be easily artifacted for movement. In addition, initial investigations of the use of qEEG data in guiding medication selection and titrating dose have revealed decreased adverse medication effects and increased treatment compliance and maintenance when these procedures are incorporated into the assessment process (Monastra, 2005b).

On a similar note, the recognition that patients with ADHD manifest impairments across multiple functional domains (beyond inattention, impulsivity, and hyperactivity) supports the need for multimodal treatment plans that are comprehensive in nature. For example, a treatment plan that includes a methylphenidate-based medication may prove helpful in promoting alerting and behavioral control in a patient whose ADHD symptoms are associated with cortical hypoarousal. However, such a treatment plan is not likely to prove sufficient if the patient has a comorbid mood disorder combined with social skill deficits and impaired speech–language processing. Effective treatment of the vast majority of patients with ADHD will require not only pharmacological treatment for core ADHD symptoms but also specific developmental, educational, and psychosocial therapies that target specific areas of functional impairment as manifested on a case-by-case basis.

3

MEDICAL CONDITIONS
THAT MIMIC ADHD

Despite a preponderance of scientific evidence that attention-deficit/ hyperactivity disorder (ADHD) is inherited and is associated with specific genetic polymorphisms; atypical anatomical development of the frontal lobes, the corpus callosum, the basal ganglia, and the cerebellum; and uniquely structured neuronal receptors and transporters, it is not uncommon to read reports in scientific journals and news releases suggesting that ADHD can be caused by allergies, sleep apnea, exposure to environmental toxins, dietary insufficiencies, birth complications, maternal exposure to cigarettes or alcohol, traumatic brain injury (TBI), or other medical conditions. Following the release of a study linking ADHD to allergies, sleep apnea, or other conditions, a debate typically ensues and is broadcast on regional and national radio and television programs.

Advocates accurately note that the treatment of allergies, apnea, or other medical conditions ameliorates what were thought to be ADHD symptoms in a significant percentage of the sample that they studied. Critics accurately cite studies that indicate that the proposed "cause" of ADHD has not been demonstrated to be responsible for these so-called ADHD symptoms in a significant number of patients. Ultimately, the brief debate is concluded, leaving adults with ADHD, parents of children with ADHD, as well as educators and health care providers, confused. After all, how could both sides be "correct"?

A comprehensive review of the scientific literature clearly reveals that there indeed are a substantial number of medical conditions that are characterized (in part) by symptoms of inattention or impulsivity/hyperactivity. One only needs to examine a standard medical textbook to confirm that reality. However, out of all of the conditions that can cause symptoms of inattention, impulsivity, and hyperactivity, only one is termed *ADHD*. The range of other medical conditions that can cause inattention, impulsivity, and hyperactivity is quite extensive, and includes conditions such as allergies; anemia; insufficiencies of zinc, magnesium, and essential fatty acids (EFAs); thyroid disorders; hypoglycemia; diabetes; exposure to environmental toxins (e.g., maternal use of nicotine, alcohol, or drugs during the pregnancy; lead or carbon monoxide poisoning during childhood); low birth weight; TBI; seizure disorders; sleep apnea; and visual and hearing impairments.

The purpose of this chapter is to provide health care professionals with a review of some of the more common "other medical conditions" that can cause symptoms of inattention, impulsivity, and hyperactivity. Throughout this section, the term *ADHD* will not be used as a descriptor of symptoms because these other medical conditions impair attention and/or behavioral control but do not cause ADHD. Estimates derived from recently conducted, large-scale clinical studies reveal that medical conditions such as allergies, anemia, hypoglycemia, thyroid disorders, exposure to toxins, vitamin and mineral deficiencies, and visual or hearing impairments were determined to be responsible for the symptoms of inattention, impulsivity, and hyperactivity exhibited by approximately 3% to 10% of patients presenting with ADHD-like symptoms (Monastra, 2005a, 2005b).

It is ironic that the use of laboratory testing for such potentially relevant medical conditions has been minimized by both the American Academy of Pediatrics (AAP; 2000) and the American Academy of Child & Adolescent Psychiatry (AACAP; 1997), who correctly asserted that there is no laboratory test that is specific for ADHD but incorrectly presumed that the assessment of other medical disorders that can cause symptoms of inattention, impulsivity, and hyperactivity is either irrelevant or can be achieved simply by interview and routine physical examination. Although certain medical conditions are characterized by easily observable symptoms (e.g., enduring or cyclical patterns of nasal congestion in a child with environmental allergies), other types of disorders associated with impairment of attention and behavioral control (e.g., food allergies, lead poisoning, dietary insufficiencies, sleep disorders) are not characterized by such overt symptoms during clinical interview.

Instead of delineating the types of common medical conditions that can mimic ADHD and emphasizing the importance of screening for such conditions, both the AAP and AACAP guidelines imply that the use of clinical history, behavioral observations, and rating scales completed by parents and teachers is sufficient to make an accurate multiaxial diagnosis. The impact of such published guidelines on clinical practice is readily evident in the results of national surveys of the diagnostic practices of primary care physicians (E. Chan, Hopkins, Perrin, Herrerias, & Homer, 2005). In their survey of 2,000 primary care pediatricians and family physicians, E. Chan et al. (2005) reported that only 26% of physicians reported using even minimal laboratory tests such as hematocrit; only 20% screened for lead levels; and 15% ordered a thyroid profile. Conversely, approximately 70% of physicians reported administering ADHD-specific rating scales to parents and teachers.

The impact of such practice guidelines on the initiation and maintenance of treatment is evident in the high percentage of parents who either do not initiate medical treatment for their child's symptoms of inattention, impulsivity, and hyperactivity or discontinue treatment within the first 3 months following a behaviorally based diagnosis. Estimates derived by systematic reviews of prescription rates for stimulants (P. S. Jensen, 2000; P. S. Jensen et al., 1999; Multimodal Treatment Study of Children With ADHD Cooperative Group, 1999) indicate that only 25% to 50% of diagnosed patients will initiate and sustain pharmacological treatment. At least half of the parents whose children have been diagnosed with ADHD using AAP and AACAP guidelines either will not initiate treatment or will discontinue treatment within 3 months. Such a high rate of treatment noncompliance or discontinuation is alarming, given the long-term adverse effects on functioning when ADHD is untreated.

Investigations of the factors contributing to parental reluctance to initiate and maintain pharmacological treatment have revealed that parents are quite concerned about administering a medication without direct assessment of attention and evaluation for other medical conditions that can cause symptoms of inattention, impulsivity, and hyperactivity. They are distrustful of professionals, fear the potential side effects of medication, and are often unsure why stimulant medications are being used to treat children who seem overly stimulated (Angold, Erkanli, Egger, & Costello, 2000; Costello et al., 1996; Monastra, 2005b). By addressing such fears through direct assessment of attention and conducting routine laboratory and medical evaluation to rule out the most common medical causes of symptoms of inattention, impulsivity, and hyperactivity (other than ADHD), Monastra (2005b) reported a compliance rate of 95% with medical treatment for ADHD that was sustained for a 2-year follow-up period.

Because of the impact of medical assessment for other relevant medical conditions on treatment compliance, a review of other disorders associated with symptoms of inattention, impulsivity, and hyperactivity appeared relevant for promoting the effective treatment of patients with ADHD. The most common medical disorders reported in published studies examining the association between ADHD-like symptoms and other medical conditions are included in this review.

PRENATAL MEDICAL CONDITIONS

In general, the greater the number of medical conditions that are present in a mother prior to or during pregnancy, the greater the risk for attention deficits and impaired behavioral control in offspring (D. E. McIntosh, Mulkins, & Dean, 1995; Milberger, Biederman, Faraone, Guite, & Tsuang, 1997). Among all the specific prenatal, maternal medical conditions that have been associated with increased risk for attention deficits and impaired behavioral control in offspring, maternal stress during pregnancy, as well as maternal smoking and other psychoactive substance abuse, have been associated with the greatest risk (D. E. McIntosh et al., 1995; Milberger et al., 1997). A higher occurrence of hypertension, anemia, and urinary tract infections was also reported in the mothers of children with ADHD.

D. E. McIntosh et al. (1995) used a discriminant function analysis to determine which prenatal factors best differentiated 130 children diagnosed with ADHD from 135 "normal children." They reported that the overall number of medical problems reported by the mother yielded a correlation of .50 with a diagnosis of ADHD. The degree of maternal stress and the number of cigarettes the mother smoked yielded correlations greater than .40. Analysis of the correlations between maternal alcohol consumption and months to term with a diagnosis of ADHD also yielded rates above .25.

In a similar manner, Milberger et al. (1997) conducted a factor analysis of 10 potential risk factors for attention deficits and impaired behavioral control, including parental age, maternal infection or illness during pregnancy (e.g., excessive nausea or vomiting for over 3 months, weight loss, infection requiring medical care), maternal substance abuse, hypertension, maternal bleeding, and type of delivery. Again, maternal substance abuse and maternal emotional problems or stress were most closely associated with presence of attentional deficits and impaired behavioral control in a child. Excessive bleeding was also associated with increased risk for such problems.

BIRTH COMPLICATIONS

Several conditions occurring at the time of birth have also been associated with increased risk for attentional deficits and impaired behavioral control. Duration of the time between onset of labor and birth and the presence of delivery complications (e.g., breach presentation, use of forceps or suction) have also been associated with greater risk for such impairments (Claycomb, Ryan, Miller, & Schnakenberg-Ott, 2004; Hartsough & Lambert, 1985; Milberger et al., 1997; Minde, Webb, & Sykes, 1968). Low birth weight (less than 5 pounds) has also been associated with increased risk for attentional deficits and impaired behavioral control (Nichols & Chen, 1981; Milberger et al., 1997), as well as other psychiatric symptoms such as depression and anxiety (Botting, Powls, Cooke, & Marlow, 1997).

MEDICAL CONDITIONS EMERGING DURING CHILDHOOD AND ADOLESCENCE

There are numerous medical conditions that occur during childhood and adolescence that have been associated with symptoms of impaired attention and behavioral control. These include repeated infection (e.g., otitis media, pediatric autoimmune neuropsychiatric disorders associated with streptococcal Group A beta-hemolytic infection [PANDAS]), exposure to environmental toxins (e.g., lead), allergies (i.e., environmental and dietary), thyroid disorders, blood sugar disorders, dietary insufficiency, deficiencies of EFAs, vitamins and minerals, poor dietary habits, sleep deprivation, seizures, and visual impairments. The primary findings are as follows.

Infectious Disease

Two types of infection have been examined relative to attention deficits and hyperactivity: otitis media (Hagerman & Falkenstein, 1987) and PANDAS (Swedo et al., 1998). Hagerman and Falkenstein (1987) reported that the rate of otitis media in hyperactive children was twice the rate of their control population. Similarly elevated rates of association were noted between a specific streptococcal infection (PANDAS) and symptoms of inattention, impulsivity, and hyperactivity, with 40% of such patients meeting diagnostic criteria for ADHD (Swedo et al., 1998). A study by Mick, Biederman, and Faraone (1996) supports further investigation of the association between infection and attentional and behavioral control disorders. In their study, Mick et al. (1996) noted a significant association between season of birth and the presence of ADHD with comorbid learning disorders. Commenting on the tendency toward higher incidence in children born in the fall and winter months, Mick et al. (1996) postulated that season of birth was perhaps a proxy for the timing of seasonally mediated viral infections and that increased exposure to such infections was responsible for the association between season of birth and ADHD.

Exposure to Environmental Toxins

The primary environmental toxin that has been examined is exposure to lead. Multiple studies have identified a significant association between elevated levels of lead (in blood or tooth samples) and inattention and impaired behavioral control (Baloh, Sturm, Green & Gleser, 1975; David, 1974; de la Burde & Choate, 1972, 1974; Gittelman & Eskinazi, 1983; Needleman et al., 1979; Needleman, Schell, Bellinger, Leviton, & Alfred, 1990). The level of correlation is approximately .10 to .19.

Efforts to reduce inattention and hyperactivity in children with elevated lead levels have yielded positive results. David, Hoffman, Sverd, Clark, and Voeller (1976) treated 13 children with hyperkinetic disorder with penicillamine. Significant improvement in level of hyperactivity and impulsivity was noted in those participants whose symptoms did not appear related to any medical cause other than elevated blood levels (> 25mcg/dcl). David, Hoffman, Clark, Grad, and Sverd (1983) subsequently conducted a double-blind, placebo-controlled study in which the effects of penicillamine were compared with methylphenidate. Participants in the study all displayed hyperactivity and minimally elevated lead levels ($M = 28$ mcg/dL; $SD = 6$ mcg/dL). The results again indicated significant improvement in patients whose symptoms were treated with penicillamine (compared with placebo) and no significant difference in the response of patients treated with penicillamine or methylphenidate. Such findings support the position that elevated lead levels are associated with symptoms of inattention, impulsivity, and hyperactivity and that screening for the physical causes of such symptoms in an individual patient should include screening for elevated lead levels.

Allergies

As noted by Marshall (1989) in his review of the relationship between ADHD and allergy, "one of the most controversial of all the proposed etiological factors in ADHD is allergy" (p. 434). Yet despite the controversy surrounding the relationship between allergies and ADHD, there are a substantial number of well-controlled, group studies that point to a significant association between allergies and symptoms of inattention, impulsivity, and hyperactivity.

The initial indicator of a possible link between allergies and symptoms of inattention, impulsivity, and hyperactivity was derived from the significantly elevated rates of food allergies in hyperactive children. Tryphonas and Trites (1979) reported that 47% of 90 hyperactive children were determined to be allergic to at least one food, as indicated by the radioallergosorbent test. Similarly, Rapp (1978) determined that 66% of a group of 24 hyperactive children being treated with Ritalin had a history of respiratory or cutaneous allergy. Such rates significantly exceed the incidence rates for food allergy of approximately 7% found in epidemiological surveys (Arbeiter, 1967; Buckley & Metcalfe, 1982) and 24% for any type of allergy (Appel, Szanton, & Rapaport, 1961; Arbeiter, 1967).

As reviewed by Arnold (2002) and Breakey (1997), over a dozen well-controlled group studies (with most using double-blind, placebo-controlled food challenges or repeated measures methodology) have been published since 1985. The findings of these studies consistently point to an association between dietary allergies and symptoms of inattention, impulsivity, and hyperactivity. Significant improvement of symptoms has been noted in patients treated with a diet that restricted intake of suspected allergens (Kaplan, McNicol, Conte, & Moghadam, 1989; Schmidt et al., 1997). Furthermore, exacerbation of symptoms has occurred following ingestion of identified allergens in placebo-controlled challenges to substances identified as allergens for a specific patient (Boris & Mandel, 1994; Carter et al., 1993; Egger, Carter, Graham, Gumley, & Soothill, 1985; Egger, Stolla, & McEwen, 1992; Pollock & Warner, 1990; Rowe & Rowe, 1994). Although both Arnold (2002) and Breakey (1997) correctly assert that such findings do not indicate a causal relationship between ADHD and allergies, they also conclude that the research clearly supports the position that allergies can and do cause symptoms of inattention, hyperactivity, and impulsivity in children and adolescents.

Dietary Habits

Over the past 35 years, substantial progress has been made in understanding the relationship between the timing and composition of meals and attention, memory, and cognitive functions. As reviewed by D. Benton and Sargent (1992); Dye, Lluch, and Blundell (2000); and Pollitt (1995), an overnight fast, extending into the late morning, as well as the selective ingestion of a high-carbohydrate, low-protein breakfast, has been shown to exert multiple adverse effects on school performance. In addition, well-controlled studies examining meal composition have revealed the beneficial effect of breakfast and the enhancement of functioning when the breakfast meal includes protein (Mahoney, Taylor, Kanarek, & Samuel, 2005; Vaisman, Voet, Akivis, & Vakil, 1996; Wesnes, Pincock, Richardson, Helm, & Hails, 2003).

Investigations of the adverse effects of skipping breakfast have consistently revealed impairment of problem-solving skills, short-term memory, and attention (Dye et al., 2000). Furthermore, when breakfast was consumed, gains in attention, arithmetic, problem solving, and logical reasoning have typically been noted. However, as reported by Mahoney et al. (2005), there is emerging evidence that the composition of meals may have a moderating effect on the benefits derived from breakfast.

Foster-Powell, Holt, and Brand-Miller (2002) provided an overview of the rates of blood glucose absorption for various foods (the Glycemic Index [GI]). This index of glucose absorption is most elevated following ingestion of low-fiber, low-protein, high-carbohydrate foods (such as most cereals). In contrast, foods that are higher in fiber and/or protein (e.g., oatmeal, eggs, cheese) cause a lower blood glucose peak and are associated with more sustained blood sugar levels. By examining the impact of various breakfast foods with a high and low GI, both Mahoney et al. (2005) and Wesnes et al. (2003) noted significant differences in attention, memory, and cognitive performance on the basis of the speed of glucose absorption.

Wesnes et al. (2003) initially examined children's attention and memory in response to four breakfast conditions: no breakfast, a glucose drink, a toasted oat cereal, and a shredded wheat cereal. They found that when children ate either toasted oat cereal or shredded wheat, they demonstrated improved attention and memory, relative to children who consumed no breakfast or a glucose drink. Wesnes et al. also noted differences in duration of attentional enhancement among the three types of breakfasts. They reported that although gains in attention and memory were noted in children who had ingested a glucose drink or ate a cereal breakfast, the beneficial effects of glucose dissipated within 2 hours of ingestion. Children who ate cereal for breakfast continued to outperform those who did not eat any breakfast for a 4-hour period following consumption of cereal.

Mahoney et al. (2005) examined breakfast composition in a more expanded manner, including a breakfast containing a higher fiber and protein composition than most breakfast cereals (oatmeal). Their study revealed that additional gains on various cognitive, memory, and attentional tasks were noted following the ingestion of the higher fiber and protein breakfast. Mahoney et al. speculated that the differences between ready-to-eat cereals and oatmeal centered on the amount of protein and fiber in oatmeal. By providing a slower and more sustained energy source, as well as protein to be used in the synthesis of essential neurotransmitters, oatmeal was able to promote a more prolonged improvement in attentional functions.

Consistent with Mahoney et al.'s (2005) hypothesis, studies examining the effects of ingesting protein, amino acids, and carbohydrates (see reviews by Fernstrom, 1994; Lieberman, Spring, & Garfield, 1986) show that meals rich in carbohydrates cause an initial increase in alertness and memory through the elevation of blood sugar levels. However, such high-carbohydrate meals also trigger an increase in the release of insulin and a shift in neurotransmitter synthesis in the brain. Instead of selectively permitting the amino acids tyrosine and phenylalanine to pass the blood–brain barrier (for use in the synthesis of the neurotransmitters dopamine [DA] and norepinephrine [NE]), ingestion of high-carbohydrate meals causes an increase in the flow of tryptophan into the brain. This amino acid is synthesized into the neurotransmitter serotonin (5-HT). Elevations in tryptophan levels have also been shown to cause increased drowsiness.

Collectively, the studies on the impact of dietary habits (particularly breakfast) indicate a significant adverse effect of sustained fast (i.e., skipping breakfast) on attention, memory, and cognitive functions. In addition, evidence supporting the beneficial effect of breakfast, particularly when it contains complex carbohydrates and protein, on these functions has also been consistently reported. It is presumed that these beneficial effects occur because of a combination of the gradual, sustained increase in blood glucose levels and the increase in brain levels of amino acids essential for the synthesis of neurotransmitters, such as DA, which are essential for alertness. Because a substantial percentage of children and adolescents (as many as 40%) do not eat breakfast (Seiga-Riz, Popkin, & Carson, 1998), examination of an individual's dietary habits would appear particularly relevant in the evaluation of patients who present with attentional deficits. Also, because impaired regulation of blood sugar levels due to medical conditions such as diabetes and hypoglycemia have been associated with impairment of attention, assessment for such conditions appears warranted.

Sleep Disorders

Among the medical conditions known to adversely affect attention, sleep-onset insomnia, frequent waking, restlessness while sleeping, and sleep inertia upon waking are noted in a significant percentage of patients diagnosed with ADHD and in the general population as well. Estimates derived from published studies indicate that as many as 56% of children with ADHD will display sleep-onset insomnia and 39% will wake repeatedly. Among "healthy" peers, a significant percentage (approximately 25%) will also exhibit insomnia (see review by Corkum, Tannock, & Moldofsky, 1998). On a similar note, over 55% of children with ADHD will exhibit excessive fatigue (i.e., *sleep inertia*) upon waking (Gruber, Sadeh, & Raviv, 2000), as will 27% of healthy peers (Trommer, Hoeppner, Rosenberg, Armstrong, & Rothstein, 1988).

The adverse effects of such sleep problems include decline in reaction time, cognitive slowing, memory impairment, and a decrease in vigilance and sustained attention (Scott, McNaughton, & Polman, 2006). In addition, the association between the quantity of sleep and teacher ratings of inattention is clear, with significant impairment of attention noted in children who have sleep-onset insomnia (Aronen, Paavonen, Fjallberg, Soininen, & Torronen, 2000). Even the occurrence of a single night in which sleep is limited to 4 hours yields significant impairment in attention the next day (Fallone, Acebo, Arnedt, Seifer, & Carskadon, 2001).

Patients with ADHD also demonstrate a higher frequency of sleep-related breathing disorders (Johnstone, Tardif, Barry, & Sands, 2001). As with other types of sleep problems, patients with sleep apnea syndrome will display symptoms of hyperactivity, inattention, impulsiveness, poor school performance, learning difficulties, and mood and behavior problems (Corkum et al., 1998; Kirk, Kahn, & Brouillette, 1998). The severity of the impairment of attention is such that as many as 30% of children with a sleep-related breathing disorder will also be diagnosed with ADHD (Chervin, Dillon, Bassetti, Ganoczy, & Pituch, 1997), and treatment for such breathing disorders (e.g., bi-level positive airway pressure therapy) can result in significant improvement in cases where sleep apnea is present (Johnstone et al., 2001).

Overall, the impact of sleep disorders is significant, immediate, and enduring with respect to attentional functions. Because such disorders are highly prevalent and cause attention deficits in a significant percentage of the general population (as well as exacerbating such symptoms in patients with ADHD), an examination of a child's sleeping patterns seems relevant as part of the assessment for ADHD.

Deficiencies of Vitamins, Minerals, and Essential Fatty Acids

In addition to revealing the adverse effects of sustained fasting on alertness and attentional functions, nutritional studies have also revealed that deficiencies of certain macronutrients (EFAs) and micronutrients (e.g., iron, zinc, magnesium, vitamin B) are associated with symptoms of inattention and hyperactivity. The association is presumably due to the specific roles that each of these nutrients contributes to healthy brain function.

Zinc Deficiency

Zinc is a mineral that serves as an essential cofactor in the production of over 100 enzymes that are essential in the metabolism of carbohydrates, fatty acids, proteins, and nucleic acids (Hambidge, 2000; Rogers et al., 1995). As such, deficiencies of this mineral would be anticipated to exert an adverse effect on brain functions. Studies examining the effects of zinc deficiency have revealed that moderate zinc deprivation adversely affected visual attention and short-term memory of monkeys (Golub et al., 1994). Atypically low levels of zinc have been identified in hair and serum assays in children presenting with symptoms of hyperactivity (Arnold, Pinkham, & Votolato, 2000; Colquhon & Bunday, 1981; Toren et al., 1996), further supporting the association between zinc deficiency and impaired behavioral control.

Zinc sulphate supplementation has been associated with reduction of symptoms of hyperactivity and impulsivity in double-blind, randomized clinical trials involving patients diagnosed with ADHD (Akhondzadeh, Mohammadi, & Khademi, 2004; Bilici et al., 2003). In addition, there is some evidence that the effects of methylphenidate and d-amphetamine may be enhanced by supplementation with zinc sulfate (Arnold et al., 2000; Azkhondzadeh et al., 2004). As with all suspected nutritional deficiencies, these findings highlight the importance of considering other medical conditions when evaluating patients who present with symptoms of inattention, hyperactivity, and impulsivity.

Iron Deficiency

Iron is a mineral that is essential in the production of tyrosine hydroxylase and tryptophan hydroxylase, the enzymes that determine the rate of catecholamine (i.e., DA, NE, and epinephrine) and 5-HT synthesis. Deficiencies of iron have been associated with diminished density of D2 DA receptors (Ashkenazi, Ben-Shachar, & Youdim, 1982; Youdim et al., 1980), as well as behavioral symptoms such as motor hyperactivity and attention deficit (Kozielec, Starobrat-Hermelin, & Kotkowiak, 1994).

Evidence of the potential benefits of iron supplementation was provided by the research of Deinard, Gilbert, Dodds, and Egeland (1981); Deinard, Murray, and Egeland (1976); and Oski, Honig, Helu, and Howanitz (1983). In these studies, improvement in cognitive development and attention was noted in nonanemic but iron-deficient infants who received iron supplement. Sever, Ashkenazi, Tyano, and Weizman (1997) also reported improvement in symptoms of inattention, impulsivity, and hyperactivity (parent ratings) in 14 boys diagnosed with ADHD following treatment with an iron supplement. However, no improvement was noted on teacher ratings. Again, such findings are not considered indicative of an etiological role of iron deficiency in ADHD, primarily because of the low rate of iron deficiencies in patients with ADHD. Rather, these findings further illustrate how certain mineral deficiencies can cause symptoms of inattention, impulsivity, and hyperactivity and how treatments targeting such deficiencies can yield positive results.

Magnesium Deficiency

Ionized magnesium is a coenzyme for over 300 enzyme activities, including the metabolism of carbohydrates, lipids, and protein (Kozielec & Starobrat-Hermelin, 1997). Magnesium plays a role in the stabilization of the electrochemical balance of the cellular membrane, exerting a moderating effect on sodium, potassium, phosphorus, and calcium ion exchanges. As reported by Kozielec and Starobrat-Hermelin (1997), deficiencies of magnesium cause symptoms of hyperactivity, poor concentration, irritability, fatigue, and difficulty sleeping.

Assessment of the rates of magnesium deficiency among patients diagnosed with ADHD has suggested an elevated rate of occurrence. Kozielec and Starobrat-Hermelin (1997) reviewed the research in this area, noting magnesium deficiencies in 77% to 87% of patients diagnosed with ADHD in Poland (compared with approximately 10% in healthy age peers on the basis of hair samples). Blood serum assays indicated that 33% of patients with ADHD had a magnesium deficiency.

Efforts to treat symptoms of inattention, impulsivity, and hyperactivity in patients diagnosed with ADHD and magnesium deficiency via magnesium supplements have yielded improvements in symptoms of hyperactivity. Starobrat-Hermelin and Kozielec (1997) reported a decrease in symptoms of hyperactivity in such children, as levels of magnesium increased over a 6-month period. Whether the children studied in their research represent patients with ADHD or were actually children with magnesium deficiencies was not directly assessed. Nevertheless, their repeated findings of an association between magnesium deficiency and symptoms of hyperactivity are note-worthy from an assessment perspective, as clinicians seek to understand the causes of hyperactivity in a specific patient.

Deficiencies of Essential Fatty Acids

The omega-3 and omega-6 EFA are necessary for the maintenance and functioning of the human nervous system. They are primary components in the synthesis of phospholipids and cholesterol esters, serving to build and maintain the integrity of the myelin sheath over dendritic membranes (Crawford, 1992; Uauy, Hoffman, Peirano, Birch, & Birch, 2001). As reported by Hallahan and Garland (2004), EFA deficiencies can be expressed as symptoms of impulsivity.

Evidence of lower blood levels of free fatty acids in ADHD versus healthy peers has been reported by Bekaroglu et al. (1996); Mitchell, Aman, Turbott, and Manku (1987); Stevens, Zentall, Abate, Kuczek, and Burges (1996); and Stevens et al. (1995). Examination of the research findings suggests that the deficiency is related to the conversion of EFA into long-chain polyunsaturated fatty acids (a process mediated by zinc), leading researchers to question whether the association was a function of EFA deficiency or was related to zinc deficiency.

Supplementation studies generally bear out the limited benefits of EFA supplementation, with respect to the treatment of ADHD. Voigt et al. (2001) did not report any significant improvement on measures of attention and impulsivity following a 4-month trial of docosahexaenoic acid (DHA). Similarly, Hirayama, Hamazaki, and Terasawa (2004) found no improvement following increase in the daily consumption of DHA-containing foods. Aman, Mitchell, and Turbott (1987) found no significant improvement following treatment with primrose oil (a source of omega-6 EFAs). Richardson and Puri (2002) did note improvement on ADHD-related symptoms in their examination of the combined effects of several EFA supplements (DHA, dihomo-gamma-linolenic acid, arachidonic acid, and eicosapentaenoic acid); however, none of the participants of their study had been diagnosed with ADHD.

Overall, although deficiencies of EFAs have been associated with symptoms of impulsivity and have been found in patients diagnosed with ADHD, there is no clear indication that EFA supplementation is beneficial in the care of ADHD. However, the relationship between EFA deficiencies; zinc deficiencies; and symptoms of inattention, impulsivity, and hyperactivity lends further support for the value of assessment for zinc levels in patient evaluation.

Thyroid Disorders

The thyroid glands are associated with the regulation of the rate of a wide range of metabolic processes, including those associated with attention and behavioral control. Consistent with the widespread role of thyroid hormone in metabolism, children with thyroid dysfunction do display significant attentional deficits, as well as hyperactivity and impulsivity (Hauser, Soler, Brucker-Davis, & Weintraub, 1997; Rovet & Alvarez, 1996).

Examinations of the benefits of thyroid hormone supplementation have yielded positive results for patients displaying symptoms of inattention, impulsivity, and hyperactivity, in combination with a thyroid disorder. In a double-blind, placebo, crossover study, in which children diagnosed with both ADHD and a thyroid disorder were treated with supplemental thyroid hormone (R. E. Weiss, Stein, & Refetoff, 1997), significant improvement in attention occurred in response to supplementation. No such improvement was apparent in children diagnosed with ADHD who did not have a thyroid disorder. Although there is no indication of an excessive rate of thyroid disorders among children with ADHD, such findings underscore the importance of identifying all other relevant medical conditions as part of the treatment of children with ADHD and support the rationale for screening for thyroid disorder.

Megaloblastic Anemias

Although not directly examined as a causative factor for ADHD, symptoms of inattention, impaired concentration, and mental fatigue can be caused by megaloblastic anemias. As noted in Beeson, McDermott, and Wyngaarden (1979), the most common causes of these anemias (occurring in about 95% of cases) are nutritional, caused by deficiency of vitamin B-12, folic acid, or both. Because of the clear evidence of impairment of attention and concentration in such anemias; the poor dietary habits of children with ADHD; and the relationship between anemia, nutritional intake, and absorption, a screening for anemia (including assessment of B-12, folic acid, and other B vitamins, including B-1 and B-6) may prove helpful in understanding the physical causes of symptoms of inattention, impulsivity, and hyperactivity in a patient.

Seizure Disorders

According to the U.S. Department of Health and Human Services Centers for Disease Control and Prevention (2006), approximately 10% of Americans will experience at least one seizure during their lifetime and 3% will be diagnosed with some form of epilepsy. Among patients diagnosed with ADHD, the occurrence of epileptiform activity appears significantly greater than in the general population, with clinical studies suggesting rates as high as 30% (Boutros, Fristad, & Abdollohian, 1998; Hughes, DeLeo, & Melyn, 2000). In their study of 176 children diagnosed with ADHD, Hughes et al. (2000) noted positive spike patterns at 6- to 7-Herz and at 14-Herz frequencies in 34% of their patients with ADHD. These abnormalities were mainly focal (appearing over occipital or temporal regions). Although EEGs obtained during brief examinations (e.g., photic stimulation, hyperventilation) tend to yield a higher degree of "false negatives" (W. J. Borkowski, Ellington, & Sverdrup, 1992), studies using overnight monitoring of EEG during sleep (with or without sleep deprivation) tend to identify a larger number of patients diagnosed with ADHD with "absence" seizures.

Attention deficits are a common symptom in children, adolescents, and adults with epilepsy and other seizure disorders. As described by Semrud-Clikeman and Wical (1999) and Weinstock, Giglio, Kerr, Duffner, and Cohen (2003) children diagnosed with simple and complex partial seizures (with or without ADHD) exhibit a wide range of deficits in attention and motor control, and demonstrate epileptiform activity on EEG recordings obtained over the frontal and temporal lobes, as well as the Rolandic cortex. Neuropsychological assessment of patients diagnosed with seizure disorders commonly reveals impairment of continuous and selective attention and immediate verbal memory (Binnie, 1994; Laporte, Sebire, Gillerot, Guerrini, & Ghariani, 2002).

Although psychostimulants can be used in the treatment of children with ADHD regardless of the presence of a seizure disorder, Feldman, Crumrine, Handen, Alvin, and Teodori (1989); Hemmer, Pasternak, Zecker, and Trommer (2001); and Weber and Lutschg (2002) advise that stimulant therapy is safe only for children with a seizure disorder once the epilepsy is stabilized via anticonvulsant therapy. Therefore, in evaluating children for ADHD, whose inattentive symptoms are characterized by reoccurring periods in which they seem to simply stare off and seem unaware of their surroundings at home or in class, an overnight EEG examination, conducted either with or without sleep deprivation, may prove helpful in determining whether an underlying seizure disorder is responsible for the child's attentional deficits.

Traumatic Brain Injury

As reviewed by Barkley (2006), children with ADHD are at higher risk for accidental injury, including injury to the head sufficient to cause TBI. Such events cause injury induced lesions to brain regions implicated in the regulation of attention and behavioral control (e.g., the frontal lobes and the basal ganglia, including the caudate nucleus, the globus pallidus, and the putamen; Gentry, Godersky, & Thompson, 1988; Herskovits et al., 1999).

As would be expected, similarities between the behavioral manifestations of TBI and ADHD are also quite apparent. Kraus (1995); Lemkuhl and Thoma (1991); Max et al. (1998); and Max, Smith, and Sata (1997) all reported the emergence of ADHD symptoms in a significant number of patients following TBI. The emergence of secondary ADHD following TBI ranges from 20% (Herskovits et al., 1999) to 56% (Max et al., 1998). Because of the high likelihood that a child will exhibit enduring ADHD symptoms within 3 months of the occurrence of a TBI, assessment of the child's history of accidental injuries to the head is advised. In my experience, asking whether a child has had any type of head injury is typically insufficient to prompt the memory of informants. Instead, I will inquire whether the child has experienced any accidental injury associated with loss of consciousness or required examination by a physician.

Visual Impairments

Although visual acuity is commonly assessed during routine physical examinations, evaluation of a child's ability to control visual fixation and saccadic eye movements is not commonly performed. Recently, there has been increased interest in examining the incidence of such impairments, as both ADHD and the ocular–motor control involve frontal–striatal pathophysiology (Borsting, Rouse, & Chu, 2005; Granet, Gomi, Ventura, & Miller-Scholte, 2005; Munoz, Armstrong, Hampton, & Moore, 2003).

As described by Munoz et al. (2003), saccadic eye movements can be divided into two classes: reflexive or sensory-triggered movements and volitional movements. Neurological studies have identified the occipital and parietal cortices, as well as their projections through the superior colliculus to the brain stem and cerebellum, as the areas controlling visually triggered saccades (Moschovakis, Scudder, & Highstein, 1996; Munoz, Dorris, Pare, & Everling, 2000; Wurtz & Goldberg, 1989). The planning of volitional saccades and the suppression of reflexive saccades is controlled by the frontal cortex and basal ganglia, which also project to the superior colliculus, the brain stem, and the cerebellum (Hikosaka, Takikawa, & Kawagoe, 2000; J. D. Schall, 1997). Impairment in a child's ability to maintain visual convergence on a target and to track objects makes it difficult for a child to concentrate while reading and working on writing tasks (Granet et al., 2005; Munoz et al., 2003).

Examinations of the association between such visual impairments and symptoms of inattention, impulsivity, and hyperactivity have revealed a high rate of visual impairment in patients diagnosed with ADHD, as well as a high rate of ADHD in children with convergence insufficiency (CI) or impairment of visual accommodation (IVA). Munoz et al. (2003) reported significant impairment in the ability of patients with ADHD to suppress unwanted saccades and control visual fixation voluntarily. Borsting et al. (2005) studied a group of 24 children diagnosed with CI or IVA (but not ADHD) and found that such children obtained significantly elevated scores on the Conners' Parent Rating Scale (CPRS; Conners, 2001) subscales of cognitive problems and inattention, hyperactivity, and the ADHD Index. Granet et al. (2005) found that 15.9% of their ADHD sample had convergence insufficiency; approximately 10.0% of their patients with CI or IVA were eventually diagnosed with ADHD.

On the basis of such findings, examination for CI and IVA appears warranted in the evaluation of patients suspected for ADHD. The inclusion of such an assessment would seem particularly relevant in evaluating children who present with delays in reading or writing skills (or marked avoidance of such tasks) in addition to symptoms of inattention, impulsivity, and hyperactivity.

Central Auditory Processing Disorder

Approximately 2% to 7% of children are estimated to have a condition termed *central auditory processing disorder* (CAPD; Chermak & Musiek, 1997; Musiek, Gollegly, Lamb, & Lamb, 1990). As described by Chermak, Hall, and Musiek (1999),

> a CAPD involves a deficit in one or more of the central auditory processes responsible for generating the auditory evoked potentials and the behaviors of sound localization and lateralization, auditory discrimination, auditory pattern recognition, temporal processing (e.g., temporal resolution, temporal masking, temporal integration, and temporal ordering), auditory performance with competing acoustic signals, and auditory performance with degraded acoustic signals. (p. 290)

Children with such disorders have difficulty comprehending spoken language in the presence of competing speech or noise backgrounds (e.g., classrooms, playgrounds, home). As a result, they seem inattentive, easily distracted, and have difficulty following directions, all of which are among the core symptoms of ADHD.

Unlike ADHD, the cause of CAPD is most commonly a history of chronic otitis media (Adesman, Altshuler, Lipkin, & Walco, 1990; Feagans, Sanyal, Henderson, Collier, & Applebaum, 1987; Pillsbury, Grose, Coleman, Conners, & Hall, 1995; Roberts et al., 1989; P. A. Silva, Kirkland, Simpson, Stewart, & Williams, 1982). Patients with chronic otitis media will continue to exhibit central auditory processing deficits, even after the otitis media has been treated and normal hearing levels have been reestablished (Adesman et al., 1990; Jerger, Jerger, Alford, & Abrams, 1983; Moore, Hutchings, & Meyers, 1991; P. A. Silva, Chalmers, & Stewart, 1986). Indeed, as noted previously in this chapter, otitis media is a medical condition that has been associated with increased risk for impairment of attention. Consequently, because of the degree of similarity between certain of the behavioral manifestations of CAPD and ADHD, screening for CAPD merits consideration, particularly for children with a history of severe otitis media during early childhood and for those children whose attentional deficits appear most evident on tasks requiring sustained listening rather than visual skills.

IMPLICATIONS FOR CLINICAL PRACTICE

Children, adolescents, and adults can exhibit chronic symptoms of inattention and impaired behavioral control due to a variety of medical conditions other than ADHD. In a similar fashion, patients can have multiple medical conditions, including ADHD, which are responsible for their attentional and behavioral problems. Because of the high prevalence rates of these other medical conditions, and the *Diagnostic and Statistical Manual of Mental Disorders* (4th ed., text rev.; American Psychiatric Association, 2000) requirement that such conditions be ruled out prior to a determination of ADHD, thorough assessment for other medical conditions associated with inattention and impaired behavioral control is essential in the determination of a diagnosis of ADHD. In addition, as reviewed in this chapter, without such a thorough assessment process, at least 50% of parents will decline treatment for their child with ADHD, even when diagnosed by a qualified health care provider.

As is presented in detail in the next chapter, such an assessment includes a thorough clinical interview to review the patient's genetic, prenatal, birth, and early childhood medical histories, as well as a careful examination to determine patient exposure to toxins, infection, and accidental injury. Particular emphasis needs to be placed on determining whether the patient has been evaluated for indicators of allergies (i.e., both environmental and dietary); seizure disorder; anemia; hypoglycemia; diabetes; thyroid disorders; and vitamin B, zinc, magnesium, and iron deficiencies. In addition, this interview process will need to examine the patient's dietary and sleep habits, as both are essential for attention and behavioral control. Finally, because attentional deficits can occur frequently in patients with certain types of visual and auditory processing disorders, examination of those abilities will be routinely conducted.

Although such a comprehensive clinical interview and review of a patient's medical, developmental, educational, and psychiatric history is a valuable component of such an assessment process, it is rarely sufficient for the purpose of evaluating each of the multiple medical causes of inattention and impaired behavioral control. Consequently, targeted blood and urine analyses, as well as assessment of impairment of visual tracking and convergence and evaluation of a patient's auditory processing abilities (particularly in the presence of competing auditory signals), appear useful in clarifying diagnostic issues.

Such a comprehensive assessment for other medical conditions also seems essential from a research perspective. To date, thousands of studies have been conducted in an effort to identify the causes of ADHD. Although researchers have developed certain insights into the factors contributing to the development of ADHD in an individual, much of the research is confounded by the absence of a process that excludes participants whose ADHD symptoms are due to other medical problems. By failing to specifically screen for the most common medical conditions associated with impairment of attention and behavioral control, we risk formulating conclusions regarding etiology and treatment response that are invalidated by the absence of well-defined clinical and control groups. Consequently, the inclusion of such a screening process in the selection criteria for participants in studies on ADHD appears necessary to ensure the validity of findings.

4

PATIENT ASSESSMENT:
A NEUROBEHAVIORAL APPROACH
FOR DIAGNOSING ADHD

According to the *Diagnostic and Statistical Manual of Mental Disorders* (4th ed., text rev.; *DSM–IV–TR*; American Psychiatric Association, 2000) the diagnosis of attention-deficit/hyperactivity disorder (ADHD) has several requirements. First, there needs to be an assessment to determine whether the individual "often" exhibits a sufficient number of symptoms of inattention and/or hyperactivity–impulsivity. Second, the individual's history needs to be examined to determine an approximate age of onset, as "some" symptoms of inattention and hyperactivity–impulsivity must be evident by the age of 7 years. Third, this historical review must reveal evidence that there is "some" functional impairment in at least two settings (home, school, work, or other social contexts) and that there is "clear evidence" of clinically significant impairment in social, academic, or work settings. Finally, the diagnostic manual requires that the clinician determine that these symptoms are not caused by another psychiatric condition.

Based on such diagnostic requirements, the assessment of individuals for ADHD needs to incorporate strategies that can identify the type and number of symptoms and age of onset, evaluate a specific individual's capacity for attention and behavioral control in comparison with healthy age peers, provide a perspective on the individual's functioning in multiple social contexts (i.e., home, school, employment, and recreational settings), and specifically assess whether the observed symptoms are caused by other medical or psychological conditions. In clinical practice, this process may include the use of a semistructured or structured clinical interview format, the completion of behavioral rating scales specific for ADHD (by parents, teachers, spouses, supervisors, or friends, depending on the age of the patient), as well as the completion of broad-spectrum psychiatric symptom screening questionnaires; direct assessment of an individual's capacity for attention and behavioral control through continuous performance tests (CPTs); and neurophysiological, blood, urine, tissue, and/or hair analyses to clarify medical factors potentially contributing to an individual's deficits in attention and behavioral control.

This chapter presents a process for conducting evaluations in an outpatient clinical setting, including the clinical history questionnaire developed at our clinic, behavioral rating scales, CPT, and quantitative electro-encephalographic (qEEG) procedures used in clinical practice, emphasizing the contribution of each in the assessment process. It also includes a presentation of patient monitoring surveys and rating scales used by us in the evaluation process. As described previously, the goals of the assessment process are to determine the number of core ADHD symptoms, evaluate the severity of symptoms (through comparisons with healthy age peers), identify symptom onset, clarify the type and degree of functional impairments, and assess the contribution of other medical conditions to symptom onset and maintenance.

THE PROCESS OF CLINICAL ASSESSMENT

The sections that follow describe the process for patient assessment that has been used in multiple studies conducted at our clinic (Monastra, 2005b; Monastra et al., 1999; Monastra, Lubar, & Linden, 2001; Monastra, Monastra, & George, 2002). They are intended to provide an overview of symptoms, areas of functional impairment, and potentially relevant medical issues, thereby providing a foundation for comprehensive patient care.

Preassessment: The Telephone Screening Interview

The process of patient evaluation proceeds from the initial telephone request made by a parent or guardian, or an adult patient. At our clinic, a licensed clinical social worker conducts the initial clinical screening, to determine the nature of the primary problems and the appropriateness for evaluation and treatment at our clinic. A copy of our Clinical Intake Form is

EXHIBIT 4.1
Clinical Intake Form

NAME OF CALLER: _____ DATE: _____

REFERRED BY: _____ PHYSICIAN: _____

PATIENT'S NAME: _____ DOB: _____ AGE: ___

PARENT(S) NAMES: _____

ADDRESS(ES): _____

_____

PHONE #: H: _____W: _____C: _____

SCHOOL: _____ GRADE: _____IEP/504 PLAN (circle)

MAIN CONCERNS:_____

_____

_____

PRIOR EVALUATION: _____

PRIOR TREATMENT:_____

MEDICATIONS: _____

PRIOR DX (circle all): 314.00; 314.01; 312; 313.81; 296; 300; 315; 299; 307

   OTHER DX: _____

NAME OF INSURED: _____ INS. CO: _____

INS. ID #: _____ INS. CO. PHONE # _____

DATES OF SESSIONS: 1st: _____ 2nd: _____

                3rd: _____

Note. DOB = date of birth; H = home; W = work; C = cell; IEP = Individual Education Plan; DX = diagnosis; INS. ID = insurance identification; INS. CO = insurance company.

provided in Exhibit 4.1. During the clinical screening interview, we ask for a description of the caller's primary concerns, the type of treatment currently being provided, whether the patient had ever been evaluated for ADHD, and whether any type of intervention or accommodation is or was being provided at their school or work setting.

As part of the telephone interview, we request educational records for all our patients, regardless of age, and ask parents or adult patients to bring such records to the first appointment. I am particularly interested in examining the report cards and academic records of adults, because the diagnosis of ADHD requires evidence of symptoms beginning in childhood. If such records are unavailable, I request permission to conduct an interview with their parents or a sibling. We also obtain necessary insurance and contact information, provide the caller with a description of the initial three-session evaluation process, and schedule appointments. A follow-up letter confirming the dates of the appointments is subsequently mailed to the caller, with a follow-up "reminder" call on the day preceding each session. Such reminder letters and phone calls are quite helpful to our families, because a significant number of callers will have ADHD (whether diagnosed or not).

A final essential aspect of the initial telephone screening interview centers on addressing parental concerns about explaining the upcoming visit to their child. When a child hears that a doctor's visit has been scheduled, there can be a certain amount of anxiety and/or confusion. To address such concerns, a simplified but accurate depiction of the purpose of the sessions can be helpful. If the primary concern centers on the fact that little Timmy is having a hard time remembering what mom and the teacher tell him to do, then the boy can be told that the family is going to see a doctor who helps kids listen and remember. If the problem is that Audrey is running around the house, jumping on furniture, and hanging from the lamps, then the girl can be told that the family is going to see a doctor who helps kids who have a hard time sitting still and concentrating on one thing at a time. Such a straightforward explanation can be quite helpful. Other explanations such as "we're going to see someone who you can talk to, play games with, and be your friend" are inaccurate and confusing at best. This rationale is also presented to the child during the initial moments of the first session.

Session 1: Clinical Interview, Visual Continuous Performance Test, Clinical History Questionnaire, and Behavioral Rating Scales

The comprehensive evaluation of an individual proceeds from a thorough clinical interview. Various formats have been developed for use in clinical and research settings, including the Diagnostic Interview for Children (Reich, 1997), the National Institute of Mental Health Diagnostic Interview Schedule for Children—Version IV (see review by Shaffer, Fisher, Lucas, Dulcan, & Schwab-Stone, 2000), and the Clinical Interview (Parent and Adult Forms) developed by Barkley and Murphy (2006). Each of these formats provides a clinician with a framework for initially examining the primary concerns precipitating a referral for evaluation. In addition, a review of the child's medical, developmental, educational, and psychiatric history is conducted through these questionnaires. Finally, areas of functional impairment are evaluated in detail.

Although each of these interview formats provides information that can facilitate diagnostic formulation and treatment planning for a patient, we found that in clinical practice, they provided insufficient information to assess certain variables that are highly relevant for understanding a child's attentional problems (e.g., the composition of meals at breakfast; the number of hours of sleep each night; the determination of whether the child had actually been evaluated for conditions such as anemia, allergies, and impairments of visual tracking and convergence). Instead of inquiring whether a child or adult had ever been specifically evaluated for medical conditions known to cause symptoms of inattention, impulsivity, or hyperactivity, most semistructured or structured interviews inquire whether the person had ever been treated for such conditions. To inquire whether a child has ever *had* a potentially relevant medical condition is quite different than determining whether the child had ever been specifically *evaluated* for such a condition. We have learned to inquire what kinds of medical evaluations a child or adult has actually undergone before we presume that a potentially relevant medical condition has been ruled out.

Because one of the primary goals of the clinical interview is to not only clarify the presence and severity of symptoms but also to investigate whether the patient's medical and developmental histories point to factors other than ADHD as causative, both interview and questionnaire formats are beneficial. As reviewed in previous chapters, ADHD is an inherited condition, hence it is quite likely that an informant (e.g., a parent or an adult patient) will have the condition (but not be diagnosed). Impairments of working memory, language processing, and word retrieval are common among patients with ADHD and their parents. As a result, reliance on information gleaned from a clinical interview is suspect. In addition, because of such word-retrieval problems, open-ended questions (requiring retrieval rather than recall) can be problematic.

Consequently, at our clinic, we conduct a clinical interview and provide the informant with a Clinical History Questionnaire (Monastra, 2006) to complete at home, after the first clinic visit. This Clinical History Questionnaire replicates the format of the interview conducted in the clinic. As I often share with parents, it is very common to leave a doctor's office and realize on the way home that you have forgotten to mention a very important piece of information. The Clinical History Questionnaire provided to our patients or their parents is intended to address such oversights. A copy of the Clinical History Questionnaire is provided at the end of this chapter (see Appendix 4.1).

In addition to conducting a thorough clinical interview, a CPT is administered during the first session. When an adult is being evaluated, a CPT is typically administered after the initial clinical interview. When a child is being evaluated, the parents will provide the information while the child's attention and capacity for behavioral control is being assessed through a CPT (e.g., Test of Variables of Attention [TOVA]: Greenberg, 1994; Intermediate Visual and Auditory Continuous Performance Test [IVA]: Sanford, 1994; the Gordon Diagnostic System [GDS]: Gordon, 1983). These tests vary in the type of stimulus presented (visual or auditory) and duration (12–23 minutes). All require the patient to respond under certain stimulus conditions and inhibit under other conditions. Measures used to assess attention and capacity for behavioral control include capacity to detect target stimuli, capacity to inhibit response to nontarget stimuli, rate of decision making, and consistency of decision-making speed.

The TOVA, the IVA, and the GDS differentiate patients with impaired attention from healthy age peers with a high degree of accuracy (see reviews by Barkley, 2006; Riccio & Reynolds, 2001; Riccio, Reynolds, Lowe, & Moore, 2002). Test sensitivity rates ranging from 70% to 100% have been reported, with specificity rates ranging from 65% to 75%. Other CPTs (e.g., Conners' Continuous Performance Test; Conners, 1995) do not appear as sensitive in clinical practice (McGee, Clark, & Symons, 2000; Monastra et al., 2001), with sensitivity rates of approximately 50%. The reported sensitivity and specificity rates for the TOVA, IVA, and GDS have prompted Barkley (2006), Riccio and Reynolds (2001), and Riccio et al. (2002) to conclude that these tests can be useful in the assessment process. However, they cannot be considered *diagnostic* for ADHD.

As clarified by Riccio and Reynolds (2001), "most current CPT paradigms are highly sensitive to most types of CNS dysfunction including all forms of ADHD" (p. 127). Nevertheless, they caution that "CPT performance is affected adversely by all forms of schizophrenia . . . and is adversely affected by metabolic disorders with cognitive sequelae" (pp. 127–128). Because of the sensitivity of CPT to a variety of medical conditions that impair attention, a "positive" finding on a CPT provides additional support for the position that a specific individual's capacity for attention and/or behavioral control is atypical for his or her age and is consistent with a diagnosis of ADHD or other medical condition known to adversely affect attention. A negative finding on a CPT is considered quite unusual in a patient with a neurologically based impairment of attention and/or behavioral control. In either event, CPT findings are to be interpreted in light of patient history and the observations of multiple informants.

At the conclusion of the interview, we provide parents and adults with behavioral rating scales specific for ADHD (e.g., Attention Deficit Disorders Evaluation Scales: McCarney, 2004; Conners' Rating Scales—Revised: Conners, 2001; Conners' Adult ADHD Rating Scales: Conners, Erhardt, & Sparrow, 1999). With children and teenagers, form(s) to be completed by a teacher(s) are provided in stamped envelopes that are addressed to our clinic (to facilitate ease in return). With adults, form(s) to be completed by a spouse, partner, and coworker or supervisor are provided. As described previously, the purpose of these rating forms is to provide a comparison with healthy age peers.

Although rating scales can provide information regarding the observations and impressions of various informants (e.g., parents, teachers), it is important to stress that the ratings provided by any informant do not determine a diagnosis of ADHD. Clinicians are well aware that the degree of interrater reliability of any of the published rating scales is quite low (approximately .30; Barkley, 2006; Swanson, Lerner, March, & Gresham, 1999). Even when an extreme cutoff score is used to identify patients scoring "positive" for ADHD (e.g., the 95th percentile), fewer than 50% of children will be rated as significant for ADHD by both parents and teachers (Swanson et al., 1999).

Concluding Session 1

After reviewing the clinical history, I present parents with the clinical history questionnaire and the behavioral rating scales (home and school) and describe what will occur during the second session. Again, it is important to prepare the child as part of this process. Because a simplified qEEG assessment (Monastra et al., 1999, 2001) will be conducted during the second session at our clinic (to monitor neurophysiological activity in the brain while the child is engaged in academic tasks), I take the time to explain this process to the child. Videotaped clinical demonstrations of techniques for explaining test procedures and results to children and adolescents have been released in DVD format by the American Psychological Association (APA; Monastra, 2005d).

In clinical settings where a qEEG assessment is not conducted, the next session will typically consist of a review of the results of the Clinical History Questionnaire, the behavioral rating scales, and the medical and educational records provided by the parent, guardian, or adult patient. During this time, a child may complete the Auditory Version of the TOVA, or an initial screening of intellectual and academic abilities may be conducted. Because of the importance of preparing the child for each session, I would describe the nature of the next session to the child at the conclusion of the first session, reviewing the kinds of tasks that they will be asked to perform.

At our clinic, we do not routinely conduct intelligence and academic testing. Instead, if a child is determined to have a diagnosis of ADHD, we refer the child to his school district's committee on special education (or office for special services). Because ADHD is recognized as a condition that qualifies a student for a comprehensive psychoeducational evaluation and the development of a 504 Accommodation Plan (504 Plan) or Individual Education Plan (IEP), we rely on the school district to conduct this evaluation. A form for requesting such an evaluation is provided in Exhibit 4.2. A detailed description of the educational rights of students with ADHD is provided in chapter 9.

Session 2: Quantitative Electroencephalographic Examination for Cortical Dysregulation

In this session, we conduct a qEEG session as described in our previously published work (Monastra et al., 1999, 2001). The purpose of this procedure is to determine whether the patient exhibits patterns of cortical dysregulation while completing academic tasks. The extensive qEEG literature, reviewed by Chabot, di Michele, and Prichep (2005) and Clarke, Barry, McCarthy, and Selikowitz (2001b), indicates that two primary types of dysregulation are evident during qEEG studies of patients with ADHD. One subtype is characterized by excessive cortical slowing over frontal and central midline regions (hypoaroused) and one is characterized by excessive cortical activation (hyperaroused). Cortical slowing (evidenced by an excessive amount of activity at 4–8 Hz relative to 13–21 Hz activity) appears the far more common variation, occurring in approximately 80% to 95% of patients diagnosed with ADHD. Hyperarousal (evidenced by lower ratios of activity at 4–8 Hz vs. 13–21 Hz) appears to occur in approximately 5% to 20% of patients diagnosed with ADHD.

Other EEG-based indicators of attention, behavioral control, and informational processing have also been extensively investigated in the literature, particularly the P300 (P3 component) noted in research examining event-related potentials (ERP). During ERP studies, stimuli are presented to participants, with the instruction to selectively attend to one stimulus while ignoring another. Both active and passive response conditions can be used. In the active response condition, participants are instructed to respond to certain stimuli (e.g., via a button push) and inhibit response to others. In the passive response condition, the participant is simply asked to notice or attend to the different stimuli.

The amplitude and latency of the P300 wave have been associated with behavioral inhibition and information processing speed. An excellent review of this literature is available (Barry, Johnstone, & Clarke, 2003). The amplitude of the P3 component has been associated with behavioral inhibition (the larger the P3, the more the inhibition; Birbaumer, Elbert, Canavan, & Rockstroh, 1990; Desmedt, 1980). The onset of the occurrence of the P3 has been associated with mental processing speed (Polich & Herbst, 2000): the more rapid the onset of occurrence, the faster the processing speed. Multiple studies have revealed that a low P3 amplitude is present in various conditions characterized by behavioral disinhibition, including substance abuse (Anokhin, Vedeniapin, Sirevaag, Bauer, & O'Connor, 2000; Biggins, MacKay, Clark, & Fein, 1997; Herning, 1996; Iacono, Malone, & McGue, 2003), conduct disorder (Iacono et al., 2003; Kiehl, Hare, Liddle, & McDonald, 1999), ADHD (Klorman, 1991; Pliszka, Liotti, & Woldorf, 2000; van der Stelt, van der Molen, Boudewijn-Gunning, & Kok, 2001), and Tourette's disorder (Johannes, Wieringa, Nager, & Rada, 2003; U. Schall, Schon, Zerbin, Eggers, & Oades, 1996).

Examinations of the sensitivity and specificity of qEEG procedures for ADHD reveal test sensitivity ranging from approximately 80% to 94%, with specificity ranging from 85% to 96% (see review by Chabot et al., 2005). Test–retest reliability is approximately 95% (Monastra et al., 2001). As described previously, the qEEG is incorporated into the assessment not as the gold standard but to provide another comparison of the patient with age peers and to evaluate whether the patient's ADHD symptoms are associated with atypical neurophysiological findings. The procedure used at our clinic provides such a comparison while the patient is performing common academic tasks (e.g., reading, listening to instructions, writing).

I consider the qEEG measure to serve the same purpose as a thermometer during a medical examination. Although a thermometer recording of elevated body temperature does not determine a specific medical condition, it is a sensitive indicator of the presence of a number of infections and disease conditions. When present, an elevated body temperature alerts the practitioner that there are physical factors contributing to the patient's symptoms. On a similar note, the presence of indicators of cortical dysregulation on the qEEG alerts the practitioner to the increased likelihood that the patient's symptoms are associated with neurophysiological abnormalities, which require additional medical evaluation and treatment.

As reported by Monastra (2005b), physical evidence of atypical brain functioning contributes to parental acceptance of the need for treatment. In addition, there is emerging evidence that patients can be matched to the type of pharmacological treatment on the basis of their qEEG profiles (i.e., stimulant medications for patients exhibiting cortical slowing and nonstimulant medications for patients exhibiting cortical hyperarousal). In initial clinical trials, such matching has been associated with improved clinical response and reduction in adverse side effects (Chabot et al., 2005; Monastra, 2005b).

Concluding Session 2

When the qEEG is completed, I usually provide several pictures of the child's EEG recordings for the child and family. These copies of EEG data illustrate what attention and inattention look like in the child (or adult patient) and will be helpful during the third session, when we review test findings and discuss the initial phases of treatment. To prepare the child for the next session, I take a few minutes to inform him or her of what we will do. Examples of such discussions have been recorded by APA and are available for review (Monastra, 2005d).

Session 3: Auditory Continuous Performance Test, Review of Clinical Findings, and Presentation of the Initial Treatment Plan

During the third session, the child or adult patient completes an auditory test of attention and we review test findings. At this point, we have the following sources of information: Clinical Interview, Clinical History Questionnaire, educational records, medical history, behavioral rating scales (home, school, work), CPT results (visual and auditory), and qEEG findings. At this point, the clinician has the ability to address several of the *DSM–IV–TR* requirements for a diagnosis of ADHD. Interview data and educational records, as well as the Clinical History Questionnaire and behavioral rating scales, enable the clinician to determine whether there are a sufficient number of symptoms of ADHD to meet Criteria A through D and whether the patient's level of symptomatology is atypical compared with age peers. CPT data provide additional comparisons with age peers with respect to attention and behavioral control. The qEEG data also serve as a basis for comparison with age peers on a neurophysiological indicator of attention and behavioral control. In addition, the Clinical Interview and Clinical History Questionnaire provide an initial indication whether there are medical conditions (other than ADHD) that can be causing presenting problems.

Despite the abundance of clinical information, a comprehensive medical evaluation has not typically been completed by this time. Furthermore, although an initial evaluation of symptoms of other psychiatric disorders has been conducted (through the Clinical History Questionnaire), the clinician cannot be certain whether such symptoms are due to another medical condition or are reflective of untreated ADHD. Therefore, although the child or adult's performance on measures of attention will be reviewed during the third session, only a provisional diagnosis will be determined at this phase. A final, multiaxial diagnosis will be made following examination of the results of medical evaluation and patient response to treatments for any identified medical condition (including ADHD).

Translating Clinical Findings Into an Initial Intervention Plan

ADHD has historically been defined from a behavioral and functional perspective. Consequently, a review of the results of the evaluation typically proceeds from a presentation of the results of the Clinical History Questionnaire, educational records, and behavioral rating scales specific for ADHD. I typically present the criteria for a diagnosis of ADHD to the parents and patient as I review test data. Initially, I review the number of symptoms of ADHD, noting that at least six symptoms of inattention and/or hyperactivity–impulsivity must be occurring "often" to meet the *DSM–IV–TR* criteria.

Next, several comparisons with age peers are made. The first comparison is made using behavioral rating scale findings. I review frequency ratings with the parents and patients, indicating the child's percentile ranking on symptoms of inattention, impulsivity, and hyperactivity. I often use percentiles because parents are familiar with such scores when they track their child's progress in developing other skills (e.g., reading, mathematics, writing). Because the interrater reliability is quite low for behavioral scales, I typically use these scales to indicate whether any symptoms of inattention, impulsivity, or hyperactivity are occurring "often" or on a daily basis in multiple settings. The presence of such symptoms in multiple settings is required for a diagnosis of ADHD.

The next comparison with age peers is made using CPT data. I provide percentile scores to the parents and patient, indicating the child's or adult's ranking relative to peers. Although impairment on the CPT does not determine that a patient has ADHD, evidence of impaired attention and/or behavioral control on a CPT such as the TOVA, IVA, or GDS is noteworthy. These tests are quite sensitive to a variety of CNS and psychiatric disorders that impede attention (including ADHD) and support the need for further evaluation to clarify the source of the child's or adult's attentional deficits.

The final comparison with age peers is made using the qEEG. As noted previously, evidence of cortical dysregulation is highly predictive of medical conditions associated with impairment of attention and behavioral control. As a result, when we interpret qEEG findings, we inform parents and patients of the degree of deviance from age peers. These comparisons again provide an indication that the behavioral symptoms evident to parents, teachers, and the patient are associated with physical evidence of impairment of cortical structures associated with attention and behavioral control.

We have found that without such evidence, parents are quite reluctant to begin treatment. Parents are often quite frightened to initiate medications for ADHD, when there is no physical evidence "that anything is wrong." Practically speaking, parents often express their hesitation in the following way: "If my child has to take a brain medication for a decade or more, then there better be some sort of medical evidence that there is a brain problem."

The qEEG data provide such evidence in clinical practice. Although evidence of cortical dysregulation on a qEEG is not specific to ADHD, the qEEG data (like CPT findings) support the need for medical evaluation to determine the cause(s) of the neurophysiological abnormalities.

Concluding Session 3

At the conclusion of the third session, we review medical history to initially discuss medical conditions that may be causing the symptoms for which the patient was referred to our clinic. Consistent with the position that there are multiple medical causes for symptoms of inattention, impulsivity, and hyperactivity (as reviewed in chap. 3), we provide parents and our adult patients with a letter to be given to the child's or their physician. This letter informs the physician that the patient meets criteria for a diagnosis of ADHD. However, before such a diagnosis can be concluded, other medical conditions need to be considered and ruled out. Consequently, this correspondence requests that the physician perform whatever medical evaluation is needed to identify other relevant medical conditions that may be present. A copy of this Request for Medical Evaluation Form is provided in Exhibit 4.3. A detailed report summarizing my findings is mailed to the physician to aid in determining what types of testing may be needed.

In addition to initiating a request for medical evaluation, a form letter (Request for Evaluation by the Committee on Special Education) requesting a psychoeducational evaluation by a child's school district is also provided to the parents. ADHD is recognized as a qualifying condition under the Individuals With Disabilities Education Act (Public Law 94-142; see http://idea.ed.gov/) and Section 504 of the Rehabilitation Act of 1973 (Public Law 93–112; see http://www.hhs.gov/ocr/504.pdf). Children diagnosed with ADHD are entitled to a thorough evaluation by their school districts to determine the presence of coexisting learning disabilities and areas of functional impairment associated with ADHD. The child does not need to demonstrate evidence of another type of disability (e.g., learning disorder) to qualify for such an evaluation. The diagnosis of ADHD is sufficient. Depending on the need for services, schools will provide assistance either through an IEP or a 504 Plan. The types of programs that are typically helpful for students with ADHD are reviewed in chapter 9. A copy of the Request for Evaluation by the Committee on Special Education is provided in Exhibit 4.2.

Session 4: Evaluation of Treatment Response

At our clinic, approximately 4 to 6 weeks transpire between the completion of the third and fourth evaluation sessions. During this time period, parents or patients meet with their physician, complete necessary medical evaluations, and initiate treatments for any other medical conditions that

EXHIBIT 4.3
Request for Medical Evaluation Form

DATE: _____

PATIENT: _____

BIRTH DATE: _____

Dear Dr. _____

This patient has recently been evaluated by me because of symptoms suggestive of attention-deficit/hyperactivity disorder (ADHD). On the basis of a comprehensive re-view of patient medical, developmental, educational, and social histories, as well as the results of behavioral rating scales and neuropsychological tests of attention and executive functions, this patient has been diagnosed with ADHD, pending medical evaluation by your office. A copy of my evaluation report will be forwarded to you.

Because symptoms of inattention and impaired behavioral and emotional control can be caused by medical conditions other than ADHD, I have recommended that _____ be evaluated by you to rule out the following medi-cal conditions that can cause inattention and loss of behavioral and emotional control:

- anemia
- thyroid disorders
- diabetes
- magnesium deficiency
- illegal psychoactive substance use (teenagers; adults)
- allergies (dietary and airborne)
- hypoglycemia
- zinc deficiency
- vitamin B deficiency

To provide effective clinical care for this patient, I would appreciate your assistance in conducting whatever laboratory and clinical assessments you consider necessary in order to rule out these conditions, prior to initiating treatment for ADHD.

Thank you for your assistance.

_____

Name of Referring Provider

****

I, _____ , authorize that the results of laboratory tests and medical evaluations for _____ be faxed to _____ at the following number _____ or mailed to _____ .

have been identified. During the fourth session, we evaluate the results of treatment for other medical conditions. Our goal is to determine whether the behavioral, neuropsychological, and neurophysiological evidence of im-paired attention and behavioral control persists despite medical treatment for other relevant medical problems, as it is quite possible for a patient to have another relevant medical condition such as allergies, as well as ADHD. If present, both will require treatment. Consequently, if evidence of ADHD persists despite effective treatment for other medical conditions (e.g., aller-gies), then treatment for ADHD will be initiated following this fourth evalu-ation session.

If no other medical conditions requiring treatment have been identi-fied, a clinical trial of a pharmacological treatment for ADHD has often been introduced by the physician prior to this fourth session. Typically, stimulant medications have been initiated for patients exhibiting cortical hypoarousal; antihypertensives or a norepinephrine-specific reuptake inhibitor such as atomoxetine have been recommended for those demonstrating hyperarousal or no evidence of cortical slowing. If medication(s) have been prescribed, CPT and qEEG tests will be repeated, in addition to examining the results of behavioral reports and ratings from parents and teachers. Scores within 1.0 standard deviations of age peers on these tests are the initial goal of treatment. When such results are evident on CPT and qEEG, our presumption is that the neurological causes of ADHD are being effectively treated. With such a foundation, we can proceed into an examination of residual psychiatric and functional problems that require psychological treatment. Such treatments may include the development of an educational support plan, nutritional counseling, parent counseling, EEG biofeedback, social skills training, marital therapy, cognitive therapy, and coaching, depending on the results of the functional analysis. If no treatment has been initiated, parent fears and reservations will be reviewed and a treatment plan will be developed.

COST ANALYSIS

A criticism of the application of techniques such as the CPT and qEEG is that they are too costly for use in clinical practice (Barkley, 2006). However, the cost of the first four sessions outlined in this chapter is approximately $600, which is well within the range for mental health care provided by a licensed psychologist or psychiatrist. If a multichannel qEEG is administered (e.g., to clarify the multiple brain regions damaged by trauma or other medical disorders and guide rehabilitative efforts using EEG biofeedback), an additional cost of approximately $300 to $700 may be incurred. However, by providing parents or patients with sufficient data to address their fears and make an informed decision about treatment options, we have found that approximately 95% of our patients initiate and maintain effective pharmacological treatment for at least a 2-year period (Monastra, 2005b). The long-term impact of such continued care on the eventual adjustment of our patients remains to be evaluated. However, given the risk for a wide range of functional problems in patients with ADHD who are untreated or insufficiently treated, it would be anticipated that early, effective care will lead to much better outcomes (and reduced long-term health care costs) in this at-risk population.

APPENDIX 4.1: CLINICAL HISTORY QUESTIONNAIRE

Copyright 2007 by Vincent J. Monastra

NAME OF PATIENT:_____ BIRTH DATE: _____
INFORMATION PROVIDED BY: _____
RELATIONSHIP TO PATIENT: _____

Over the years, doctors have learned that children, teenagers, and adults can develop symptoms of inattention, impulsivity, and restlessness for a variety of reasons. They have also learned that it is rare that these symptoms occur in isolation. Usually, patients with these problems will also have difficulty controlling their emotional reactions and functioning effectively at home, school, work, and other social settings. The purpose of this questionnaire is to help your doctor or therapist better understand the kinds of problems that you want to overcome and to begin to determine possible causes for these problems. By answering these questions, you will be providing important information to guide this process.

Take your time in answering; there is no rush. If you do not understand a question, please circle it, and your doctor or therapist will discuss it with you. If you have difficulty writing your responses, please let your therapist or doctor know so that they can assist you. Thank you for taking the time to complete this form.

PRIMARY REASON(S) THAT YOU DECIDED TO SEEK A CONSULTATION

Please check all that apply:
_____ Problems paying attention while listening
_____ Problems paying attention while reading
_____ Problems paying attention while completing homework
_____ Problems paying attention while completing writing tasks at work
_____ Failure to pass subjects at school
_____ Truancy or excessive absence from classes
_____ Problems organizing paperwork
_____ Problems organizing personal belongings
_____ Time management (procrastination, missing deadlines)
_____ Restlessness or hyperactivity
_____ Acting impulsively (without considering the consequences)
_____ Problems controlling anger or temper
_____ Depression
_____ Anxiety
_____ Alcohol or drug abuse
_____ Difficulty falling or staying asleep
_____ Poor response to medication or medication side effects

_____ Family conflicts
_____ Other; please describe:

I. AREAS OF CLINICAL CONCERN
Your answers to the following questions will give your doctor or therapist a comprehensive perspective of the types of problems that caused you to seek a consultation.

A. Problems of Attention, Impulsivity, and Hyperactivity
Please circle Y (yes) or N (no) if the problem described is a cause of concern to you:

a.	Problems giving close attention to details, careless mistakes in school tasks, work assignments or other activities	Y	N
b.	Problems sustaining attention in tasks or play activities	Y	N
c.	Problems listening when spoken to directly	Y	N
d.	Problems following through on instructions. Failure to complete schoolwork, chores, or duties in the workplace	Y	N
e.	Problems organizing tasks and activities	Y	N
f.	Problems engaging in tasks that require sustained mental effort (e.g., schoolwork, homework, or job assignments) because of avoidance or dislike for the activity	Y	N
g.	Problems losing things necessary for tasks or activities	Y	N
h.	Problems with distractibility	Y	N
i.	Problems with forgetfulness	Y	N

Critical Number (CN) = 6

j.	Problems controlling fidgeting with hands or feet; squirming	Y	N
k.	Problems leaving seat in classrooms or in other situations in which remaining seated is expected	Y	N
l.	Problems controlling an urge to run about or climb excessively in situations in which it is inappropriate. A sense of restlessness (teens and adults)	Y	N
m.	Problems playing or engaging in leisure activities quietly	Y	N
n.	Problems associated with excessive activity. Often "on the go" or seems/feels "driven by a motor"	Y	N
o.	Problems controlling the urge to talk excessively	Y	N
p.	Problems controlling the urge to blurt out answers before questions have been completed	Y	N
q.	Problems waiting turn	Y	N
r.	Problems controlling the urge to interrupt or intrude on others (e.g., butts into conversations or games)	Y	N

CN = 6
At what age did these problems begin? _____
Have any of these problems gotten better over the course of time? (list by letter) _____

_____

Have any of these problems gotten worse over the course of time? (list by letter) _____

_____

B. Problems of Oppositionalism and Defiance
    a. Problems controlling temper   Y   N
    b. Problems controlling the urge to argue with adults   Y   N
    c. Problems controlling the urge to defy or refuse adult   Y   N
    d. Problems controlling the urge to deliberately do things
        that annoy other people   Y   N
    e. Problems taking responsibility for own mistakes: tends to
        blame others   Y   N
    f. Often "touchy" or easily annoyed by others   Y   N
    g. Often angry or resentful   Y   N
    h. Often spiteful or vindictive   Y   N
    i. Problems controlling the urge to swear or use obscene
        language   Y   N

CN = 4
At what age did these problems begin? _____
Have any of these problems gotten better over the course of time? (list by letter) _____

_____

Have any of these problems gotten worse over the course of time? (list by letter) _____

_____

C. Problems of Conduct
    a. Problems controlling the urge to bully, threaten, or
        intimidate others   Y   N
    b. Problems controlling the urge to initiate physical fights   Y   N
    c. Problems controlling the urge to use a weapon that can
        cause serious physical harm to others   Y   N
    d. Problems controlling the urge to be physically cruel
        to others   Y   N
    e. Problems controlling the urge to be physically cruel
        to animals   Y   N
    f. Problems controlling the urge to steal while confronting
        the victim   Y   N

g. Problems controlling the urge to force someone into
    sexual activity   Y   N
h. Problems controlling the urge to set fires with the
    intention of causing serious damage   Y   N
i. Problems controlling the urge to deliberately destroy
    another's property (other than by fire)   Y   N
j. Problems controlling the urge to break into someone
    else's house, building, or car   Y   N
k. Problems controlling the urge to lie to obtain goods or
    favors or to avoid obligations ("cons" others)   Y   N
l. Problems controlling the urge to steal items of nontrivial
    value without confronting the victim (e.g., shoplifting)   Y   N
m. Problems controlling the urge to stay out at night,
    despite parental prohibition (before the age of 13)   Y   N
n. Problems controlling the urge to run away from home
    overnight (at least twice while living in the home of
    a parent or guardian or once without returning for a
    lengthy time period)   Y   N
o. Problems controlling the urge to be truant from school
    (beginning before the age of 13)   Y   N

CN = 3

At what age did these problems begin? _____

Have any of these problems gotten better over the course of time? (list by
letter) _____

_____

Have any of these problems gotten worse over the course of time? (list by
letter) _____

_____

D. Problems of Mood Control
    a. Feeling depressed or irritable most of the day, nearly
        every day   Y   N
    b. Decreased sense of pleasure during activities   Y   N
    c. Decrease or increase in appetite or weight   Y   N
    d. Difficulty falling asleep or sleeping excessively, nearly
        every day   Y   N
    e. Feelings of restlessness   Y   N
    f. Feeling "slowed down"   Y   N
    g. Feeling fatigued; lack of energy   Y   N
    h. Feeling worthless or guilty   Y   N
    i. Decrease in ability to concentrate   Y   N
    j. Suicidal ideas or a suicide attempt   Y   N
    k. Low self-esteem   Y   N

l. Feelings of hopelessness   Y   N

CN = 5 (2 weeks); a + 2 (2 years)
At what age did these problems begin? _____
Have any of these problems gotten better over the course of time? (list by
letter) _____
_____

Have any of these problems gotten worse over the course of time? (list by
letter) _____
_____

E. Problems of Anxiety
    a. Excessive anxiety and worry   Y   N
    b. Avoidance of being alone   Y   N
    c. Anxiety about sleeping alone   Y   N
    d. Worry and excessive distress in anticipation of separation
        from parent or guardian   Y   N
    e. Excessive distress when separated from parents or
        guardian   Y   N
    f. Unrealistic worry about future events   Y   N
    g. Excessive need for reassurance   Y   N
    h. Marked inability to relax   Y   N
    i. Marked self-consciousness   Y   N
    j. Repeated nightmares   Y   N
    k. Repetitive nonfunctional rituals to reduce anxiety (e.g.,
        hand washing, counting, checking)   Y   N
    l. A specific fear or phobia (e.g., public places, animals,
        elevators). Please list: _____   Y   N
    m. Panic attacks   Y   N
    n. Discomfort with textures of specific foods or clothing
        Please list: _____   Y   N

CN = 1
At what age did these problems begin? _____
Have any of these problems gotten better over the course of time? (list by
letter) _____
_____

Have any of these problems gotten worse over the course of time? (list by
letter) _____
_____

F. Problems of Socialization and Communication
    a. Problems maintaining eye contact during social
        interactions   Y   N

b. Problems developing peer relationships as would be expected for the patient's age   Y   N

c. Lack of behaviors that show a desire to share enjoyment, interests, or achievements with others   Y   N

d. Lack of social or emotional reciprocity   Y   N

e. Delay in (or total lack of) the development of speech   Y   N

f. Problems starting and maintaining a conversation with others (even though the patient is able to speak)   Y   N

g. Conversation consists of repetition of the same topics   Y   N

h. Problems in engaging in make-believe play or imitative social play that is appropriate for the patient's age   Y   N

i. Preoccupation with one (or a relatively few) area of interest. The preoccupation is unusual in either intensity or focus.   Y   N

j. Rigid adherence to nonfunctional routines or routines. Patient will become agitated with even minor changes in routine.   Y   N

k. Repetitive, nonfunctional motor mannerisms (e.g., hand or finger flapping, twisting, or more complex total body posturing)   Y   N

l. Preoccupation with the parts of objects   Y   N

CN (Autism) = 6; CN (Asperger's disorder) = 2 (a–d) + 1 (i–l)

At what age did these problems begin? _____

Have any of these problems gotten better over the course of time? (list by letter) _____

_____

Have any of these problems gotten worse of the course of time? (list by letter)

_____

G. Problems in Learning Academic Skills

a. Problem recognizing words when reading   Y   N

b. Problem comprehending when reading   Y   N

c. Problem maintaining visual focus when reading (skips from one line to another; words blur or move)   Y   N

d. Problem learning basic mathematics facts (adding, subtracting, multiplication tables)   Y   N

e. Problem recognizing how to solve word problems in mathematics   Y   N

f. Problem learning how to form letters when writing   Y   N

g. Problem learning how to spell words   Y   N

h. Problem with spacing of words when writing   Y   N

i. Problem expressing ideas in writing   Y   N

CN = 1
At what age did these problems begin? _____
Have any of these problems gotten better over the course of time? (list by letter) _____

Have any of these problems gotten worse over the course of time? (list by letter)

_____

H. Problems of Language and Motor Coordination
Were there any concerns about the patient's
    a.   rate of learning to sit, crawl, walk, or run?   Y   N
    b.   rate of learning to use toilet for urinating or bowel
          movements?   Y   N
    c.   rate of learning to speak?   Y   N
    d.   rate of learning how to tie shoelaces, button shirts
          dress self, hold eating utensils, assemble puzzles, or
          build with blocks?   Y   N
Does the patient show signs of motor or verbal tics?   Y   N
    If yes, describe: _____

    _____
    _____

Does the patient urinate or defecate in their pants during the day
or in their bed at night?   Y   N
    If yes, how often? _____

CN = 1
At what age did these problems occur? _____
Have any of these problems improved over the course of time? Describe:
_____
Have any of these problems gotten worse over the course of time? Describe:
_____

++

II. TREATMENT HISTORY
Please indicate the types of treatment that you have tried to overcome the problems listed above.
    a.   Consulted with a physician   Y   N
          Name: _____ Year: _____
          Type of treatment:_____

          _____
          Name: _____ Year: _____
          Type of treatment:_____

Name: _____ Year: _____
Type of treatment: _____

b. Consulted with a psychologist, social worker, psychiatric
    nurse, or counselor   Y   N
    Name: _____ Year: _____
    Type of treatment: _____

    Name: _____ Year: _____
    Type of treatment: _____

    Name: _____ Year: _____
    Type of treatment: _____

c. Consulted with a speech therapist, occupational therapist,
    or physical therapist   Y   N
    Name: _____ Year: _____
    Type of treatment: _____

    Name: _____ Year: _____
    Type of treatment: _____

    Name: _____ Year: _____
    Type of treatment: _____

d. School intervention   Y   N
    1. Meeting with teacher and instructional support team
        (Grade[s]: _____)   Y   N
    2. Collaboration with the teacher(s) and school
        psychologist to develop a behavioral intervention plan
        (Grade[s]: _____)   Y   N
    3. Evaluation for learning disabilities by the school
        psychologist (Grade[s]: _____)   Y   N
    4. The development of an Individual Education
        Plan (IEP; Grade[s]: _____)   Y   N
    5. The development of a 504 Plan
        (Grade[s]: _____)   Y   N
Other types of treatment (e.g., career counseling,
coaching)   Y   N
    Please describe: _____
    _____

+++

III. MEDICAL HISTORY

The following sections are intended to provide your doctor or therapist with information about the potential causes of your problems.

A. PRENATAL HISTORY

The following questions relate to the health of the patient's mother during pregnancy. Please circle your answers.

1. Did the mother experience
   - a. a high level of stress during pregnancy?   Y   N
   - b. high blood pressure during pregnancy?   Y   N
   - c. anemia during pregnancy?   Y   N
   - d. excessive bleeding during pregnancy?   Y   N
   - e. urinary tract infections during pregnancy   Y   N
   - f. toxemia?   Y   N
   - g. eclampsia?   Y   N
   - h. accidental injury that caused bleeding or loss of consciousness?   Y   N
   - i. carbon monoxide or lead poisoning?   Y   N
   - j. seizures?   Y   N
   - k. diabetes?   Y   N
   - l. any other medical problems?   Y   N

   Please list: _____

   _____

2. Did the mother
   - a. take any type of prescription medication for a psychiatric condition during pregnancy?   Y   N

     Please list: _____

   - b. take any type of prescription medication for any other disease or illness during pregnancy?

     Please list: _____

   - c. smoke cigarettes during pregnancy?   Y   N

     How often? _____
   - d. drink alcoholic beverages during pregnancy?   Y   N

     How often? _____
   - e. drink coffee, tea, or other caffeinated beverages?   Y   N

     How often? _____
   - f. smoke marijuana during pregnancy?   Y   N

     How often? _____

g. use any other illegal drugs during pregnancy?   Y   N
   What drugs? _____
   How often? _____

B. BIRTH HISTORY

1. How old was the mother at the time of birth? _____
2. Was the pregnancy considered "full term"?   Y   N
   If no, duration of the pregnancy: _____
3. Were there birth complications due to Rh factor
   incompatibility?   Y   N
4. How long was labor (initial labor pains to childbirth)? _____
5. How was the patient delivered? (circle)
   Vaginal planned   C-section   Emergency C-section
6. Were instruments used? (circle)   Forceps   Suction
7. Did the patient present in the breech position?   Y   N
8. Was there fetal distress (variable heart rate with
   contraction)?   Y   N
9. Was the umbilical cord wrapped around the patient's
   neck?   Y   N
10. Did the patient ingest meconium?   Y   N
11. What was the patient's birth weight? _____ lbs. _____ oz.
12. Were there any problems with the patient's color at
    birth?   Y   N
    Blue? (cyanotic)   Yellow? (jaundice)
13. Did the patient have any difficulty beginning to breathe? Y N
14. Was there any evidence of heart problems (irregular
    heart beat)?   Y   N
15. Did the patient have seizures?   Y   N
16. Did the patient develop any type of infection in the
    hospital?   Y   N
    If yes, describe: _____
17. Did the patient require treatment in the NICU for any
    reason?   Y   N
    If yes, what type of treatment? _____
    _____
18. How long did the patient remain in the hospital before
    release? _____

C. MEDICAL HISTORY: INFANCY

1. Was the patient breast fed?   Y   N
   If yes, were there difficulties tolerating breast milk? Y N
   Describe: _____
   How long was the child breast fed? _____

2. Was the patient fed a formula after birth?   Y   N
    What type? (circle)   milk based   soy based   rice based
    If yes, were there difficulties tolerating formula?   Y   N
    Describe: _____

3. Did the patient contract any type of disease or develop
any medical condition during the first 3 months
after birth?   Y   N
    Describe: _____

_____

D. MEDICAL HISTORY: CHILDHOOD, ADOLESCENCE, ADULTHOOD

1. Did the patient experience more than two ear infections per year
during the first 5 years of life?   Y   N
    If yes, how many? _____
    Were tubes inserted?   Y   N
    Were tonsils surgically removed?   Y   N
    Were adenoids surgically removed?   Y   N

2. Did the patient experience any significant side effects
following any immunization vaccinations?   Y   N
    If yes, describe: _____

3. Did the patient ever ingest a toxic substance (e.g., lead)?   Y   N
    If yes, what substance? _____

4. Did the patient ever become ill from exposure to toxic
vapors (e.g., carbon monoxide)?   Y   N
    If yes, what toxin? _____

5. Did the patient contract a strep infection more than
twice per year during the first 5 years of life?   Y   N
    If yes, how many? _____

6. Is the patient allergic to any airborne allergen?   Y   N
    If yes, describe: _____

7. Is the patient allergic to any food?   Y   N
    If yes, describe: _____

8. Has the patient ever had a fever high enough to cause
loss of consciousness or seizure?   Y   N

9. Has the patient ever had an injury to the head sufficient
to cause nausea, vomiting, or loss of consciousness?   Y   N

10. Has the patient ever experienced a seizure for reasons
other than a fever?   Y   N

11. When was the patient's last hearing examination?
    Who conducted the examination?
    Was there any evidence of hearing loss?   Y   N
    If yes, describe: _____

How is the loss being treated? _____

Has the patient ever been tested by an audiologist in
order to evaluate auditory processing?   Y   N

Was a central auditory processing disorder identified?   Y   N

How is the CAPD being treated? _____

12. When was the patient's last vision examination?

Who conducted the examination? _____

Was there any evidence of visual impairment?   Y   N

  If yes, describe: _____

Were corrective lenses prescribed?   Y   N

Has the patient ever been tested by an optometrist or
ophthalmologist to evaluate impairment of visual
tracking or convergence?   Y   N

Were problems in tracking or convergence identified?   Y   N

  If yes, how were they treated: _____

13. Aside from "colds" and common infections, has the patient
required medical treatment for any other disease or
medical condition?   Y   N

  If yes, describe: _____

  _____

  _____

MEDICAL EVALUATIONS

Has the patient's physician ever ordered laboratory tests for:

anemia?	Y	N	thyroid disorders?	Y	N
zinc deficiency?	Y	N	magnesium deficiency?	Y	N
iron deficiency?	Y	N	vitamin B deficiency?	Y	N
hypoglycemia?	Y	N	diabetes?	Y	N
estrogen?	Y	N	progesterone?	Y	N
lyme disease?	Y	N	celiac disease?	Y	N
amino acids?	Y	N	growth hormones?	Y	N
illegal drugs?	Y	N	food allergies?	Y	N
airborne allergies?	Y	N			

Other tests? Please list: _____

_____

Any significant results? Describe: _____

_____

++

DIETARY, SLEEP, AND EXERCISE HABITS

Diet

1. What does the patient eat for breakfast (i.e., between 6 a.m. and 10:30
    a.m.)?

Meal Type 1: _____ How many days per week? ___
Meal Type 2: _____ How many days per week? ___
Meal Type 3: _____ How many days per week? ___
2. What does the patient eat for lunch (i.e., between 11 a.m. and 2 p.m.)?
Meal Type 1: _____ How many days per week? ___
Meal Type 2: _____ How many days per week? ___
Meal Type 3: _____ How many days per week? ___
3. What does the patient eat in the evening (i.e., after 5 p.m.)?
Meal Type 1: _____ How many days per week? ___
Meal Type 2: _____ How many days per week? ___
Meal Type 3: _____ How many days per week? ___
Snacks? _____ How many days per week? ___

Sleep
1. What time does the patient go to bed? _____
2. How long does it usually take for the patient to fall asleep? _____
3. Does the patient wake during the night? _____
   If yes, how often? _____
4. At what time does the patient wake in the morning? _____
5. How many hours of sleep does the patient typically obtain at night? _____
6. Is the patient tired and difficult to wake in the morning?   Y   N
7. Does the patient move excessively while sleeping?   Y   N
8. Does the patient walk during sleep?   Y   N
9. Does the patient snore during sleep?   Y   N
10. Has the patient ever been evaluated for sleep apnea?   Y   N
    If yes, describe results: _____
    _____

Exercise
1. How many days per week does the patient engage in at least 30 minutes of exercise? _____
2. What types of exercise does the patient do? Describe: _____
   _____
   _____
   _____
3. Does the patient experience shortness of breath or chest pains when exercising?   Y   N
   If yes, has the patient been evaluated by a physician?   Y   N
   Describe the results of such an evaluation: _____
   _____

++

PSYCHOACTIVE SUBSTANCE USE

Please indicate any substance that the patient uses:

Substance	Current use per day	Current use per week
Caffeine	_____	_____
Nicotine	_____	_____
Beer	_____	_____
Wine	_____	_____
Liquor	_____	_____
Marijuana	_____	_____
Cocaine	_____	_____
Other drugs:		
_____	_____	_____
_____	_____	_____
_____	_____	_____

Has the patient ever used any substance more frequently than currently used?
   If yes, please describe: _____

_____

_____

Has the patient ever participated in treatment for drug or substance abuse problems?
   Please describe: _____

_____

++

EDUCATIONAL AND WORK HISTORY

1.   What is the highest grade completed by the patient?
     Name of high school: _____
     Name of college or university: _____
     Name of graduate school: _____
     Was the patient ever retained in a grade?   Y   N
     Did the patient ever have to attend summer school due to
     academic failure?   Y   N
        If yes, list subject(s): _____
     Did the patient ever need tutoring or remedial instruction? Y   N
        If yes, list subject(s): _____
3.   What is the patient's current occupation? _____
4.   How many jobs has the patient held in the past 10 years? _____
5.   Has the patient ever been terminated from a job due to
     problems related to attention, accuracy, organization, or
     timely completion of tasks?   Y   N
6.   Has the patient ever quit a job due to problems related to
     attention, accuracy, organization, or timely completion of tasks?Y   N

++

FAMILY HISTORY

Has any blood relative of the patient (e.g., grandparents, parents, brothers, sisters, aunts, uncles, cousins) ever shown symptoms of

a. alcoholism (e.g., intoxication more than six times per year; problems controlling drinking habits; blackouts)?   Y   N

b. drug abuse (e.g., "getting high" more than six times per year; problems controlling use of drugs like pot)?   Y   N

c. obesity (e.g., weight control problems)?   Y   N

d. depression (e.g., a pervasive sense of sadness that lasts for weeks, months, or years)?   Y   N

e. ADHD (e.g., difficulty concentrating while listening or reading, disorganization, procrastination, forgetfulness, or impulsivity and restlessness)?   Y   N

f. compulsive gambling (e.g., inability to control the urge to wager more than the person could afford; needing to borrow money to repay gambling debts; inability to pay household bills because of gambling losses)?   Y   N

g. frequent loss of temper (e.g., yelling, cursing, swearing, throwing things, or hitting others when frustrated on a daily or weekly basis)?   Y   N

h. learning disorders (e.g., difficulty learning to read, write, or solve math problems; retention in a grade; special education class)?   Y   N

i. anxiety (e.g., experiencing a sense of nervousness and tension that lasts for weeks, months, or years)?   Y   N

j. panic disorder (e.g., experiencing a sudden, intense state of anxiety that is so intense that the patient is unable to function)?   Y   N

k. sexual addiction (e.g., engaging in sexual behavior that is dangerous from a health perspective or threatens the stability of a relationship)?   Y   N

l. criminal actions (e.g., arrest and conviction for activities other than driving)?   Y   N

++

MARITAL HISTORY

1. Has the patient ever been married?   Y   N
   If yes, how many times? _____
   Is the patient currently married?   Y   N
2. Is there a history of divorce in the patient's family?   Y   N
   If yes, did the patient experience the divorce of parents?   Y   N
   At what age? _____

+++

Thank you for completing this questionnaire. If there are any questions or problems that you would like to discuss with your doctor or therapist in more detail, please list here:

_____

_____

_____

_____

5

NUTRITION, SLEEP, AND EXERCISE: THE FOUNDATION OF ATTENTION AND BEHAVIORAL CONTROL

Although there is little scientific support for the hypothesis that attention-deficit/hyperactivity disorder (ADHD) is caused by nutritional deficiencies, sleep deprivation, or insufficient exercise, there is considerable evidence that dietary, sleep, and exercise habits exert a demonstrable impact on attention, mood, and capacity for behavioral control. The purpose of this chapter is to provide an overview of research examining the cognitive and behavioral effects of nutritional deficiencies, inadequate sleep habits, and insufficient exercise and to present a model for integrating these findings into clinical practice.

Included in this chapter is a presentation of the biosynthesis of those neurotransmitters implicated in mediating attention, behavioral control, and other executive functions (i.e., dopamine [DA], norepinephrine [NE], and serotonin [5-HT]), the relationship between carbohydrate and protein intake and neurotransmitter levels in the blood and in the brain, and the impact of meal composition and timing on brain neurotransmitter levels. The section on the relationship between dietary factors and attention and behavioral control also includes a comparison of the effects of high-carbohydrate, high-protein, and balanced meals on neurotransmitter levels and performance on tasks requiring attention and behavioral control in school.

Following this review of diet and executive functions, an examination of the relationship among (a) exercise; sleep habits; and attention, mood, and performance on tasks of memory and cognitive functions is presented. Once again, this review is not intended to imply that ADHD is caused by insufficient sleep or exercise. Rather, it is directed at addressing the question, Do nutrition, exercise, and sleep really make a difference in an individual's capacity to sustain attention, concentrate on cognitive tasks, and function effectively in work and school settings?

NUTRITION AND ATTENTION

The ability of the brain to perform essential life tasks is dependent on the bioavailability of neurotransmitters. As reviewed in earlier chapters of this book, genetic and biochemical research has suggested that the catecholamines, DA, and NE, as well as another monoamine neurotransmitter (i.e., 5-HT) are essential for attention and behavioral control. During the past 40 years, an extensive body of research has been published that has clarified the process by which foods are processed to yield amino acids (e.g., tryptophan, tyrosine, phenylalanine), how neurotransmitters are synthesized from such amino acids by brain cells, and how meal composition affects the rate at which certain neurotransmitters are synthesized. In addition, this research has examined the impact of nutritional factors on alertness, mood, and concentration. Much of this research has been conducted by Fernstrom, Wurtman, and their colleagues at the Laboratory of Brain and Metabolism, within the Department of Nutrition and Food Science at the Massachusetts Institute of Technology. Reviews of the research literature provide an overview of the relationship between food intake, the biosynthesis of neurotransmitters, and the impact of dietary habits on functioning (e.g., Fernstrom, 1976, 1977, 1981, 1994; Fernstrom & Wurtman, 1974; Lieberman, Spring, & Garfield, 1986). A summary of the primary findings of this extensive research literature follows.

The Biosynthesis of Neurotransmitters

The biosynthesis of the neurotransmitters DA, NE, and 5-HT occurs at the brain cell level, with the greatest amounts of these neurotransmitters being produced by brain cells in the ventral tegmental region of the brain stem (see Figure 2.1 in chap. 2, this volume). The biosynthesis of DA begins when the amino acid tyrosine (derived from ingested protein) is hydroxylated to become dihydroxyphenylaline (DOPA) by the enzyme tyrosine hydroxylase. DOPA is then decarboxylated to DA by aromatic L-amino acid decarboxylase. NE is synthesized by the beta-hydroxylation of DA, which is mediated by the enzyme DA beta-hydroxylase. The biosynthesis of 5-HT proceeds from the hydroxylation of the amino acid tryptophan by the enzyme tryptophan hydroxylase to form 5-hydroxytryptphan (5-HTP). 5-HTP is then decarboxylated to form 5-HT by the enzyme aromatic L-amino acid decarboxylase.

The rate of biosynthesis of each of these neurotransmitters is determined by dietary factors. Amino acids are derived from the proteins found in food sources such as meats, poultry, fish, legumes, and dairy products. They are readily absorbed into the bloodstream and enter the brain by moving across the blood–brain barrier. This barrier is constituted of endothelial cells that line the capillaries that supply blood to the brain. These cells mediate the transport of compounds into and from the brain. One set of transport mechanisms regulates the movement of the large neutral amino acids (LNAA) such as tryptophan and tyrosine.

The transport of LNAAs such as tryptophan and tyrosine into the brain is competitive. The transport of any given LNAA into the brain after food ingestion depends not only on the blood level of a specific LNAA but also on the blood levels of other LNAAs. On a similar note, the transport of any given LNAA into the brain following amino acid supplementation will be impacted by the blood levels of other LNAAs. Therefore, efforts to increase brain levels of a specific LNAA or neurotransmitter is not a linear process.

The impact of ingesting specific meal compositions is as follows. Following consumption of a high-carbohydrate meal (e.g., cereals, muffins, donuts), insulin is secreted from the pancreas. This release of insulin causes large reductions in the blood levels of other LNAAs that compete with tryptophan for uptake into the brain. The ratio of tryptophan to other LNAAs increases. As a result, more tryptophan passes into the brain, leading to increase in the synthesis of 5-HT.

In contrast, when a meal containing a moderate amount of protein is ingested, no such preference for tryptophan occurs. Instead, the blood levels of a variety of LNAAs increase, with a greater proportional increment in the level of serum tyrosine occurring (compared with other LNAAs). This is due to the fact that protein foods contain significantly higher amounts of the amino acids tyrosine and phenylalanine than other LNAAs, including tryptophan. As the blood ratio of tyrosine to the sum of LNAA competitors increases, brain levels of tyrosine and DA also increase rapidly.

As emphasized by Lieberman et al. (1986), it is not so much the blood level of a specific LNAA that is a critical determinant of neurotransmitter metabolism. Rather, it is the ratio of a specific LNAA to the other LNAAs that determines selective brain absorption and the biosynthesis of specific neurotransmitters.

The Behavioral Effects of Administering Tryptophan and Tyrosine

The ingestion or administration of pure tryptophan or tyrosine has the same neurochemical effect as consuming a high-carbohydrate or high-protein meal, respectively. When tryptophan is introduced in a "pure" state, blood and brain levels of this LNAA increase, as does the biosynthesis of 5-HT. When pure tyrosine is introduced, blood and brain levels increase, as does the biosynthesis of DA. As tryptophan levels increase, evidence of fatigue and reduced alertness is commonly reported. Similar results have been reported when protein or carbohydrate meals are consumed, with evidence of sedation and reduced alertness noted following carbohydrate meals. High-protein meals (like the administration of pure tyrosine) produce no such decline in alertness.

Breakfast Composition, Attention, and Educational Performance

Given the demonstrated relationship between meal composition and sedation or alertness, it is not surprising that a substantial body of research exists that examines the impact of dietary habits on attention and educational performance. Initially, studies examining the impact of skipping breakfast were conducted. As reviewed by Pollitt (1995) and Pollitt and Mathews (1998), the deleterious effects of breakfast omission have been consistently reported in the scientific literature. The types of impairment have included diminished response rate and accuracy on tests of visual and auditory short-term memory, immediate recall, delayed recall, recognition memory, and spatial memory. In addition, adverse effects on measures of verbal fluency and calculation speed and accuracy have also been reported.

Studies examining the impact of skipping breakfast have revealed that such impairments can be reversed by consumption of breakfast. Much of the early nutritional research (reviewed by Dye, Lluch, & Blundell, 2000; Pollitt, 1995; Pollitt & Mathews, 1998) examined the functioning of children who skipped breakfast in comparison with those who had breakfast. As noted by these reviewers, improvements on multiple measures relating to working memory have consistently been reported when children consume breakfast, although factors such as time of day, circadian rhythms, type of task, and habitual diet appear to be significant moderators of effect size. In general, performance on tasks requiring sustained attention is impaired in the early afternoon compared with late morning, in children who fail to eat breakfast. However, greatest impairment is noted following consumption of a high-carbohydrate lunch (Dye et al., 2000).

Because of evidence that increased sedation and decreased alertness occurs following consumption of high-carbohydrate meals, multiple studies have been conducted investigating the relationship between meal composition and performance on tasks requiring alertness, sustained attention, and working memory (K. Fischer, Colombani, Langhans, & Wenk, 2001, 2002; Mahoney, Taylor, Kanarek, & Samuel, 2005; Spring, Maller, Wurtman, Digman, & Cozolino, 1982; Wesnes, Pincock, Richardson, Helm, & Hails, 2003). Specifically, these researchers have investigated the impact of meals varying in composition of carbohydrates and protein, hypothesizing that a breakfast higher in protein would enhance functioning. In general, their findings have supported the beneficial effects of including protein at breakfast and lunchtime meals.

Spring et al. (1982) studied the effects of high-carbohydrate and high-protein meals consumed by 184 adult men and women (ages 40–65) at breakfast and lunch. They found that participants felt "calmer" and "less tense" after eating a high-carbohydrate breakfast (coffee and pastry) or lunch (nondairy sherbet) but performed significantly poorer on tests of selective attention after eating a high-carbohydrate meal. When adults were tested following ingestion of a protein meal (turkey breast), they demonstrated better performance on tests of attention and concentration.

Similar findings have been reported in studies of children and younger adults. Wesnes et al. (2003) compared the performance of children (ages 9–16) on computerized tests of attention and memory following consumption of a commercially available cereal with milk (Cheerios or Shreddies), a glucose drink, or no breakfast. They found that when children consumed the glucose drink or failed to eat breakfast, significant declines in attention and memory were noted. However, no such declines were noted when a breakfast including carbohydrates and protein was ingested.

Mahoney et al. (2005) expanded this research by comparing two different types of breakfast foods (instant oatmeal and commercially available cereal with 8 oz of milk) to a no-breakfast condition. Participants were children ages 6 to 11 years. Again, both of the breakfasts that included carbohydrates and protein (milk) yielded gains on tasks of spatial memory, auditory memory, and auditory attention.

Analysis of the relative merits of various ratios of protein and carbohydrates was conducted in a study performed by K. Fischer et al. (2002). In this study, the amounts of carbohydrate and protein in a breakfast mixture were systematically controlled. The breakfasts consisted of creamlike suspensions, which contained varying ratios of protein and carbohydrates. The effects of a high-carbohydrate meal (carbohydrate-to-protein ratio = 4:1) was compared with the impact of balanced (carbohydrate-to-protein ratio = 1:1) and protein rich (carbohydrate-to-protein ratio = 1:4) breakfasts on tests of attention and memory. In addition, analysis of the duration of effects was conducted for a 3.5-hour postbreakfast period.

K. Fischer et al. (2002) reported that the beneficial effects of a high-carbohydrate meal on measures of reaction time lasted for approximately 1 hour postingestion. During the 1st hour, the reaction times were faster following the high-carbohydrate breakfast than after consumption of the balanced and protein-rich breakfasts. Thereafter, the beneficial effects of the high-carbohydrate meal dissipated. After 1 hour, reaction time was slowest following the high-carbohydrate meal and fastest in the high-protein meal. This pattern persisted for the duration of the 3.5-hour period.

On measures of memory and attention, the high-carbohydrate meal yielded greater improvement on a measure of attention for the 1st hour. However, it did not yield any evidence of superiority to the high-protein or balanced meals beyond the 1st hour. In contrast, following consumption of the high-protein meal, children demonstrated better accuracy on tests of short-term memory and attention. Again the superiority of the high-protein meal endured for 3.5 hours.

To test the hypothesis that the variations in reaction time, memory, and attention were associated with different rates of glucose metabolism and fluctuations in blood sugar levels, K. Fischer et al. (2001) tested the impact of pure carbohydrate, protein, and fat on tests of short-term memory and attention. They administered creamy mixtures with similar sensory properties to 15 male college students. Like all of the previous studies, they used a randomized design in which each of the students ingested each of the various breakfasts on multiple occasions. Effects were monitored for a 3-hour period following breakfast.

The results of this study confirmed their hypothesis that fluctuations in glucose level were related to changes in performance on tests of memory and attention, as overall performance on tasks was best after fat ingestion. Again, these researchers noted that the pure carbohydrate meal yielded brief (1-hour) gains on measures of short-term memory and the pure protein meal yielded better results on measures of attention for a sustained time period. The researchers interpreted these findings as supporting the hypothesis that "good and stable cognitive performance is related to a balanced glucose metabolism and metabolic activation state" (K. Fischer et al., 2001, p. 393).

Consistent with prior research linking fluctuations in glucose levels with changes in insulin levels and alterations in the availability of tryptophan and tyrosine, Wurtman et al. (2003) examined the impact of high-carbohydrate and high-protein breakfasts on plasma tryptophan and tyrosine ratio in eight adults, ages 20 to 30. As anticipated, Wurtman et al. (2003) demonstrated that these two types of breakfasts yielded quite different changes in insulin levels over a 4-hour period, with significant increases occurring after the carbohydrate, but not the protein, meal. In addition, they demonstrated that the high-carbohydrate breakfast caused a significant rise in the tryptophan-to-LNAA ratio (ranging from 7%–14%). The high-protein breakfast was associated with a significant decline in the tryptophan-to-LNAA ratio (between 17% and 35% reduction).

Collectively, the studies on the relationship between diet, attention, and memory implicate the significance of fluctuations in blood sugar levels and the ratio of tryptophan to other LNAAs. Increases in blood sugar levels are associated with the release of insulin, an increase in the permeability of the blood–brain barrier to tryptophan, with resultant increase in the biosynthesis of 5-HT. The behavioral effects of such biochemical processes have been associated with short-term improvement in reaction time and certain measures of short-term memory. However, these gains dissipate within 60 minutes, to be followed by a sense of sedation and poorer performance on tests of attention and memory. In contrast, high-protein meals do not significantly increase blood sugar, insulin, or the tryptophan-to-LNAA ratio. Although such meals do not appear to prompt a rapid improvement in reaction time or short-term memory, they appear to contribute to the maintenance of attention and memory functions over a 3- to 4-hour period postingestion.

Such findings support the importance of consuming simple and complex carbohydrates, fats, and protein at breakfast and lunch. The rationale is that simple carbohydrates prompt an immediate boost in alertness; complex carbohydrates provide a more enduring source of sugars (promoting sustained mental energy); and proteins provide the amino acids necessary for the biosynthesis of essential neurotransmitters (i.e., DA, NE, and 5-HT). Fats are essential for the development and maintenance of the myelin sheath that surrounds brain cells and permits rapid neural transmission. Vitamins (particularly B vitamins) and minerals such as iron, zinc, and magnesium are found in substantial levels in high-protein foods, grains, vegetables, and fruits and are also essential for the biosynthesis of the enzymes that determine the rate of neurotransmitter biosynthesis (e.g., tryptophan hydroxylase, tyrosine hydroxylase, aromatic L-amino acid decarboxylase). Skipping breakfast or eating a high-carbohydrate breakfast simply does not provide the brain with the nutrients needed for tasks requiring attention, concentration, and working memory for the 4 hours between breakfast and lunch. Likewise, skipping lunch or eating high-carbohydrate or other low-protein lunches (e.g., fruit and vegetable salads) will not be sufficient to sustain attention, concentration, and working memory during the afternoon hours.

Teaching Parents, Children, Teenagers, and Adult Patients About Nutrition

At our clinic, we begin discussing the relationship between food and attention and memory during the assessment phase. By the third session, our patients have learned that brain cells need protein to make neurotransmitters (which we refer to as "brain juice") and that without this "juice" the brain simply cannot do its job. We teach our patients that foods such as cereals are like straw or kindling: They start up the fire in our brain and help us to concentrate for brief periods. However, the protein foods that we eat are the logs that keep the fire in our brain going, helping us to concentrate all morning (or afternoon).

TABLE 5.1
Recommended Dietary Allowances for Protein, Magnesium, Iron, and Zinc

Group	Age (years)	Protein (g)	Magnesium (mg)	Iron (mg)	Zinc (mg)
Children	4–6	24	120	10	10
Children	7–10	28	170	10	10
Males	11–14	45	270	12	15
Males	15–18	59	400	12	15
Males	19+	58	350	10	15
Females	11–14	46	280	15	12
Females	15–18	44	300	15	12
Females	19+	46	280	15	12

Note. Data from Food and Nutrition Board of the National Academy of Sciences (1989).

Because patients with ADHD tend to be picky eaters, with limited appetite in the morning, we emphasize the importance of consuming the recommended dietary allowances (RDAs) for protein, as published by the Food and Nutrition Board of the National Academy of Sciences (1989), at breakfast and lunch. Such foods, even in low quantity, provide a wide range of nutritional benefits. A summary of these recommendations is provided in this section (see also Table 5.1).

Children, teenagers, and adults are required to perform tasks demanding sustained attention, concentration, and memory during school and work periods lasting approximately 8 hours. Therefore, we encourage our patients to consume at least 80% of these dietary recommendations at breakfast and lunch. This translates to approximately 10 grams of protein for young children at breakfast and lunch, increasing to approximately 20 to 25 grams of protein for teenagers and adults at these meals. The ingestion of the RDAs for protein provides an ample supply of essential amino acids, as well as a substantial amount of iron, magnesium, and zinc. An example of the nutritional content found in a number of commonly consumed foods is presented in Table 5.2.

To reduce the complexity of figuring out how much protein is contained in specific foods, I simplify the process by teaching our patients the "Rule of Sevens": Approximately 7 grams of protein can be obtained by consuming the following portions of the following foods: 1 ounce of beef, pork, poultry, or fish; 1 egg; 1 ounce of cheese; 7 ounces of milk (regardless of fat content); 2 tablespoons of peanut butter; and 1 slice of pizza. Although I can provide comprehensive lists of the nutritional contents of various foods from sources such as *Bowes & Church's Food Values of Portions Commonly Used* (J. A. Pennington & Douglass, 2004), I typically teach our patients to estimate the protein content of foods using the Rule of Sevens.

TABLE 5.2

Nutritional Content of Foods Commonly Consumed
at Breakfast and Lunch

Food	Protein (g)	Tyrosine (mg)	Phenylalanine (mg)	Tryptophan (mg)	Iron (mg)	Zinc (mg)	Magnesium (mg)
Cheerios	4.3	153	233	58	4.4	0.79	39
Cap'n Crunch	1.5	59	76	12	4.8	2.37	10
Raisin Bran	3.0	68	105	39	6.2	2.00	58
Oatmeal	6.0	205	320	84	1.6	1.15	56
White toast	2.0	0	0	0	0.7	0.15	5
Wheat toast	2.4	0	0	0	0.9	0.42	23
Egg	6.3	257	334	76	0.6	0.52	5
Cheese (1 oz)	6.3	344	319	92	0.1	0.85	6
Sausage	5.3	153	177	42	0.3	0.68	5
Pancakes (3)	8.3	318	402	102	2.6	1.03	48
French toast (2)	10.3	345	536	143	1.9	0.60	16
Milk (8 oz)	8.0	388	388	113	0.1	0.95	34
Yogurt (8 oz)	9.0	456	493	51	0.1	1.52	30
Taco (small)	20.7	759	883	230	2.4	3.90	71
Pizza (1)	7.7	348	366	91	0.6	0.82	16
Chicken nugget (6)	16.9	567	709	203	1.3	1.06	20
Cheeseburger (4 oz)	30.1	1,045	1,278	379	5.5	5.54	38
Hot dog (1)	10.4	277	409	96	2.3	1.98	13
Peanut butter (2 tbsp)	7.9	320	408	76	0.5	0.80	50
Peanuts (1 oz; 15–20 nuts)	6.6	270	344	64	0.6	0.93	49

Note. Data from J. A. Pennington and Douglas (2004).

During our initial meetings, I demonstrate to parents and children how little food actually constitutes an ounce. For example, I show a quarter-pound burger and demonstrate how each quarter of a quarter-pounder (which is just a little bit of food) provides 7 grams of protein. I'll repeat the process with foods such as chicken nuggets, cheese sandwiches, and other easy-to-digest foods. I also try to simplify the process by teaching patients to stop thinking about only "breakfast" foods for breakfast.

Most of my patients associate foods such as cereals, pastry, granola bars, and the like with breakfast. Many are quite surprised when I begin to tell them about my breakfast habits, which often include a chicken sandwich or a ham and cheese sandwich on a bagel, with a glass of milk, juice, and some fruit. However, they seem to catch on pretty quickly. I teach our patients that their brains are looking to fuel up on protein at breakfast and lunch, not at dinner. Children have little difficulty understanding the irony of tanking up on a lot of food and then trying to go to sleep.

During these initial three meetings, I also help them to understand one of our mantras: Cereal is the dessert of breakfast. I would no more expect them to simply eat a bowl of cereal for breakfast than I would expect them to only eat a piece of chocolate cake for dinner. If you compare the nutritional contents of a slice of cake and a bowl of any cereal, you will find that they are quite similar. The only difference is that the manufacturers of cereals decided to sprinkle a multivitamin into their batter. Consequently, I teach children and parents that cereals are fine as part of a balanced breakfast. The only difference is that I emphasize that cereals are the dessert part, not the main course. Kids and parents understand this concept quite readily but typically need assistance in establishing dietary habits that can help them and their children sustain attention and concentration throughout the day.

Nutritional Supplements

As reviewed in chapter 3 of this book, there are several specific nutritional deficiencies that have been associated with inattention, impulsivity, and hyperactivity. Among these medical conditions are anemias; hypoglycemia; diabetes; thyroid disorders; and deficiencies of iron, zinc, magnesium, and essential fatty acids. Consequently, screening for such deficiencies is routinely recommended by our clinic. When any of these conditions are diagnosed, nutritional counseling, dietary modifications, pharmacological treatment, and supplementation are initiated. However, as reviewed by Arnold (2002), there appears to be little rationale for the routine use of amino acid, vitamin, mineral, or other supplements in the treatment of disorders of attention and behavioral control in the absence of demonstrated deficiencies or dietary inadequacy.

SLEEP, ATTENTION, MEMORY, AND COGNITIVE FUNCTIONING

Sleep is a period when the body is involved in a variety of activities, including the biosynthesis of protein, the repair and regeneration of tissue (including bone and muscle), the strengthening of our immune system, and the consolidation of memory. During sleep, such changes in body function are reflected in variations of brain activity (measured on electroencephalographs [EEGs], heart rate, body temperature, and muscle tone). The human body transitions between five *sleep stages*, classified as periods with or without rapid eye movements (REM and non-REM, respectively). Each of the four non-REM stages lasts approximately 5 to 15 minutes. During Stage 1 of non-REM sleep, there is a reduction in body activity, the eyes close, the rate of brain activity begins to slow, and individuals may begin to experience a sense of falling. During Stage 2, the body alternates between periods of muscle tone and relaxation. There is a decline in heart rate and a decrease in body temperature. Stages 3 and 4 (termed *delta sleep*) are periods characterized by the predominance of slow EEG wave forms (delta waves). It is within these periods that the body repairs and regenerates tissue, builds bones and muscle, and strengthens the immune system.

Stage 5 (REM) sleep occurs approximately 90 minutes after onset of Stage 1. During this stage, the EEG reflects patterns of brain activity that mimic the waking state. During REM sleep, the body is immobile as the brain processes and consolidates memories. The first REM period of the night is about 10 minutes in duration. Subsequent periods of REM during an evening increase in duration, with the final REM period extended to approximately 1 hour.

The amount of sleep required for effective daytime functioning varies with age. Infants may require 16 to 18 hours of sleep, whereas children appear to require approximately 10 hours of sleep. Adolescents need about 9 hours of sleep, and adults benefit from 7 to 8 hours of sleep. The beneficial effects of sleep, and the detrimental effects of sleep deprivation, have been examined in numerous scientific studies (see reviews by Blissitt, 2001; Durmer & Dinges, 2005). A summary of the primary findings is provided in the next section.

Effects of Sleep Deprivation

Studies of the effects of sleep deprivation can be categorized into three groups, based on the degree of sleep disruption: long-term total sleep deprivation (> 45 hours consecutively), short-term total sleep deprivation (< 45 hours of consecutive sleep loss), and partial sleep deprivation (< 7 hours of sleep in a 24-hour period). As noted by Durmer and Dinges (2005), all types of sleep deprivation are associated with feelings of fatigue, loss of vigor, daytime sleepiness, and mental confusion. On cognitive measures, the performance of individuals subjected to any of the three types of sleep deprivation is poorer than approximately 90% of non–sleep-deprived individuals (ranging from 84%–98%), with cognitive performance becoming progressively worse as the duration of the task is increased.

Individuals subjected to any type of sleep deprivation have demonstrated the following types of functional impairments: involuntary "microsleeps" during the daytime, increased frequency of errors of omission and commission on continuous performance tests, slowing of response time, decline in short-term recall and working memory, slowing of rate of learning new tasks, deterioration of performance on tasks requiring divergent thinking, and perseveration of ineffective solutions to complex problems.

As noted in multiple studies (Deming, Zhenyun, & Daosheng, 1991; Gieseking, Williams, & Lubin, 1957; Williams, Gieseking, & Lubin, 1966; Wimmer, Hoffmann, Bonato, & Moffitt, 1992), impairment of memory (immediate word recall) and divergent (creative) thinking occur following even one night of sleep deprivation. Because it is common for children, teens, and adults to develop patterns of chronic partial sleep deprivation (i.e., > 4 days) studies examining the effects of such habits appear particularly relevant for clinical practice. As reviewed by Durmer and Dinges (2005), individuals who have 4 or more consecutive days of partial sleep deprivation (i.e., < 7 hours of sleep) exhibit a wide range of cognitive deficits, including decreased cognitive speed and accuracy on working memory tasks and increased errors on vigilance tasks, such as continuous performance tests (Belenky et al., 2003; Carskadon & Dement, 1981; Dinges et al., 1997; Drake et al., 2001; Van Dongen, Maislin, Mullington, & Dinges, 2003).

Neurological Manifestations of Sleep Deprivation

It is not surprising that neuroimaging and electrophysiological studies have revealed adverse effects of sleep deprivation in brain regions involved in the mediation of attention, concentration, and memory functions. Positron emission tomography (PET) studies have shown decreased glucose metabolism in the prefrontal cortex, the anterior cingulate gyrus, and the basal ganglia following sleep deprivation (Thomas et al., 2000; Wu et al., 1991). Animal analog studies indicate that additional structural changes in hippocampal pyramidal neurons occur after sleep deprivation, which "profoundly inhibit hippocampal functioning" (McDermott et al., 2003, p. 9687). On a similar note, EEG studies have consistently revealed decreases in the amplitude of band frequencies associated with alertness (Gevins, Smith, McEvoy, & Yu, 1997; Smith, McEvoy, & Gevins, 1999, 2002) and a decline in the amplitude of the P300 wave following varying degrees of sleep deprivation. Such findings provide further substantiation that the subjective reports of fatigue and impaired performance on various tests of alertness and memory are associated with atypical patterns of activation of brain structures essential for these functions.

Parent and Patient Education

When examination of a patient reveals that partial sleep deprivation is present, intervention to improve sleep habits seems advisable prior to a determination of a diagnosis of ADHD and the initiation of pharmacological treatments that can increase insomnia. At our clinic, we determine sleep patterns through parent and patient interview and intervene at several levels.

First, because sleep onset is triggered by elevated blood levels of the protein-derived neurotransmitter melatonin, we closely examine the patient's dietary intake of protein. Melatonin is a neurotransmitter that is derived from the amino acid tryptophan. As noted previously, tryptophan is an essential amino acid, derived from protein and synthesized into 5-HT. Within the pineal gland, 5-HT is converted into N-acetylserotonin by the enzyme N-acetyl transferase and subsequently to melatonin, via the enzyme hydroxyl-O-methyl transferase. The activity of the pineal gland is highly sensitive to external light, and secretion of melatonin by the pineal gland increases in the darkness and subsides in daylight. Increase in the blood level of melatonin has been associated with drowsiness and sleep onset.

Consequently, I encourage our patients and their parents to take steps to ensure that the patient is consuming RDAs of protein each day. To further enhance sleep onset, I encourage patients to consume foods likely to cause increased brain availability of tryptophan in the early evening (e.g., cereals, warm milk, turkey, cheese) prior to bed. Ingestion of foods or drinks containing caffeine (e.g., colas, chocolates, teas) is discouraged.

Establishment of a pattern of early evening physical activity, followed by a consistent pattern of bathing and quiet activities with a parent (e.g., reading a book together) is also recommended. Highly stimulating activities (e.g., playing a video game, watching television) are likely to interfere with sleep onset. Use of a low dose of a time-release or two-stage supplement of melatonin can also be helpful (1–3 mg; administered 1.5–2.0 hours prior to intended hour of sleep). However, such an intervention is intended to interrupt a pattern of sleep deprivation so that healthy dietary and activity patterns can be established and should not be considered a long-term solution.

Most of the kids that I treat are willing to figure out a simple strategy to eat high-protein breakfasts and lunches, once they realize that I am not talking about a ton of food and that they can eat their favorite foods (e.g., pizza, chicken nuggets, beef jerky) for breakfast. Other kids find out that protein powders can be mixed into a variety of "yummy" foods (e.g., puddings, yogurt) or baked into brownies, breads, and muffins. The key is that the patient comes to understand that sleep is connected to dietary habits and patterns of activity during the day and that there are strategies that they can use. I provide patients and their parents with a variety of forms to help them keep track of their dietary habits. See Figure 5.1 and Exhibit 5.1 for samples of these forms.

EXERCISE, ATTENTION, AND COGNITIVE FUNCTIONS

Exercise, defined as physical activities that involve "large muscle groups at an intensity requiring 60% or greater of an individual's cardiovascular capacity for 20 to 30 minute periods from three to five days a week" (Keays & Allison, 1995, p. 62), has been associated with a wide range of health and functional benefits. Studies of school-aged children have noted gains on measures of academic performance, cognitive abilities, self-esteem, and classroom behavior (Tomporowski & Ellis, 1986; Worsley, Coonan, & Worsley, 1987). Other researchers have noted gains on tests of alertness, memory, observation, problem solving, rate and accuracy of decision making, and reading and mathematics (Dwyer, Coonan, Leitch, Hetzel, & Baghurst, 1983; Martens & Grant, 1980; Tomporowski & Ellis, 1986).

In adolescents and adults who exercise regularly, lower levels of depression and anxiety, and improved quality of sleep, have also been reported (Benloucif et al., 2004; Craft & Landers, 1998; Field, Diego, & Sanders, 2001; Mutrie & Biddle, 1995). Although a variety of factors appear to moderate the level of benefit noted in an individual (e.g., age, genetics, body weight, diet, and smoking; Keays & Allison, 1995; Kesaniemi et al., 2001; U.S. Department of Health and Human Services, 2000), the consensus is that participation in regular moderate to vigorous physical activity (MVPA) holds the potential for helping an individual maintain alertness, concentration, and a variety of other cognitive abilities (U.S. Department of Health and Human Services, 2000).

The process by which participation in regular MVPA produces such improvements has been investigated in human and animal analog studies. For example, Nakamura, Nishimoto, Akamutu, Takahashi, and Maruyama (1999) studied event-related potentials (ERPs) in an investigation of the relationship between acute, self-paced jogging and performance on tests of executive functions. They found improved performance associated with increased amplitude in P300 at central midline and posterior brain sites. Similarly, Magnie et al. (2000) found elevated P300 amplitude and decreased latency over the left parietal region of the brain. Because the amplitude and latency of the P300 has been associated with improved alertness and attention, these authors hypothesized that physical activity increases performance by causing an increase in cortical arousal. Research conducted by Hillman, Snook, and Jerome (2003) further illustrated that the beneficial effects of

Remember
Cereals, pastas, fruits, and vegetables—
although good food choices—are a **POOR
SOURCE** of protein.

Food	Protein (g)
Granola bar	2.0
Cap'n Crunch, 1 serving	1.5
Pop-Tart	1.0
Potato chips (1 oz); small bag	2.0
Apple	0.0
1 slice of white toast	3.0
1 donut	1.0
Banana	1.0

General protein content of different foods:

1 oz of meat = 7 g
3 oz of meat = the size of a deck of cards = 21 g
8 oz of milk = 8 g
1 oz of cheese = 7 g
1 grain serving = 1 slice of bread, 1/2 cup cooked
vegetables or 1 cup raw vegetables = 3 g

Fruits = no protein

All food groups provide nutrients and minerals
but **PROTEIN PROVIDES BRAIN JUICE!!!**

- Children 11 years old or younger need to eat
  15–20 g of protein at both breakfast and
  lunch.

- Children 12 years old or older need to eat
  20–30 g of protein at both breakfast and
  lunch.

- It is important that these meals be consumed
  before 3 p.m.!!!

COMMON PROTEIN-RICH FOODS

Food name	Protein (g)
BREAKFAST	
1 slice of American cheese	6
1 glass of milk (8 oz)	8
Yogurt—fruit flavor (8 oz)	9
Carnation Instant Breakfast with 8 oz of 1% milk	14
1 large egg	7
Bagel with 2 Tbsp of cream cheese	8
Oatmeal made with milk	6
English muffin with egg & cheese, Canadian bacon	20
3 pancakes with butter & syrup	8
Sausage, 1 patty	5
1 slice of toast with peanut butter	10
3 slices of bacon	4
Canadian bacon, 2 slices	11
LUNCH	
1 hot dog	10
Turkey breast, 1 slice	5
Ham, 1 slice	5
Peanut butter and jelly sandwich	13–15
Tuna salad, 1/2 cup	33
Burrito with beans	14
6 chicken nuggets	17
Hamburger	12
Cheeseburger	16
1 slice of cheese pizza	8
1 slice of pizza with pepperoni	10
Roast beef sandwich	22
Taco, small (6 oz)	21
1 cup of chocolate milk	8

Figure 5.1. Quick Nutritional Reference Guide.

exercise appear to be greatest on tasks that are more demanding of attention
and mental effort.

The biochemical process by which such arousal is mediated appears
related to changes in plasma and cortical levels of catecholamines (e.g., epinephrine) that occur during exercise (Chmura, Krysztofiak, Ziemba, Nazar,
& Kaciuba-Uscilko, 1998; Chmura, Nazar, & Kaciuba-Uscilko, 1994). During acute periods of physical exercise, the release of catecholamines increases
heart rate, blood flow, oxygen uptake, and activation of multiple cortical
pathways (as noted during ERP studies). Gains in alertness, attention, and

EXHIBIT 5.1
Healthy Life Chart

Name: _____

Medication: _____

Type: _____

Dosage: _____

	EXERCISE (What exercise did you do today and for how long?)		SLEEP (How much sleep?)	FOOD CONSUMPTION (What did you eat today?)	
	Type	Duration (how long)	No. of hours per day	Breakfast	Lunch
MONDAY					
TUESDAY					

WEDNESDAY				
THURSDAY				
FRIDAY				
SATURDAY				
SUNDAY				

the performance of various cognitive and motor tasks are the products of this process.

Polich and Kok (1995) reviewed evidence that such changes in biological arousal are enduring. They note that the resting EEGs of individuals who exercise regularly are characterized by increased P300 amplitude and reduced latency. Similarly, Kubitz and Mott (1996) and Kubitz and Pothakos (1997) observed increased levels of alpha activity (9–11 Hz) following exercise. Such increases in alpha activation have been associated with increased P300 amplitude and decreased P300 latency (Bashore, 1989; Hillman et al., 2003; Lardon & Polich, 1996). Dustman, Emmerson, and Shearer (1990) and Isaacs, Anderson, Alcantara, Black, and Greenough (1992) observed an association between cerebral blood flow and exercise, noting improved blood flow and shorter diffusion distances in the blood vessels of the cerebellum of rats. These findings support the hypothesis that the long-term, beneficial effects of exercise are derived from increased vascularization and enhanced blood flow to the brain, although additional research is clearly required to clarify the mechanisms by which exercise produces beneficial effects.

On the basis of findings that participation in 20 to 30 minutes of MVPA for 3 to 5 days per week can exert a beneficial effect on alertness, concentration, and problem solving, clinical efforts to increase patient awareness and involvement in such activities are clearly supported. In our clinical practice, discussion of the specific gains associated with exercise begins during our third session with the patient and continues during each contact. Our treatment plan includes specific targets for exercise, as well as dietary and sleep goals to support the physical foundations of attention and behavioral control. Part of this process includes instructing patients how to calculate a threshold and a ceiling heart rate per minute. This calculation is performed as follows:

> *Step 1*. Subtract the patient's age from 220.
> *Step 2*. Multiply number by 0.6. That number represents the suggested minimum heartbeats per minute for training effects, which is termed the *threshold*.
> *Step 3*. If you subtract age from 200 and multiply by 0.8, that is the ceiling number for the maximum heart rate per minute.

The goal is to sustain heart rate between the threshold and ceiling level for at least 20 minutes to achieve the desired gains in cardiovascular functions, decrease in blood glucose levels, and boost attention and concentration.

Once we calculate the threshold and ceiling rates, I typically experiment with the patient (and family). We practice several activities (e.g., push-ups, sit-ups) and track changes in heart rate. Then we discuss different activities at home and ask the family to check out which activities get their hearts pumping the most (e.g., swimming, riding a bike, skateboarding, walking, jumping rope, running, jumping on a trampoline, roller-blading, skiing) and work out a plan to start doing 20 minutes of exercise every day.

IMPLICATIONS FOR CLINICAL PRACTICE

Although ADHD is not caused by dietary, sleep, or exercise habits, a review of the current scientific literature indicates such factors constitute the foundation of attention and behavioral control. Without sufficient amounts of dietary protein, sleep, and exercise, a patient will not be able to sustain attention, concentration, and behavioral control throughout the day, regardless of the type of pharmacological treatment. Consequently, the following recommendations are suggested as guidelines for patients seeking treatment for attentional problems:

Nutrition
> Children ages 4 to 10: At least 10 grams of protein at breakfast and at lunch.
> Children ages 11 to 14: At least 20 grams of protein at breakfast and at lunch.
> Males ages 15 to 18: At least 25 grams of protein at breakfast and at lunch.
> Females ages 15+: At least 20 grams of protein at breakfast and at lunch.
> Males ages 19+: At least 25 grams of protein at breakfast and at lunch.

Sleep
> Children: At least 10 hours sleep per night.
> Adolescents: At least 9 hours sleep per night.
> Adults: At least 7 hours sleep per night.

Exercise
> At least 3 days per week, 20 minutes of exercise sufficient to increase heart rate by at least 50% above resting heart rate. The target is 60% to 80%.

6

PHARMACOLOGICAL TREATMENTS FOR ADHD

The treatment of children, adolescents, and adults diagnosed with attention-deficit/hyperactivity disorder (ADHD) typically proceeds from a consideration of the benefits and risks of medication. At this time, there are several types of medications that are prescribed to treat symptoms of inattention, impulsivity, and hyperactivity, as well as symptoms of depressed mood, anxiety, and impaired anger control that commonly occur in patients with ADHD. When data analysis is collapsed across the three types of ADHD, reviews of the scientific literature have consistently revealed that clinical improvement is noted in 65% to 75% of patients with ADHD (Barkley, 2006; Greenhill, 2002; Jacobvitz, Sroufe, Stewart, & Leffert, 1990; Spencer et al., 1996; Swanson, 1993).

The varying types of medications for ADHD exert their beneficial effects through quite divergent mechanisms of action, supporting the position that ADHD represents a common symptomatic consequence of multiple neurological conditions. As discussed in chapter 2 (this volume), patients with ADHD frequently exhibit atypical genetic characteristics on regions of chromosomes associated with the development of dopamine (DA) receptors and reuptake transporters. However, other genetic markers, such as those

117

associated with the formation of norepinephrine (NE) and serotonin (5-HT) receptors and reuptake transporters, have also been associated with ADHD in certain patients.

Such genetic variations appear to be reflected in the divergent patterns of dysregulation of cortical arousal manifested during quantitative electroencephalographic (qEEG) examinations (i.e., cortical hypoarousal, cortical hyperarousal). As is discussed in this chapter, these markers of cortical arousal have served as a basis for identifying stimulant responders versus nonresponders (as reviewed by Chabot, di Michele, & Prichep, 2005) and have been applied in a large-scale clinical study to match patient to type of pharmacological treatment on the basis of qEEG markers (Monastra, 2005b), with enhanced clinical response rates. This chapter presents a description of the most commonly used pharmacological treatments and describes a process for improving medication response that includes examination and treatment for other relevant medical conditions; matching patient to type of medication on the basis of neurological markers of level of cortical arousal; and adjusting dosage on the basis of a combination of behavioral, neuropsychological, and neurophysiological measures.

MEDICATIONS FOR TREATING THE CORE SYMPTOMS OF ADHD

Stimulants (e.g., methylphenidate, dextromethylphenidate, dextroamphetamine, mixed amphetamine salts), antidepressants (e.g., imipramine, atomoxetine, buproprion), antihypertensives (e.g., clonidine, guanfacine), and anticonvulsants (e.g., carbamazepine) have been shown to be effective in the treatment of the core symptoms of ADHD and associated mood and conduct disorders. However, the pharmacokinetics of these medications varies markedly, as does the duration of clinical benefits and side-effects profiles. In the following sections, the pharmacokinetics of the commonly prescribed medications for ADHD is presented. In addition, the range of dosage associated with clinical benefits in controlled studies and types of side effects are reviewed.

Stimulant Medications

At present, there are four primary types of stimulants that are prescribed for the treatment of ADHD: methylphenidate (e.g., Ritalin, Ritalin-SR, Methylin, Methylin ER, Concerta, Metadate CD), dextromethylphenidate (e.g., Focalin, Focalin XR), dextroamphetamine (e.g., DextroStat, Dexedrine), and mixed amphetamine salts (e.g., Adderall, Adderall XR). These medications are available in tablet, capsule, and liquid (e.g., Methylin) preparations, as well as in a skin patch application (e.g., Daytrana). Immediate release (IR), intermediate release, and sustained release (SR) types of stimulants are available, providing clinical benefits for 4 to 6 hours, 6 to 8 hours, and 10 to 12 hours, respectively. In general, peak medication effects occur approximately 1 to 2 hours postingestion. To sustain benefits for more extended periods, intermediate-release preparations (e.g., Metadate CD, Ritalin-LA) and SR preparations (e.g., Concerta, Adderall XR) have been developed. These medications exhibit a bimodal pattern of absorption characterized by an initial peak of medication levels within the first 2 hours, followed by a second peak in medication levels occurring 4 to 6 hours postingestion.

Stimulant medications are rapidly absorbed into the bloodstream, with onset of clinical effects noted within 20 minutes for IR medications (e.g., Ritalin, Focalin, DextroStat) and within 30 minutes for mixed amphetamine salts (e.g., Adderall), intermediate preparations (e.g., Metadate CD, Ritalin-LA), and certain SR preparations (e.g., Concerta). More delayed onset of clinical effects occurs with the SR type of dextroamphetamine (i.e., Adderall XR; approximately 1 hour). As reviewed by Barkley (2006) and Greenhill (2002), there is substantial evidence that stimulant medications can be beneficial for patients with ADHD beginning in early childhood (ages 4–6 years) and extending into adulthood.

Clinically effective dosages vary widely, depending on type of stimulant used. Dosages as low as 5.0 milligrams, three times daily (methylphenidate), and 2.5 milligrams, twice daily (b.i.d.) (mixed amphetamine salts), have been associated with positive response, although dosages extending to 75 milligrams per day (methylphenidate), 40 milligrams per day (mixed amphetamine salts), and 35 milligrams per day (dextroamphetamine) have been required to attain clinical benefits. As reviewed by both Barkley (2006) and Greenhill (2002), there is little evidence that increased dosages are needed as the patient proceeds from childhood into adulthood.

Because of the unique delivery systems of certain medications (e.g., Concerta, Metadate CD), it is important for practitioners to realize that an 18-milligram dose of Concerta does not represent a threefold increase in the dose of methylphenidate found in Ritalin nor does a 20-milligram dose of Metadate CD deliver 4 times the amount of methylphenidate available in Ritalin. Concerta (18 mg) delivers the equivalent of 5 milligrams of methylphenidate extended for a 10- to 12-hour period; Metadate CD (20 mg) provides 5 milligrams of methylphenidate for approximately 6 to 8 hours, rather than for 3 to 4 hours. On a similar note, Adderall XR (10 mg) does not constitute a dose of mixed amphetamine salts that is twice as great as Adderall (5 mg). Instead, Adderall XR provides the equivalent of 5 milligrams of mixed amphetamine salts for an extended period (10–12 hours vs. 4–6 hours). Because of the need for sustained improvement of attention and behavioral control throughout the daytime, afternoon, and early evening hours, it is not uncommon for a patient to be treated with a combination of SR and IR stimulants.

Neurochemistry

In general, stimulant medications exert their beneficial effects by increasing the availability of the catecholamines in the synaptic cleft (Fowler et al., 1999; Solanto, 1998; Volkow et al., 1995, 1998, 2001). However, the specific neuronal structures affected by stimulant medications vary, depending on type of stimulant. Methylphenidate and dextromethylphenidate exert their clinical benefits by blocking the reuptake of DA. By binding to the reuptake transporters for DA, medications such as Ritalin and Focalin permit increased concentration of DA in the synaptic cleft, triggering increased neurotransmission within dopaminergic pathways.

Dextroamphetamine (e.g., DextroStat) stimulates the release of DA from presynaptic storage vesicles within brain cells but does not appear to block reuptake. However, the increased release from presynaptic storage also elevates DA availability at the synaptic cleft. Mixed amphetamine salts (e.g., Adderall) stimulate the release of DA and NE from presynaptic storage vesicles and block the reuptake of these neurotransmitters, enhancing the neurotransmission in multiple catecholamine pathways.

Evidence of the varying degrees of cortical stimulation provided via each of these types of stimulant is reflected in dosage levels required to attain clinical benefits. Methylphenidate-based preparations block the reuptake of the neurotransmitter DA and appear to require higher doses than the amphetamine-based preparations, which increase release of multiple neurotransmitters (e.g., DA, NE) from storage and also block reuptake. Dextromethylphenidate (i.e., [d]-methylphenidate and Focalin) is derived from the active enantiomer of methylphenidate, hence is more potent than (dl)-methylphenidate preparations (e.g., Ritalin). Mixed amphetamine salts appear twice as potent as methylphenidate. In clinical research and practice, a 5-milligram dose of mixed amphetamine salts yields a response equivalent to approximately 10 milligrams of methylphenidate (Shire Pharmaceuticals, 2002). On a similar note, dextromethylphyenidate appears more potent than methylphenidate, with a 2.5-milligram dose of Focalin yielding benefits comparable to 5.0 milligrams of Ritalin (Novartis Pharmaceuticals, 2002a, 2002b).

Clinical Benefits

As reviewed by Barkley (2006), Greenhill (2002), and Swanson (1993), patients who respond to stimulants typically demonstrate improved performance and functioning across multiple domains. Symptoms of hyperactivity and impulsivity (e.g., disruptive behavior in the classroom, noncompliance, interrupting classroom instruction, leaving seat in the classroom, restlessness when seated) will decrease in frequency and intensity. Performance on measures of vigilance, fine motor coordination, and reaction time improves, and children who respond to stimulants typically demonstrate gains in academic productivity. Despite such gains, there is little evidence that stimulant medication enhances functioning on measures of intelligence and academic ability (Barkley, 2006; Swanson, McBurnett, Christian, & Wigal, 1995).

In social contexts, reduction in aggressive behavior and increased compliance have generally been noted. However, as emphasized by Pelham (2002), there is little evidence that medications alone will effect long-term changes in interpersonal relationships. Such an impression is supported by the findings of the Multimodal Treatment Study of Children With ADHD (MTA) Cooperative Group (1999), which indicated that children with ADHD benefit from the addition of behavioral treatments to their treatment program (e.g., parent counseling, social skills training), particularly when evidence of anxiety, depression, or oppositionalism is present (P. S. Jensen, Hinshaw, Swanson, et al., 2001).

Side Effects

Reviews of the scientific literature indicate that many patients treated with stimulant medications will exhibit at least one type of adverse side effect (Barkley, 2006; Greenhill, 2002). The most common side effects include appetite suppression, weight loss, headaches, abdominal pain, sleep-onset insomnia, sleep discontinuity disturbance, nervousness, and irritability. The frequency rates of each of these side effects range from approximately 5% to 15% when patients are treated with a methylphenidate type of stimulant to 5% to 22% when treated with an amphetamine. Although neuromuscular tics can develop in children treated with stimulants (Law & Schachar, 1999; Palumbo, Spencer, Lynch, Co-Chien, & Faraone, 2004; Shapiro & Shapiro, 1981; Wilens et al., 2005), the results of multiple, controlled, group studies have not indicated increased risk with low-to-moderate doses of stimulant (medication vs. placebo groups). However, it is noteworthy that in studies comparing the rates of tics in medicated versus placebo-treated groups of patients with ADHD, 2% to 20% of participants receiving stimulant therapy developed neuromuscular tics. Overall, it is evident that neuromuscular tics can and do develop in children, and the management of such symptoms is commonly required following treatment with stimulants.

Controversial Side Effects

Cancer. In recent years there has also been concern regarding the toxicology of stimulant medications, particularly the risk of chromosomal aberrations and cancer risk. Although there are no epidemiological data indicating increased risk for cancer in children treated with stimulants, findings reported by El-Zein et al. (2005) and the National Toxicology Program (1995) support caution with respect to the long-term use of stimulant medications as the primary treatment for ADHD.

In the National Toxicology Program (1995) study, one strain of rats and one strain of mice were fed diets containing varying concentrations of methylphenidate for 14 days, 13 weeks, or 2 years. The results of the study revealed no increased risk for carcinogenic activity in either group at 14 days and 13 weeks. However, increased risk for neoplasms in the liver cells of the mice was reported at 2 years. El-Zein et al. (2005) examined the risk for cytogenetic abnormalities in 12 children treated with therapeutic doses of methylphenidate for a 3-month period. They found significant increase in the development of chromosomal aberrations in all participants. Although such reports do not establish a relationship between stimulant use and cancer, these findings support the need for further investigation into the long-term consequences of such aberrations, given the relationship between elevated frequencies of chromosome aberrations and increased cancer risk.

Sudden Death. During the completion of clinical trials for Food and Drug Administration (FDA) approval of the medication Adderall XR, 12 cases of sudden death occurred in children and adolescents (Shire Pharmaceuticals, 2002). Case analysis revealed that 5 of these patients had structural heart defects; 1 patient appeared to die from a toxic overdose; and 5 others either had family histories of tachycardia, had diabetes, or were exposed to rigorous exercise, heat exhaustion, dehydration, or near drowning. The report of death in the final patient was difficult to interpret, as the incident was reported over 3 years later.

Analysis of the data by the FDA indicated that the rate of sudden death was no greater in patients treated with Adderall XR than those treated with methylphenidate. Furthermore, the incidence of sudden death in patients treated with Adderall XR was no greater than in the untreated population. Consequently, the FDA concluded that this type of stimulant could be used in clinical practice. However, the FDA also advised that this type of medication should not be used by individuals with structural defects of the heart. In clinical practice, discussion of the patient's history of cardiac symptoms (e.g., arrhythmias, chest pain) and ongoing monitoring of cardiac functions should be conducted when stimulant medication is being considered.

Treatment of Side Effects

In clinical practice, appetite suppression, insomnia, headaches, gastric pain, irritability, and so-called stimulant rebound (the rapid exacerbation of symptoms of hyperactivity and impulsivity after a time period of adequate symptom control) represent the most common side effects. Barkley (2006) and Monastra (2005b) reported that dietary intervention (ingestion of food with medication) can be helpful for symptoms of gastric pain and headache. Monastra (2005b) observed reduction of insomnia, headaches, gastric pain, irritability, and stimulant rebound when dietary intake of protein at breakfast and lunch met the guidelines set forth in *Recommended Dietary Allowances* (Food and Nutrition Board of the National Academy of Sciences, 1989). Nonstimulant medications (atomoxetine, clonidine, guanfacine) also appear helpful in reducing irritability, insomnia, and rebound effects (Barkley, 2006; Monastra, 2005b; Prince, Wilens, Biederman, Spencer, & Wozniak, 1996). Use of a dietary supplement (melatonin), administered 1 to 2 hours before bedtime, (in time-release or two-stage preparations of doses ranging from 1–3 mg) can also reduce sleep onset insomnia and sleep discontinuity. Both guanfacine and clonidine are effective in the treatment of neuromuscular tics (Connor, Barkley, & Davis, 2000; Prince et al., 1996; Tourette's Syndrome Study Group, 2002).

Antidepressant Medications

Pharmacological agents such as the tricyclic antidepressants (TCAs) imipramine, desipramine, and nortriptyline, as well as buproprion and atomoxetine have been associated with beneficial effects in patients diagnosed with ADHD. In general, the antidepressants imipramine, desipramine, and nortriptyline all target reuptake transporters for the catecholamines NE and DA, presumably increasing the availability of these neurotransmitters at the synaptic cleft. Atomoxetine inhibits the reuptake of NE. Buproprion is a mild inhibitor of the reuptake of DA, NE, and 5-HT. In contrast to stimulants, these medications have a half-life of approximately 12 hours. However, the beneficial effects are not typically noted for 2 to 4 weeks after treatment is initiated.

The effectiveness of these medications in treating the core symptoms of ADHD has been supported in multiple, controlled, group studies (see reviews by Biederman & Spencer, 2002; Spencer, 2006). Response rates are similar to that noted with stimulants, with approximately 65% to 75% of patients exhibiting a significant reduction in core ADHD symptoms following treatment with antidepressant therapy. Dosage levels required to achieve clinical effects vary considerably, based on type of medication.

Atomoxetine

This medication is typically administered in a 25- to 40-milligram dose (children, adolescents, adults), titrating upwards to a target of 1.2 milligrams/kilograms per day but no greater than 100 milligrams per day.

Imipramine

The medication imipramine is initially administered in doses of 10 to 25 milligrams per day, typically titrating to a dose of 30 to 40 milligrams per day for children and adolescents (maximum dose: 100 mg/day).

Desipramine

This medication is likewise initiated at relatively low doses (25–50 mg/day) with daily dosage of 25 to 100 milligrams needed to treat adolescents (maximum 150 mg) and 100 to 200 milligrams (maximum 300 mg) needed to treat symptoms in adults.

Buproprion

The medication buproprion is available in both an IR and an SR preparation for the treatment of adults. The initial dose for the IR is 100 milligrams, b.i.d., with clinical benefits typically noted between 300 and 450 milligrams per day. The SR preparation is initially administered at the 150-milligram dosage level each day (maximum 400 mg).

Clinical Benefits

Similar to outcome studies examining the efficacy of stimulants, each of these medications has been associated with significant improvement on measures of attention and behavioral control. In addition, multiple studies of the effects of TCAs have revealed reduction of symptoms of depression, anxiety, and oppositionalism. Investigations of atomoxetine have revealed reduction in anxiety. Buproprion is recognized as an effective treatment for depression.

Side Effects

Despite the multiple beneficial effects of TCAs, buproprion, and atomoxetine, these medications are generally considered to be second-line treatments for ADHD because of the presence of serious side effects. In addition to dry mouth, nausea, and appetite suppression, the TCAs have been associated with elevated risk for increased heart rate, cardiac arrhythmias, and on rare occasion, cardiac arrest. Buproprion is metabolized in the liver and has been associated with increased risk for liver complications. Buproprion also increases risk for seizures. Atomoxetine has also been associated with increased gastric pain and appetite suppression. Increased irritability and moodiness has also been reported. With all of these medications, daytime sedation can occur.

Treatment of Side Effects

Because of the association between TCAs and cardiac arrhythmias, screening for cardiac conditions (prior to treatment) and monitoring of cardiac functions is advisable. With buproprion, monitoring of liver functions and assessment of history of seizures is necessary. To address daytime sedation associated with atomoxetine and the other nonstimulant medications, late-afternoon or early-evening administration has proven beneficial (Monastra, 2005b).

Antihypertensive Medications

Two antihypertensive medications have demonstrated positive clinical effects in the treatment of ADHD in children: clonidine and guanfacine. Although other antihypertensives (e.g., beta, noradrenergic blockers such as propranolol and pindolol) have yielded positive response on symptoms of aggression and hyperactivity (Biederman & Spencer, 2002; Connor, 2006), side effects (e.g., nightmares, hallucinations, and parasthesias) have precluded their use in clinical practice. The alpha-2 adrenergic receptor agonists (i.e., clonidine and guanfacine) appear to stimulate alpha-2-adrenergic (i.e., NE) receptors in the brain stem (i.e., locus ceruleus) and in the prefrontal cortex, essentially slowing the output from the brain stem to the cortex and enhancing the working memory and behavioral inhibition functions of the brain (Arnsten, Steere, & Hunt, 1996; Cornish, 1988; Halperin, Newcorn, McKay, Siever, & Sharma, 2003).

Clonidine and guanfacine are absorbed into the bloodstream, reaching peak plasma concentrations between 1 and 3 hours after administration. The half-life of these medications ranges from 8 to 14 hours, with duration of clinical effects lasting approximately 3 to 6 hours, hence two to four daily doses may be required. A transdermal patch administration of clonidine is available (lasting 5 days), which reduces the need for multiple daily administrations. As noted by Connor (2006), the standard daily dose range of clonidine for ADHD, Tourette's, and adrenergic overarousal is 0.10 to 0.30 milligram per day. Guanfacine has yielded clinical benefits in doses ranging from 0.75 milligram per day to 6.00 milligrams per day (Connor, 2006; Monastra, 2005b).

Clinical Benefits

Consistent with predictions based on such an understanding of the biochemical mechanisms of action, multiple studies have supported the use of these medications in the treatment of ADHD (see reviews by Biederman & Spencer, 2002; Connor, 2006). A total of eight studies investigating the efficacy of clonidine have been reviewed. Positive effects were noted in six of the eight studies (75%), with improvements noted on measures of hyperactivity, impulsivity, aggression, and frequency of tics. In a similar fashion, four studies have examined the effects of guanfacine. Each of these studies noted positive response, with improvement noted on measures of ADHD (inattention and hyperactivity) in three of the four studies (75%). Reduction in the frequency of tics was noted in the fourth study, despite the lack of improvement in symptoms of ADHD. These medications also appear to reduce excessive worry and ruminative features and improve sleeping patterns (Carskadon, Cavallo, & Rosekind, 1989; Monastra, 2005b).

Side Effects

Like the antidepressant medications, potentially life-threatening side effects can occur with the use of antihypertensives. The first of these is the rebound of adrenergic effects that can occur if guanfacine or clonidine is abruptly withdrawn. This condition is characterized by symptoms of hypertension, agitation, fever, headache, chest pain, sleep disturbance, agitation, nausea, and vomiting. A secondary potentially life-threatening condition can occur in the presence of excessive dosage and/or prolonged usage of these medications. This condition is associated with cardiac arrhythmias, fatigue, lethargy, and hypotension. Other less threatening side effects include drowsiness and sedation (noted in 10%–33% of patients using clonidine and 8%–13% of those treated with guanfacine in controlled studies).

Treatment of Side Effects

Guidelines for the treatment of antihypertensive side effects have been developed by Cantwell, Swanson, and Connor (1997). When side effects caused by adrenergic rebound are identified, treatment typically consists of the gradual reintroduction of clonidine. When the adverse effects are due to excessive medication dose, withdrawal from the antihypertensive is advised. To reduce risk of hypotension during the withdrawal process, reduction by .05 milligrams of clonidine every 3 days (or 1.00 mg of guanfacine every 3 days) has been recommended (Connor, 2006).

Anticonvulsants

Among the various anticonvulsant medications considered potentially useful in the treatment of ADHD (e.g., carbamazepine, valproic acid, gabapentin), the use of carbamazepine (Tegretol) has been supported by the findings of multiple studies (see reviews by Connor, 2006; R. R. Silva, Munoz, & Alpert, 1996). Carbamazepine is available as a suspension and tablet. Although the anticonvulsant effects of this medication appear to be mediated by partial agonistic effects on adenosine receptors (inhibiting seizures emanating from the amygdala), the mechanisms of action in ADHD are unknown. It is hypothesized that the reduction of ADHD symptoms may be achieved by suppressing central nervous system activation via facilitation of the action of the neurotransmitter gamma-amino-butyric acid, thereby inhibiting the neurotransmission of excitatory amino acids (by blocking N-methyl-D-aspartate–2A receptors), and/or by influencing calcium channels and transport of sodium and other ions (Connor, 2006).

Once administered, plasma levels of carbamazepine peak within 1 hour (suspension) and within 4 to 5 hours after ingestion of the oral tablet. However, because carbamazepine is metabolized into several active agents in the liver, the half-life is variable, averaging 12 hours. The transformation of carbamazepine into the active metabolites occurs more quickly in prepubertal children than adolescents and teens, hence, serum levels must be monitored and dose adjusted during the first few months of treatment.

Positive response to carbamazepine has been reported to be 70% in open clinical trials and 71% in controlled studies (R. R. Silva et al., 1996). Doses required for effective treatment ranged from 50 to 800 milligrams per day. Carbamazepine is typically introduced at 50 milligrams, b.i.d., and increased by 100 milligrams on a weekly basis until a dosage of 10 to 30 milligrams/kilograms per day is attained. Serum monitoring is considered to be essential, with doses ranging from 4 to 12 micrograms per milliliter considered therapeutic for epilepsy. No optimal blood level ranges are currently available for ADHD.

Clinical Benefits

In clinical practice, carbamazepine is primarily administered for the treatment of hyperactivity and aggressive behavior, particularly when such symptoms are nonresponsive to stimulants and antihypertensives. As reviewed by Connor (2006) and R. R. Silva et al. (1996), there are both open and controlled group studies that indicate carbamazepine can reduce symptoms of aggression, impulsivity, hyperactivity, and restlessness in children and adolescents. There is little evidence that significant improvement of attention or cognitive functions occurs. However, no systematic studies examining such effects have been published, to date.

Side Effects

Multiple neurological, gastrointestinal, dermatological, and hematological side effects are reported in patients being treated with carbamazepine, particularly at serum levels above 9 micrograms/milliliter. Approximately 50% of patients will report dizziness and headaches, with drowsiness, blurred vision, and fatigue noted in 25%. Nausea, vomiting, and gastric pain are reported by approximately 25% of patients. Rashes occur in nearly 50% of patients and reduction in levels of white blood cells can occur in half of those treated. Increased hyperactivity, aggression, and impulsivity have also been reported in children and adolescents treated with carbamazepine (Pleak, Birmaher, Gavrilescu, Abichandani, & Williams, 1988).

Treatment of Side Effects

Efforts to minimize side effects typically proceed from a gradual introduction of a low dose of carbamazepine, with monitoring of serum levels of medication and monitoring of liver functions to guard against toxicity. When rash or hematological symptoms are noted, medication should be withdrawn slowly.

Potentially Beneficial Combinations of Medications

Although a variety of other medications are used in clinical practice, at present there is insufficient evidence to support the use of selective serotonin reuptake inhibitor (SSRI)–type antidepressants (e.g., fluoxetine, sertraline, paroxetine), antipsychotics (e.g., clozapine, risperidone, olanzapine, sertindole), or benzodiazepines (chlordiazepoxide or diazepam) as primary treatments for ADHD. As reviewed by Connor (2006), there are a few studies examining the combined effects of stimulants and other pharmacological agents. To date, combinations of stimulants and TCAs, noradrenalin-specific reuptake inhibitors, SSRIs, and antihypertensives have shown beneficial effects in a limited number of studies.

Rapport, Carlson, Kelly, and Pataki (1993) noted that a combination of methylphenidate and desipramine yielded improved performance on certain learning tasks. Gammon and Brown (1993) reported that a combination of methylphenidate and fluoxetine yielded enhanced therapeutic effects in children and adolescents with ADHD and comorbid depression. Brown (2004) noted improved response to a combination of methylphenidate and atomoxetine in four patients who were unresponsive to stimulant alone. Hazell and Stuart (2003) and Hunt, Capper, and O'Connell (1990) noted improved control over aggressive behaviors in children treated for ADHD and comorbid outbursts of temper, when clonidine was administered in combination with a psychostimulant. Despite the promising results of these initial studies, more research is clearly required to assure the safety of patients when response to monotherapy is insufficient and medication combinations are considered.

THE SELECTION OF MEDICATION TYPE
AND DOSE IN CLINICAL PRACTICE

Because of the robust effects of stimulant medications on the core symptoms of ADHD in the majority of patients treated, methylphenidate, dextromethylphenidate, mixed amphetamine salts, and dextroamphetamine are considered first-line treatments for ADHD. Therefore, following a comprehensive assessment, a clinical trial of one of these medications would be considered to be consistent with current practice guidelines (American Academy of Child & Adolescent Psychiatry, 1997; American Academy of Pediatrics, 2000). An assessment of pretreatment levels of attention and functioning across multiple domains (e.g., core ADHD symptoms; behavioral symptoms requiring treatment through systematic environmental modification; skills deficits in academic, social, or athletic abilities, which required specialized remediation) is recommended to monitor medication effects and guide treatment planning (American Academy of Child and Adolescent Psychiatry, 1997), as there is no type of medication that effectively treats symptoms across all areas of functional impairment.

As reviewed in chapter 4, pre- and posttreatment assessment routinely involves input from multiple informants (e.g., parents, teachers, employers, counselors, and the patient). Clinical interview and behavioral rating scales are useful in clarifying symptoms and frequency of occurrence. Other types of assessment procedures (e.g., intelligence tests, tests of academic achievement, neuropsychological tests of attention, behavioral inhibition, and other executive functions) are considered helpful in evaluating specific areas of functional impairment requiring additional intervention. The application of more recently developed qEEG-based assessment techniques has not yet been widely

EXHIBIT 6.1
Medication Evaluation Form: School Rating Version

Student: _____ **Grade:** _____

Rater: _____ **Date of Rating:** _____

Relationship With Patient (circle one):
  Teacher   Therapist   Aide   **Hours/Day:** _____

This student has been evaluated by me and diagnosed with attention-deficit/hyperactivity disorder (ADHD). One aspect of this student's care consists of medication to treat the core symptoms of this disorder. At present, this student is being treated with

_____.

Because medications for ADHD can cause a variety of beneficial and adverse effects, your observations can be quite helpful in determining an effective type and dose of medication. Please complete this form and fax it to me at _____ or mail it to me at _____

_____

Thank you for your help!

1. Has there been any improvement in this student's attention, ability to listen, follow directions, or complete seat work?
2. Is this student's ability to attend, concentrate, and complete seatwork consistent with expectations for his or her grade? If not, please specify areas of concern.
3. Has there been any improvement in this student's ability to remain seated, not interrupt or intrude on others, and follow class rules?
4. Is the student able to demonstrate age-appropriate levels of behavioral control in the classroom during specials, at lunch, and during transitions? If not, please specify areas of concern.
5. When does this student appear to have the most difficulty attending and/or maintaining behavioral control? Does the problem seem related to a particular subject or task?
6. Side effects: Have you observed any increase in sedation, irritability, moodiness, restlessness, or loss of attention? If so, when is this occurring?

Note. Copyright 2007 by Vincent J. Monastra.

recognized. However, the application of such techniques in the assessment process has yielded beneficial effects in several applied clinical studies and is reviewed later in this chapter.

Titration of dosage is typically accomplished by initiating a low dose of stimulant and monitoring response and side effects through daily or weekly reports from multiple informants. Dosage is subsequently adjusted or type of treatment is changed on the basis of behavioral report. An alternative strategy (used in the 1999 MTA study) consists of a systematic trial of several different doses with ratings of efficacy and side effects. In this approach, dosages are randomly administered (in either open or single-blind trials), to determine the optimal dose. The Medication Evaluation Forms that can be used by parents, guardians, patients, and teachers to monitor medication effects are shown in Exhibits 6.1 and 6.2.

As is emphasized in current practice guidelines, it is important to recognize that a medication that is effective during the daytime hours may not be effective in the late afternoon and evening. Because it is important that

EXHIBIT 6.2
Medication Evaluation Form: Home Rating Version

Patient: _____ **Date of Rating:** _____
Rater: _____
Relationship With Patient (circle one):
  Self   Parent/Guardian   Spouse   Friend

Medications for ADHD can provide a number of beneficial effects. However, to be most helpful, medications need to be taken as prescribed. In addition, sleep and dietary habits can also help medications yield optimal results. To help determine an effective dose of medication and minimize side effects, your observations are quite important. Please take a few minutes and complete this form prior to your consultation. You can fax the form to me at
_____ or mail it to _____
_____

Current Medication: **Dose**_____ **Time(s) taken:** _____
Current Medication: **Dose**_____ **Time(s) taken:** _____
Current Medication: **Dose**_____ **Time(s) taken:** _____

1. Has the patient taken each medication prescribed for ADHD every day?
   Yes _____ No _____
   If no, how many days was medication not taken as prescribed? _____
2. Has there been an improvement in the patient's ability to pay attention and concentrate while completing reading and writing tasks? Yes _____ No _____
   Describe: _____
3. Has there been an improvement in the patient's ability to listen and follow directions? Yes _____ No _____
   Describe: _____
4. Has there been a reduction in the patient's activity level or sense of restlessness? Yes _____ No _____
   Describe: _____
5. Has the patient been more able to organize time and complete chores, homework, or other responsibilities? Yes _____ No _____
   Describe: _____
6. Has there been any type of improvement in mood or temper? Yes _____ No _____
   Describe: _____
7. Has there been any increase in sedation, loss of appetite, sleep problems, frequency of headaches, or other unpleasant side effect? Yes _____ No _____
   Describe: _____
8. How many days per week is the patient eating protein at breakfast and lunch? _____
   Describe typical breakfast: _____ Lunch: _____
9. How many hours of sleep is the patient attaining each night? _____
   Describe any sleep problems: _____
10. How many minutes of exercise is the patient engaged in each day? _____
   Describe physical activities: _____

Note. Copyright 2007 by Vincent J. Monastra.

the patient experience success not only at school but also in their family and social relationships, effective pharmacological treatment often requires multiple doses per day or a combination of medications, even when SR stimulants are prescribed. The need for such combinations is illustrated in a study of 658 patients diagnosed with ADHD and treated at our clinic (Monastra, 2005b).

In this study, medications were monitored for a 2-year period following initial diagnosis. Approximately 33% of our patients required treatment with both stimulant and nonstimulant medications (e.g., atomoxetine, clonidine, guanfacine) to address problems of attention, behavioral disinhibition, and emotional control (e.g., temper, anxiety, depressed mood). It is noteworthy that none of the patients treated in this study were effectively treated by using a single dose of any one type of medication for the duration of the 2-year period. Approximately 25% of our patients also required melatonin supplements (1–3 mg, administered 1.5–2.0 hours before bedtime) or were treated with an antihypertensive medication to address sleep onset insomnia or discontinuity.

In conducting our study, we found that it was common for patients to experience a declining medication effect in the late afternoon, even when treated with an SR type of stimulant (e.g., Concerta, Focalin-XR, Adderall XR). Such patients had difficulty concentrating while completing homework and exhibited impaired focus while participating in team sports, gymnastics, drama, dance, and other recreational activities. Because of diminished clinical benefits, the majority of our patients required treatment with a low dose of methylphenidate (i.e., Methylin, Ritalin, or Focalin) administered after school. When Adderall XR was prescribed for a child, we found it useful to have the child treated with a booster pill of Adderall prior to dismissal from school. Otherwise, it was difficult for the child to sustain attention during the late afternoon. Adolescents and adults treated with Adderall XR were able to tolerate a late afternoon dose of Adderall without significant adverse effect on sleep onset.

NEUROPSYCHOLOGICAL TESTS AND QUANTITATIVE ELECTROENCEPHALOGRAPHY IN MEDICATION SELECTION AND MONITORING

Although not yet routinely used in the determination of type and dose of medication, there is mounting evidence that certain neuropsychological and neurophysiological procedures may be helpful in the assessment process. Among the neuropsychological procedures that have been investigated, various forms of continuous performance tests (CPT; e.g., Greenberg, 1994: Test of Variables of Attention; Sanford, 1994: Intermediate Variables of Attention; Conners' Continuous Performance Test; Gordon, 1983: Gordon Diagnostic System) have been used in at least 45 randomized, placebo-controlled studies of the effects of stimulant medications (see review by Riccio, Waldrop, Reynolds, & Lowe, 2001), including the MTA (Epstein et al., 2006). Significant improvements on measures of alertness (i.e., target identification), impulse control (i.e., response inhibition to nontargets), processing speed (i.e., response rate), and vigilance (i.e., consistency of decision-making speed) are consistently reported following administration of psychostimulant medications and other stimulants (including nicotine and caffeine).

Furthermore, there is emerging evidence that qEEG examination can provide data that are useful in predicting medication response. Initially, researchers studied qEEG differences between stimulant responders and nonresponders (see reviews by Chabot et al., 2005; Loo, 2003; Monastra, 2005b). The predominant qEEG finding was that electrophysiological indicators of cortical hypoarousal were commonly found over frontal and central midline regions in the qEEGs of stimulant responders (e.g., elevated amplitude of slow-wave activity, reduced fast EEG activity, elevated theta and beta power ratios; Chabot, Orgill, Crawford, Harris, & Serfontein, 1999; Clarke, Barry, McCarthy, & Selikowitz, 2001a, 2001b; Clarke, Barry, McCarthy, Selikowitz, & Croft, 2002; Satterfield, Schell, Backs, & Hidaka, 1984). Nonresponders tend to exhibit cortical hyperarousal or no evidence of cortical slowing on qEEG examination (Chabot et al., 1999; Clarke et al., 2001a, 2001b).

Investigations of the effects of stimulants on qEEG measures have revealed that reduction of such electrophysiological hypoarousal is a commonly observed effect of both methylphenidate and amphetamines (Bresnahan, Barry, Clarke, & Johnstone, 2006; Clarke, Barry, Bond, McCarthy, & Selikowitz, 2002; Clarke et al., 2003; Loo, Hopfer, Teale, & Reite, 2004; Loo, Teale, & Reite, 1999; J. F. Lubar, White, Swartwood, & Swartwood, 1999; Monastra, 2005b; Monastra, Monastra, & George, 2002; Song, Shin, Jon, & Ha, 2005; Swartwood et al., 1998). The primary findings of these studies indicated that both methylphenidate and amphetamines increase beta activity and reduce evidence of slow-wave activity, particularly over frontal brain regions.

The clinical application of such findings has been explored in several studies (Clarke, Barry, Bond, et al., 2002; Hermens, Williams, et al., 2005; Monastra, 2005b; Monastra et al., 2002). In each project, titration of dose was adjusted until normalization of the qEEG was attained. As anticipated, such normalization of neurophysiological indicators of cortical dysregulation was associated with robust clinical response, particularly when patients were examined during task-related brain activity (Hermens, Williams, et al., 2005; Monastra et al., 2002).

In the Monastra et al. (2002) study, 100 patients diagnosed with ADHD were treated with methylphenidate. Each of these patients had displayed frontal, cortical hypoarousal on qEEG examination during task-related activities (e.g., reading, writing, listening). Normalization of the qEEG indicators of cortical hypoarousal was achieved in all of the patients, with significant clinical improvement reported by parents and teachers, and reflected in improved scores on neuropsychological tests of attention. Please refer to Table 6.1 for a listing of critical values for the qEEG examination used in the Monastra et

TABLE 6.1
Critical Values for ADHD on the Basis of Power Ratio

Age (years)	M	1.0 SD	1.5 SD	2.0 SD
6–11	3.03	4.36	5.03	5.69
12–15	2.06	2.89	3.31	3.72
16–20	2.00	2.24	2.36	2.48
21–30	1.50	1.92	2.13	2.34

Note. Data From Monastra, Lubar, and Linden (2001). Ratios compare electrophysiological power recorded at frequencies ranging from 4 to 8 hertz versus 13 to 21 hertz at the vertex. ADHD = attention-deficit/hyperactivity disorder; M = mean; SD = standard deviation.

al. (2002) study. Medications were titrated until the power ratio was within 1.0 standard deviation of the mean for age peers.

In a similar manner, Hermens, Williams, et al. (2005) examined 34 unmedicated adolescents diagnosed with ADHD and 34 age- and sex-matched control participants. Following treatment with methylphenidate, significant reduction in theta activity (across fronto-central sites) and normalization of cortical activation in this region was attained (using database comparisons drawn from their extensive research samples of healthy age peers). These researchers also reported increase in the amplitude of the P300 component during examination of event-related potentials, a finding also noted by Seifert, Scheurpflug, Zillessen, Fallgatter, and Warnke (2003).

Two additional clinical studies examining medication selection and qEEG indicators are also noteworthy. Hermens, Cooper, Kohn, Clarke, and Gordon (2005) recently used a combination of neuropsychological and qEEG measures and were able to correctly classify 85% of stimulant responders and 95% of nonresponders in their study of 40 patients with ADHD. Monastra (2005b) used a qEEG screening to determine the presence of cortical hypoarousal in 658 patients diagnosed with ADHD. Monastra (2005b) hypothesized that by prescribing stimulant medications to patients with ADHD who exhibited cortical hypoarousal and nonstimulants (e.g., antihypertensives, atomoxetine) to those exhibiting cortical hyperarousal or no cortical slowing, improved medication response and compliance rates would be noted. Consistent with this hypothesis, Monastra (2005b) reported that this type of matching of patient to medication type on the basis of qEEG data resulted in a medication compliance rate of 95% for a 2-year period.

Such treatment maintenance rates far exceed the national rates of 25% to 50% reported by P. S. Jensen (2000) and the 66% reported by the MTA Cooperative Group (1999). These findings are even more noteworthy when Jensen's report and that of the MTA Cooperative Group are examined more closely. Jensen estimated that among the children who were pharmacologically treated for ADHD, only four to eight prescriptions were written per year for each child. The MTA Cooperative Group reported that among the

66% of patients who used medications in their study, 8 months represented the average number of months in which medications were used.

Several factors appear to contribute greatly to this lack of treatment compliance. As noted previously, in a study of 856 families who had either refused to initiate medication or discontinued medication use in their child within 6 months (Monastra, 2005b), fear of medication side effects and discomfort with the use of medication without direct assessment of attentional abilities were cited as primary reasons for refusal in over 90% of families. As described in chapter 4, we use both CPT and qEEG measures in our assessment of medication effects to address such concerns. In addition to behavioral indicators of improvement, we monitor CPT and qEEG measures, adjusting dose until performance on both measures is within 1.5 standard deviations of age peers. Our goal is to essentially normalize the underlying pathophysiology of ADHD. Once that step is achieved, we can proceed to an analysis of areas of residual functional impairment.

Consequently, in clinical practice the use of CPTs and qEEG appears to have several benefits. First, the inclusion of objective measures appears to reduce patient and parental fears of medication side effects, increases the likelihood of compliance with treatment, and provides an unbiased measure of medication response. Second, because qEEG measures differentiate potential stimulant responders and nonresponders, neurophysiological measures have been able to improve the response rate to pharmacological treatments, further improving medication compliance rates. Third, because clinically effective dosages of medication are reflected in improvement (normalization) on both types of measures, these tests can be used to help determine optimal dose. Although Barkley (2006) correctly noted that none of the qEEG measures can be considered diagnostic for ADHD, given the multiple benefits of CPTs and qEEGs in clinical practice, inclusion of such procedures appears to be in the best interest of patients at this time, as was recently recognized by the American Neuropsychiatric Association (Coburn et al., 2006).

7

CONDUCTING THE FUNCTIONAL ASSESSMENT OF PATIENTS WITH ADHD

As emphasized in the practice guidelines published by the American Academy of Child & Adolescent Psychiatry (AACAP; 1997) and the American Academy of Pediatrics (AAP; 2000), pharmacological treatments for attention-deficit/hyperactivity disorder (ADHD) commonly constitute the initial stage of the treatment process. However, as stressed by AACAP and AAP, this is only one of many facets of the multimodal treatment for ADHD. As noted by these professional societies, multiple types of functional impairment are likely to persist, despite initiation of effective pharmacological treatment. On the basis of such a perspective, the AACAP proposed that

> one way to conceptualize treatment planning is to consider core symptoms of inattention, impulsivity, and hyperactivity, which are likely to require and respond to medication; behavioral symptoms to be addressed by environmental modification; and skill deficits in academic, social, or sports domains, which require specific remediation and do not respond to either medication or behavior modification. (p. 87)

In this chapter, procedures for conducting a functional assessment of patients diagnosed with ADHD is reviewed. As noted in chapter 1, patients diagnosed with ADHD can exhibit impairments of the following skills: alerting, concentration, behavioral inhibition, affective control, socialization, memory, language processing, word retrieval, and motor coordination. Most outpatient clinical settings (e.g., individual or group practices, public or private psychiatric clinics) can conduct assessments of alerting, concentration, behavioral inhibition, affective control, memory, and socialization (e.g., at home, school, community). Assessment of language processing, word retrieval, and motor coordination is commonly conducted by speech–language therapists and physical or occupational therapists but can be conducted by a neuropsychologist as well.

CONDUCTING THE FUNCTIONAL ASSESSMENT

When the core symptoms of ADHD have been treated, evaluation of the residual areas of functional impairment can be initiated. Interviews with the patient, parents, teachers, employer, and coworkers can be useful in developing an accurate perspective of the patient's current level of functioning. Questionnaires, such as the Life Skills Questionnaires (LSQ; Monastra, 2005c; see also Exhibits 7.1 and 7.2, this volume) and the Functional Assessment Checklist for Teachers (FACT; Monastra, 2005c; see also Exhibit 7.3, this volume) can be helpful as well. When impairments of working memory, language processing, and motor coordination persist, neuropsychological testing can provide a quantitative appraisal of the degree of impairment and help guide the treatment process. As reviewed in the practice guidelines published by AACAP (1997), the types of functional problems that are commonly noted include affective control, socialization, memory, language processing, word retrieval, and motor coordination.

Affective Control

As noted in chapter 1, impaired anger control, depressed mood, and anxiety are common in patients with ADHD. Although the severity of such symptoms is often reduced by effective treatment for the core symptoms of ADHD, evidence of impaired affective control is often reflected in the medication evaluation forms completed by teacher, parents, and patients. To determine the degree of variance from age expectations, the administration of a multidimensional measure of psychopathology, such as the Child Behavior Checklist (Achenbach & Edelbrock, 1983) or the Minnesota Multiphasic Personality Inventory—II or IIA (Hathaway & McKinley, 2001), may prove useful. Such questionnaires help to clarify whether the patient symptoms are

EXHIBIT 7.1
Life Skills Questionnaire: Child–Adolescent Form

Patient: _____ **Parent/Guardian:** _____ **Date:** _____

Although medications, electroencephalograph (EEG) biofeedback, and other types of treatment for attention-deficit/hyperactivity disorder (ADHD) can help reduce symptoms of inattention, impulsivity, and hyperactivity, it is likely that your child will continue to have certain kinds of problems in his or her daily life despite such treatments. To help identify those skills that you would like to teach your child, I would like you to complete the following checklist. Simply mark the goals that you have for your child. We will review this list together and begin to develop strategies that you can use to teach your child these important life skills.

****

I'd like my child to
1. _____ wake up in the morning without battling with me.
2. _____ get dressed in clean clothes in the morning.
3. _____ eat breakfast that includes some kind of protein (e.g., eggs, meat, cheese, yogurt).
4. _____ take his or her medication.
5. _____ brush his or her teeth, wash up, comb hair.
6. _____ make his or her bed, pick up room.
7. _____ pack his or her school bag with books, homework, and so on.
8. _____ not argue with me or his or her brothers and/or sisters in the morning.
9. _____ get to the school bus on time.
10. _____ get to his or her classes on time.
11. _____ remember to bring the necessary books and materials to class.
12. _____ remember to turn in homework.
13. _____ sit in his or her seat at school.
14. _____ do his or her schoolwork in class.
15. _____ speak when called on in class.
16. _____ not interrupt the teacher or other students.
17. _____ eat a lunch that contains some kind of protein.
18. _____ copy down his or her homework assignments.
19. _____ remember to bring home the books and materials he or she needs for homework.
20. _____ learn how to have conversations with other kids.
21. _____ learn how to play and solve disagreements without getting into fights.
22. _____ come home after school.
23. _____ do his or her homework without a battle.
24. _____ organize books and school materials so that his or her work doesn't get lost.
25. _____ listen and obey parental instructions.
26. _____ come home for dinner.
27. _____ eat a dinner that includes protein, fruit, and vegetables.
28. _____ do his or her chores with minimal prompting.
29. _____ play cooperatively with siblings and neighborhood kids.
30. _____ put away his or her toys, papers, clothes, and so on.
31. _____ make his or her bed, clean his or her room.
32. _____ not argue with parents.
33. _____ learn to solve problems by negotiating.
34. _____ spend some time reading, painting, building, practicing word processing skills, or engaging in any activity that requires thinking.
35. _____ express his or her ideas or feelings without using obscene or vulgar language.
36. _____ wash up, brush teeth in the evening.

(continues)

EXHIBIT 7.1
(Continued)

37. _____ go to his or her bedroom at bedtime and rest quietly.
38. _____ stay in his or her bedroom and let me sleep until morning.
39. _____ apologize, accept responsibility for mistakes, and make an effort to make up.
40. _____ do something kind or thoughtful for another person.

Other lessons? _____

_____

_____

Note. From *Parenting Children With ADHD: 10 Lessons That Medicine Cannot Teach* (pp. 42–43), by V. J. Monastra, 2005, Washington, DC: American Psychological Association. Copyright 2005 by Vincent J. Monastra. Reprinted with permission of the author.

situation specific or are more representative of a comorbid mood, anxiety, or anger control disorder.

Instances in which the expression of affective symptoms is situation specific are common in patients diagnosed with ADHD. It is not unusual for a child or adult to exhibit symptoms of impaired anger control or to make comments suggestive of depression (e.g., "I wish I was dead") when goals are frustrated (e.g., "Mom won't let me play on the computer"; "Dad told me I had to clean my room before I could play my video games") or when facing frustrating or threatening social contexts (e.g., being teased or bullied by another student). Other contexts that could drive such behaviors and statements include tasks that require sustained concentration (e.g., homework) or time of day (e.g., evening, when medication effects are declining). The medication evaluation form is often helpful in identifying such patterns.

When affective control problems are related to situation-specific factors, clinical intervention may consist of instruction in self-calming, problem-solving, conflict resolution, or other social skills, in either group or individual counseling sessions. As reported by Beelmann, Pfingsten, and Losel (1994); Frankel, Myatt, and Cantwell (1995); and Pelham and Hoza (1996) and reviewed by Barkley (2006), such systematic instruction, combined with reinforced practice, has yielded mild to moderate gains on measures of assertion and emotional control, as well as reduction in aggression in children diagnosed with ADHD. Although the long-term benefit of such training has yet to be demonstrated, the studies conducted to date support the position that patients with ADHD can be taught specific mood, anxiety, and anger control skills, with at least short-term benefits in the reduction of emotional distress.

If there is evidence that the affective symptoms are not situation specific and persist for extended periods (i.e., hours, days, or weeks, compared with the 5 to 30 minutes commonly noted when symptoms are situation specific), pharmacological treatment for the combination of ADHD and affective disorder will be initiated. Because of the evidence that stimulants can be combined effectively with TCAs and antihypertensives (Prince, Wilens, Spencer, & Biederman, 2006; Wilens, Spencer, & Biederman, 2002), con-

EXHIBIT 7.2
Life Skills Questionnaire: Adult Form

Patient: _____ **Date:** _____

When you first sought help for attention-deficit/hyperactivity disorder (ADHD), you described a number of life problems that were occurring because of problems of inattention, poor concentration, or impulsivity. Since your initial evaluation, you have hopefully begun to feel and function better. It is common for patients to begin to experience improvement after the initiation of treatment for ADHD and the establishment of healthy dietary, sleeping, and exercise habits.

Despite such improvements, it is likely that you are continuing to experience certain problems in your daily life. This is not unusual. Although medications can help improve attention and concentration and reduce restlessness and impulsive decision making, they cannot teach skills. Adjustments in medication may provide additional benefits; however, it is likely that you will need to learn new skills to overcome these problems. To help me better understand the kinds of problems that you are still experiencing, I would like you to complete the following questionnaire.

****

I would like to be able to

1. _____ wake when my alarm goes off.
2. _____ get out of bed so that I have enough time to eat a breakfast that contains protein.
3. _____ organize my clothes so that I can find an appropriate outfit for the morning.
4. _____ eat a balanced breakfast that includes protein, carbohydrates, and fruits.
5. _____ establish a routine so that my children are dressed, fed, and out the door on time.
6. _____ exercise in the morning.
7. _____ wash the morning dishes.
8. _____ make bed(s), pick up strewn clothes, toys, and so on.
9. _____ arrive at work on time.
10. _____ prioritize and schedule work tasks (at home or in a place of employment).
11. _____ remember work assignments.
12. _____ remember meeting times and deadlines.
13. _____ remember how to perform tasks.
14. _____ complete work tasks when due.
15. _____ organize my paperwork.
16. _____ remain current on e-mail correspondence.
17. _____ listen and remember conversations.
18. _____ express my opinions during conversations.
19. _____ think of topics to talk about during social conversations with others.
20. _____ make eye contact during conversations.
21. _____ not feel so worried or stressed.
22. _____ not become so angry.
23. _____ not get so discouraged.
24. _____ take time to eat a healthy lunch that contains protein, carbohydrates, fruits, and vegetables.
25. _____ exercise at some point in my day.
26. _____ sort the mail each day—discarding nonessential paper and filing essential bills and correspondence.
27. _____ keep my house clean and clear of clutter.
28. _____ remember to pay my bills on time.
29. _____ do something each day that I enjoy.
30. _____ plan and engage in an enjoyable activity with friends or family each week.
31. _____ fall asleep within 30 minutes and sleep through the night.

(continues)

EXHIBIT 7.2
(Continued)

32. _____ obtain at least 7 to 8 hours of sleep each night.

Other goals? _____

_____

_____

sideration of TCAs with a stimulant may prove helpful when depression occurs comorbidly with ADHD and antihypertensives seem useful with ADHD and comorbid anxiety and anger control problems. Buproprion and desipramine have also seemed helpful in our clinical work in adults presenting with ADHD and comorbid depression. These pharmacological treatments are combined with efforts to instruct the patient in techniques for affective regulation, problem-solving, conflict resolution, and other essential life skills (Rostain & Ramsay, 2006; Safren et al., 2005).

Socialization

Social skills deficits are commonly reported in patients diagnosed with ADHD (see reviews by Barkley, 2006; Pelham, 2002). The types of deficits include difficulty maintaining eye contact during conversation, difficulty remaining on topic when speaking with others, difficulty recognizing the interest level of the audience and adjusting the topic of conversation accordingly, difficulty expressing needs and resolving frustration in nonaggressive ways, impaired emotional control, avoidance of novel situations, and impaired ability to respond to teasing. A variety of self-care (e.g., hygiene, diet, sleep) and organizational problems (e.g., procrastination, forgetfulness, losing possessions and important papers) are also included among the social skills deficits demonstrated by patients with ADHD.

The assessment of such deficits proceeds from targeted questionnaires (e.g., LSQ) as well as more comprehensive, norm-related instruments (e.g., Social Skills Rating System; Gresham & Elliott, 1990), which can be completed by patients, parents, and teachers. As with the evaluation of affective problems, the goal of this type of assessment is to identify those skill deficits requiring instruction and remediation.

Both intensive summer camp experiences (Pelham, 2002) and community-based life skills programs (Monastra, 2007) have been developed, and the results of long-term follow-up studies have supported the position that children and adolescents can be taught a wide range of social skills, including anger control, cooperation, nonaggressive problem-solving, and self-calming skills (Arnold et al., 2004; P. S. Jensen, Hinshaw, Swanson, et al., 2001; Multimodal Treatment Study of Children With ADHD Cooperative Group, 2004). Although the results of these follow-up studies have indi-

EXHIBIT 7.3
The Functional Assessment Checklist for Teachers (FACT)

Student's Name: _____

Teacher's Name: _____

Date of Rating: _____

Dear _____

As you are aware, children with attention-deficit/hyperactivity (ADHD) have a health impairment that can adversely affect their ability to function effectively at school. To develop comprehensive intervention programs that can promote the success of these children, functional assessment of the child's behavior at school is essential. Your assistance in this process would be greatly appreciated.

The following statements relate to specific functional areas that are commonly affected by ADHD. Please read each statement and assign a numerical rating from 1 to 5 or an *N* per the following scale:

     1. Far worse than peers
     2. Slightly worse than peers
     3. About the same as peers
     4. Slightly better than peers
     5. Much better than peers
     N. Not expected at this age

ORGANIZATION
_____ arrives to class on time
_____ has necessary materials (textbook, paper, etc.)
_____ brings homework assignments to class
_____ records homework assignments in planner or agenda
_____ brings home the materials necessary to complete homework

CLASSROOM FUNCTIONING
_____ sits in seat, does not disrupt class with extraneous movements or verbalization
_____ follows written directions
_____ follows verbal directions
_____ accurately copies notes from chalkboard and overheads
_____ completes seat work during the allowed time
_____ takes accurate notes from lectures or instructional presentations
_____ participates appropriately in class discussion (does not interrupt; stays on topic)

SOCIAL SKILLS
_____ maintains eye contact while speaking
_____ maintains eye contact while listening
_____ engages in social conversations with peers
_____ is able to maintain a conversation that is of interest to the other person
_____ is invited by peers to join social activities
_____ is involved in school-based extracurricular activities (e.g., sports, music, drama)

AFFECTIVE CONTROL
_____ tolerates frustration
_____ is verbally aggressive with peers
_____ is verbally aggressive with staff
_____ complies with rules
_____ is physically aggressive with peers
_____ is physically aggressive with staff
_____ seems anxious or worried
_____ seems sad or depressed
_____ is irritable or angry

(continues)

EXHIBIT 7.3
(Continued)

ACADEMIC SKILLS

Reading
_____ reading speed and accuracy
_____ ability to comprehend the content of passages
_____ ability to reach conclusions based on inference
_____ ability to prepare outlines or study guides based on reading of textbook

Mathematics
_____ knowledge of number facts (addition, subtraction)
_____ knowledge of multiplication facts
_____ computational accuracy
_____ ability to understand word problems and calculate the correct answer

Written Expression
_____ writing speed
_____ writing legibility
_____ spelling skills
_____ ability to write answers requiring a single sentence
_____ ability to write short essays (1–3 paragraphs)
_____ ability to write compositions (3+ paragraphs)

Note. From *Parenting Children With ADHD: 10 Lessons That Medicine Cannot Teach* (pp. 116–118), by V. J. Monastra, 2005, Washington, DC: American Psychological Association. Copyright 2005 by Vincent J. Monastra. Reprinted with permission of the author.

cated that provision of social skills training does not enhance the beneficial effects of carefully titrated pharmacological treatment on core ADHD symptoms, additional benefits on a variety of social measures have been shown to persist for at least 24 months.

Despite these encouraging findings, it is important to recognize that teaching social skills to children, teens, and adults is a highly complex undertaking that can be impeded by the patient's inability to maintain instructional set, impaired retention of information, residual impairment in working memory and word fluency, insufficient practice, and lack of reinforcement for efforts to practice skills. At this time, although there is considerable support for the concepts of "social skills" or "life skills" training (e.g., AACAP, 1997; AAP, 2000), it is clear that the development of viable skill development programs that can be administered in school and outpatient clinical settings are in the preliminary stages of development. A description of the model program that was developed at our clinic is provided in chapter 11 (this volume), as a guide for clinicians seeking to begin investigating the effectiveness of such training programs in their practices.

Memory

As noted in previous chapters of this book, patients diagnosed with ADHD can demonstrate a wide range of deficiencies in memory. They may struggle to recall digits, syllables, words, sentences, and paragraphs after presentation. They are likely to forget important dates and lose track of possessions. In clinical practice, attempts to survey such deficits commonly consist of questionnaires such as the LSQ. However, when there is evidence of multiple impairments of memory, administration of tests that target specific functional deficits can be useful in guiding the development of accommodation plans at school or work settings. In clinical settings, tests of letter, number, word, sentence, and paragraph recall can be helpful in securing accommodations such as calculators or multiplication tables, note takers during class lectures, provision of desktop copies of notes, provision of written summaries of business meetings, and written copies of the nursing report in hospital settings. A summary of such procedures is provided in the reviews by Lezak (1976) and Reitan and Wolfson (1985).

Remediation of those memory deficits that are not responsive to pharmacological treatment has included efforts to coach individuals in retention strategies (e.g., Ratey, 2002) and computerized training systems such as Captain's Log (Sanford & Browne, 1988) and electroencephalogram (EEG) biofeedback. At present, there are no controlled studies that support coaching as a treatment for the core symptoms or associated functional problems of ADHD. There is preliminary support for the benefits of Captain's Log (Kotwal, Burns, & Montgomery, 1996; Slate, Meyer, Burns, & Montgomery, 1998) and multiple, controlled group studies in support of EEG biofeedback as a treatment of the core symptoms of ADHD (see reviews by Hirshberg, Chiu, & Frazier, 2005; Monastra, 2005a). However, direct examination of the impact of such treatment on memory functions has not yet been conducted. Consequently, at this time, our assessment of memory functions is primarily intended to contribute to the development of an appropriate plan of accommodation (e.g., use of electronic memory devices, visual cues, and prompts).

Language Processing and Fluency

When a patient diagnosed with ADHD presents with difficulties in word retrieval in social or academic settings that do not respond to pharmacological treatment, neuropsychological assessment may prove helpful in supporting the need for accommodation, as well as evaluation and potential treatment for a coexisting central auditory processing disorder. In clinical practice, several tests of oral fluency (reviewed by Lezak, 1976) may prove helpful, including the Token Test (Boller & Vignolo, 1966), the Stroop Word–Color Test (Stroop, 1935), the Word Naming Task (Terman & Merrill, 1960), and the Controlled Word Association Test (A. L. Benton, 1973).

The Token Test and the Stroop Word–Color Test are tests of selective attention while processing auditory information. The Token Test assesses the ability of the patient to process a series of auditory directions requiring them to touch or pick up specific colored shapes. The Stroop Word–Color

Test requires that a patient attend to the language content (rather than the color property) of printed words. In this test, the patient views words naming specific colors that are printed in an incorrect color (e.g., the word *red* is printed in the color blue). The patient is to respond with the printed word, not the color. Norms are commercially available for both of these tests.

The Word Naming Task and the Controlled Word Association Test require patients to speak words as rapidly as possible. In the Word Naming Task, the patient is simply required to say as many words as they can generate in 1 minute (sentences and number series are excluded). Terman and Merrill (1960) reported that by the age of 10, over half of their sample could generate a minimum of 28 words. In the Controlled Word Association Test, the patient is to say as many words that begin with a given letter of the alphabet (excluding proper nouns, numbers, and the same word with a different suffix). Borkowski, Benton, and Spreen (1967) published normative data for specific letters. The cutoff for brain damage was below 9 (Letters A, C, D, G, H, W), below 11 (Letters B, F, L, M, R, S, T), and below 12 (Letter P).

When evidence of impairment is evident on such measures, referral to a speech–language pathologist or therapist is recommended. Children, teens, and adults who experience neurologically based word fluency deficits will have considerable difficulty profiting from social skills and other types of communication training that ignores their essential neurologically based language deficits. In such cases, the initiation of speech–language therapy to promote word fluency skills appears to constitute an essential component of the treatment program of patients who are diagnosed with ADHD.

Motor Coordination

Although there is evidence that significant improvement in certain fine motor functions can occur following initiation of a clinically effective dose of stimulant therapy (see review by Barkley, 2006), residual impairments of fine and gross motor impairment often persist. Among the enduring deficits are impairments in the quality of handwriting (Marcotte & Stern, 1997; Sleator & Pelham, 1986), lower levels of physical fitness, and greater risk for a developmental coordination disorder (Harvey & Reid, 2003).

In clinical settings, initial evidence suggestive of impaired motor functioning is found in parent reports on the LSQ and teacher reports on report cards and the FACT that indicate marked impairment in the quality of handwriting. In addition, children who live highly sedentary lifestyles and manifest characteristics of childhood obesity are likely to have underlying coordination disorders. Intervention is needed to help children with either type of coordination disorder.

Although school districts can provide evaluations by an occupational therapist to assess fine motor coordination, children with ADHD do not typically perform poorly on tasks of simple motor tasks. Rather, it is during the performance of complex motor tasks (i.e., writing, paper-and-pencil mazes, and pursuit rotor tasks) where impairment is noted. Consequently, tasks that directly assess such abilities, such as the Written Expression subtest of the Wechsler Individual Achievement Test—II (Wechsler, 2004), are often helpful in identifying such children. When such fine-motor impairments are noted, the use of adaptive pencil grips and permission to use assistive technology (e.g., word processing programs, voice recognition programs) are more helpful than participation in occupational therapy.

In children and teens presenting with obesity, referral to a physical therapist is recommended on the basis of concerns about motor coordination and risk for serious health impairments. If these patients have significant gross motor (i.e., balance) disorders, referral for physical therapy merits consideration. In addition, the physical therapist can begin to prescribe a series of exercises to improve muscle tone and cardiovascular health, both of which have beneficial effects on mood and attention.

IMPLICATIONS FOR CLINICAL PRACTICE

Despite the initiation of effective pharmacological treatments for ADHD, patients often continue to exhibit impairments of attention, behavioral and affective control, social functioning, memory, language processing and retrieval, and motor coordination. As a result, patients with ADHD can benefit from a comprehensive functional assessment, following the establishment of medical treatment for their core symptoms. Such an assessment is likely to lead to the development of an integrative program that includes specific accommodations and referral to developmental therapists to support the emergence of underlying skill deficits in language and motor functions. In addition, the persistence of significant problems of behavioral and emotional control, as well as a variety of social skills deficits, will require targeted interventions for each of these enduring areas of functional impairment. The remainder of the book is devoted to a review of those interventions that have been associated with enhancement of treatment effectiveness in studies of children, teens, and adults with ADHD.

8

ELECTROENCEPHALOGRAPHIC BIOFEEDBACK IN THE TREATMENT OF ADHD

During the past 30 years, there has been considerable interest in examining the effectiveness of nonpharmacological treatments that have been developed to improve the attention and behavioral control of patients diagnosed with attention-deficit/hyperactivity disorder (ADHD) and other medical conditions associated with cognitive impairment (see reviews by Fox, Tharp, & Fox, 2005; J. F. Lubar, 2003; Monastra, 2005a; Monastra et al., 2005; Riccio & French, 2004). Proceeding from a perspective that ADHD is a neurologically based disorder limiting capacity for attention and behavioral control, two types of training strategies have been developed, electronic training devices (ETDs) and electroencephalographic (EEG) biofeedback (referred to as *neurofeedback therapy* [NFT] or *neurotherapy*).

ETDs seek to improve functioning through the repeated practice of tasks that require attention, memory, behavioral control, and concentration. Examples of this modality include the Attention Training System (ATS; Rapport & Gordon, 1987), the Captain's Log (Sanford & Browne, 1988), Attention Training (Wells, 1990), Attention Process Training (Sohlberg & Mateer, 1989), and Pay Attention! (Thomson, Seidenstrang, Kerns, Sohlberg, &

147

Mateer, 1994). EEG biofeedback (NFT or neurotherapy), seeks to improve attention and behavioral control by attempting to teach the patient to regulate levels of cortical arousal in brain regions that control such functions (J. F. Lubar, 2003; Monastra, 2005a).

A variety of ETDs have been developed for the treatment of ADHD, ranging in complexity from a simple response when a tone sounds (auditory training systems) to highly stimulating and challenging games involving auditory discrimination, color discrimination, and various visual search tasks (e.g., Captain's Log). During such training procedures, the patient is instructed to respond to specific target(s) and inhibit response to other stimuli, presumably reinforcing alerting, vigilance, selective attention, and behavioral inhibition skills. To date, several studies examining the effectiveness of these training programs have been published.

The ATS was initially found to yield improvement on measures of attention and behavioral control in a series of case studies (DuPaul, Guevremont, & Barkley, 1992; Evans, Ferre, Ford, & Green, 1995; Gordon, Thomason, Cooper, & Ivers, 1991). However, the only published double-blind, placebo-controlled study (Rapport et al., 1996) found that this type of treatment was significantly less effective than methylphenidate and there was no evidence of long-term improvement when medication was discontinued.

On a similar note, improvements on measures of attention and persistence have been reported in studies investigating the effectiveness of programs such as Pay Attention! (Semrud-Clikeman et al., 1999) and Captain's Log (Kotwal, Burns, & Montgomery, 1996). However, standards for determining efficacy of an intervention require positive findings from at least two controlled group studies using random assignment and (when possible) comparison with a bona fide treatment (Chambless & Hollon, 1998; LaVaque et al., 2002). None of the studies examining any of the ETDs have demonstrated beneficial effects that were comparable to stimulant therapy or were sustained when training was discontinued. Therefore, at the present time the identification of effective ETDs is considered to be at a preliminary stage of development. As ongoing systematic evaluations of the effectiveness of such devices are conducted, it is hoped that attention training protocols that can be administered at home via ETDs will be identified.

In contrast to findings with ETDs, research investigating the effectiveness of EEG biofeedback has included case and multiple-case studies, controlled group studies with comparisons to stimulant therapy, and controlled group studies using random assignment and comparison to a waiting-list condition. The three most comprehensive and recent reviews (Hirshberg, Chiu, & Frazier, 2005; Monastra, 2005a; Monastra et al., 2005) have concluded that there is sufficient evidence to support use in clinical practice, particularly in patients who are unresponsive to pharmacological treatment, who develop significant adverse reactions, or who have family histories of addiction (prompting parents to reject use of psychostimulants). In addition, two subsequent studies (using random assignment and waiting-list control conditions) further bolster support for use of this type of treatment in the treatment of patients with ADHD (Foks, 2005; Levesque, Beauregard, & Mensour, 2006). Consequently, this chapter focuses on the use of NFT in clinical practice.

THE APPLICATION OF ELECTROENCEPHALOGRAPHIC BIOFEEDBACK (NEUROTHERAPY) IN CLINICAL PRACTICE

In chapter 2, the neuroscience of ADHD was reviewed. Collectively, neuroimaging and neurophysiological studies support the perspective that ADHD is associated with dysregulation of cortical arousal (in brain regions responsible for attention, concentration, and behavioral inhibition and planning) and founded in multiple, atypical, genetically determined structural variations in the density of receptors and reuptake transporters for the catecholamines (dopamine and norepinephrine) and possibly other neurotransmitters (e.g., serotonin, acetylcholine). Evidence of such dysregulation has been consistently and reliably reported in numerous studies using quantitative electroencephalographic (qEEG) techniques (see reviews by Chabot, di Michele, & Prichep, 2005; Monastra, 2005a).

Emerging from the existing qEEG literature is the perspective that patients with ADHD exhibit at least two types of dysregulation. The most common type (noted in 80%–90% of patients) is characterized by evidence of cortical hypoarousal that appears in the form of dominant patterns of slow cortical activity over brain regions responsible for alertness, vigilance, and behavioral control. The second type of cortical dysregulation, exhibited in approximately 10% to 20% of patients, is characterized by hyperarousal on qEEG examination, as evidenced by an increase in fast EEG frequency waveforms over these regions. Patients exhibiting cortical hypoarousal tend to respond positively to medications intended to increase level of cortical activity (i.e., stimulants), whereas those who do not exhibit such slowing tend to be nonresponders (see review in chap. 6). It is considered noteworthy that the percentage of patients who do not exhibit cortical slowing on qEEG examination approaches the percentage of patients who do not respond to stimulants.

As noted by Monastra (2005a) and Chabot et al. (2005), the evidence of hypoarousal on the qEEG is consistent with reports of hypoperfusion during positron emission tomography (PET) examinations of the prefrontal cortex and basal ganglia (Lou, Henriksen, & Bruhn, 1984, 1990) and the decreased cerebral blood flow noted during single photon emission computed tomography (SPECT) studies of the right lateral prefrontal cortex, the right middle temporal cortex, and the orbital and cerebellar cortices (bilaterally;

Kim, Lee, Shin, Cho, & Lee, 2002; Sieg, Gaffney, Preston, & Hellings, 1995). In addition, PET examinations of children during cognitive challenge tasks revealed further reduction in glucose metabolism in prefrontal regions and the basal ganglia, rather than the anticipated increase in metabolic response to such tasks (Ernst et al., 1994; Zametkin et al., 1990).

As reviewed by J. F. Lubar (1991) and Sterman (1996), patterns of cortical activation on qEEG examination reflect the arousal of the prefrontal cortex and basal ganglia. Moreover, as clarified by Sterman (1996), variation in alertness and behavioral control reflects the activity of specific thalamo-cortical generator mechanisms, which are expressed in surface EEG recordings. A description of how such state fluctuations are reflected on the EEG is provided by Monastra (2005a):

> When a person is in an inattentive, unfocused state, evidence of slow EEG frequencies (3.5–8 Hz or "theta") is predominant over the prefrontal and frontal cortex and at certain midline locations (e.g., the vertex or C_z). In relaxed, wakeful states, alpha rhythms (9–11 Hz) begin to be noted in these same locations. As an individual shifts into a state of increased awareness and is preparing to engage in a planned or purposeful action, evidence of increased amplitude of the sensorimotor rhythm (SMR:12–15 Hz) is apparent over the Rolandic (motor) cortex. Finally, during tasks that require focused attention and sustained mental effort, "beta" (16 to more than 20 Hz) is noted over prefrontal, frontal, and central midline regions. (p. 60)

Because patterns of hypoarousal and hyperarousal have been identified on qEEG evaluations of patients diagnosed with ADHD, studies of NFT have sought to determine whether individuals could learn to self-regulate specific EEG frequency bands (e.g., theta, SMR, beta), thereby improving attention and behavioral control. Initial case studies demonstrated that children with ADHD could learn to decrease theta and increase SMR (J. F. Lubar & Shouse, 1976), as well as decrease theta and increase beta activity (J. O. Lubar & Lubar, 1984). Furthermore, they provided initial demonstration that such changes were associated with improvement in the core symptoms of ADHD, providing the foundation for investigations of the effectiveness of NFT as a treatment for ADHD.

Neurotherapy Protocols for ADHD

During the subsequent 2 decades, multiple controlled group studies have been conducted. Included among these studies are open trials with comparison to bona fide treatment (i.e., stimulant medications; Monastra, Monastra, & George, 2002; Rossiter & LaVaque, 1995) and randomized controlled trials (Levesque et al., 2006; Linden, Habib, & Radojevic, 1996), in addition to early case study reports. As is reviewed later in this chapter, improvements have been noted on measures of intelligence, alertness, vigilance, behavioral inhibition, and decision-making speed, as well as on scales assessing the core behavioral symptoms of ADHD. In addition, indicators of change in the neurological structures responsible for attention and behavioral control have also been presented (Levesque et al., 2006; Monastra et al., 2002). Monastra et al. (2002) reported a significant reduction in theta/beta power ratios following EEG biofeedback that was sustained following a 1-week medication washout period. Levesque et al. (2006) demonstrated increased activation of the right anterior cingulated cortex on functional magnetic resonance imaging (fMRI) examination of children treated with NFT. To date, no other type of behavioral therapy has demonstrated evidence of such improvements in the core symptoms of ADHD and associated neurophysiological and neurochemical processes.

Neurofeedback: A Brief Description

During NFT, the patient sits in a comfortable chair as sensors are attached to the scalp over specific cortical locations (see Figure 8.1, an illustration of the International 10–20 System of Electrode Placement). This process is painless, as sensors remain in place because of the adhesive quality of the conductive paste used in EEG recordings. One or two pairs of sensors are attached to the ear lobes as reference points. Once the sensors are attached and the integrity of sensors and quality of skin preparation assured, training is initiated.

During training, the patient is instructed to look at a computer monitor that will present a variety of displays. On certain displays, the patient and therapist are able to directly observe the EEG signal in the form of brain waves, or graphic displays (e.g., bars, dials). On other displays, the EEG signal is not directly observable; however, indicators of activation state are present in the form of lights and/or sounds that turn on or off (depending on production of desired or undesired brain patterns, respectively), graphic designs that change shape, and video characters that move in a variety of directions and engage in a variety of activities depending on the production of targeted brain waves. In addition, to promote generalization of training to academic tasks, neurofeedback may also be provided as the patient is engaged in performing tasks such as reading, writing, and solving mathematics problems.

Training is conducted during sessions lasting approximately 45 to 60 minutes in duration. During sessions, multiple short training periods (ranging from 2–9 minutes) are conducted. Duration of each training period is adjusted on the basis of the endurance displayed by the patient. At our clinic, we begin with five training periods (2-minute warm-up, followed by four 5-minute periods). The goal is for the patient to demonstrate a level of cortical activation consistent with age peers for a 45-minute training period (approximately the duration of a class period in school). Significant reduction in core ADHD symptoms has been noted in as few as 15 to 20 sessions con-

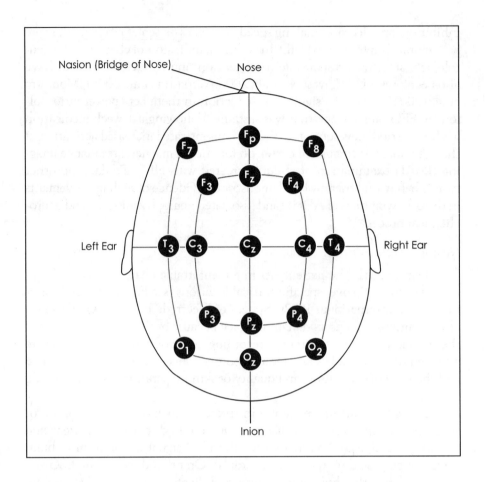

Figure 8.1. International 10–20 System. Brain regions are identified as follows: F = frontal; T = temporal; C = central; P = parietal; and O = occipital. Illustrated by Bridget Monastra.

ducted on a weekly or biweekly basis; the average number of sessions needed to obtain "normalization" of qEEG activation for three consecutive 45-minute training periods has been reported to be 43 (range = 34–50 sessions; Monastra et al., 2002).

In NFT, the desired brain frequencies are termed *reward frequencies* (REEG); the undesired frequencies are *inhibit frequencies* (IEEG). In certain training protocols, the desired REEG is beta; in others, SMR is reinforced. IEEG frequencies can include theta (in the case of hypoarousal) or high beta frequencies (in patients with hyperarousal).The patient is reinforced for producing REEG by a tone, movement of a character, and so on. No such tone or movement occurs when the patient is producing IEEG. The patient is required to maintain the desired qEEG state for 0.5 seconds to be rewarded. A counter displays the number of half-second periods of targeted neural activity.

Determination of the specific amplitudes of activity within the REEG and IEEG proceeds from a review of the results of a qEEG assessment. Such examinations provide essential information regarding cortical regions exhibiting underarousal, hyperarousal, or other qEEG abnormalities. The statistical analysis provided by current NFT systems enables the practitioner to establish frequencies and amplitudes for initial training. In our clinical research and practice, we use the process described by J. F. Lubar (2003) to determine the amplitudes for initial training. Typically, the amplitudes of the REEG frequency band and IEEG frequency band are adjusted until the patient is demonstrating the REEG approximately 40% of the time and the IEEG 60% of the time. Most systems also provide an electromyographic channel, to encourage the patient to remain relatively still during training. The goal is to help patients develop, as they are told, "active mind and a still body."

Neurofeedback Training Protocols

Although a variety of types of training have been explored, the controlled group studies that have been published to date have provided evidence in support of three training protocols. A brief description of each follows.

Protocol 1: Enhancement of the Sensorimotor Rhythm; Suppression of Theta. This training protocol seeks to reduce symptoms of hyperactivity and impulsivity by reinforcing the production of the SMR (12–15 Hz) at one of two sites positioned over the motor cortex (C_3 or C_4; see Figure 8.1, this volume) while suppressing the production of theta activity (4–7 Hz or 4–8 Hz). EEG recordings are obtained from one active site, referenced to linked earlobes, with a sampling rate of at least 128 Herz. Visual and auditory feedback (i.e., reinforcement) is contingent on the patient controlling microvolt output of theta and SMR. Rossiter and LaVaque (1995) used this protocol in the first published controlled group study of EEG biofeedback for ADHD, as did Foks (2005). It also constituted the first treatment phase in the Levesque et al. (2006) study.

Protocol 2: Enhancement of Beta 1; Suppression of Theta. This protocol was developed to treat symptoms of inattention, as well as impulsivity and hyperactivity, and the effects of this protocol have been examined in four controlled group studies of patients with ADHD, Predominately Inattentive Type, or ADHD, Combined Type (Levesque et al., 2006; Linden et al., 1996; Monastra et al., 2002; Rossiter & LaVaque, 1995). In Protocol 2, patients are reinforced for increasing production of Beta 1 activity (16–20 Hz) while suppressing theta activity (4–8 Hz). EEG activity is monitored at C_z with linked ear references, at FC_z and PC_z (midline frontal, midline parietal) with single ear reference, or at C_z and PC_z (midline central, midline parietal) with ear reference. A variation of this protocol has also been reported in the treatment of patients with ADHD, Predominately Inattentive Type (Fuchs, Birbaumer, Lutzenberger, Gruzelier, & Kaiser, 2003, who trained patients to suppress theta and enhance beta at C_3).

Protocol 3: Enhancement of the Sensorimotor Rhythm; Suppression of Beta 2. This protocol was developed to reduce symptoms of hyperactivity and impulsivity and was examined by Fuchs et al. (2003) in the treatment of patients diagnosed with ADHD, Predominately Hyperactive–Impulsive Type. In this protocol, patients are reinforced for increasing SMR (12–15 Hz) while suppressing Beta 2 activity (22–30 Hz). Recordings are obtained at C_4, with linked ear reference. Fuchs et al. (2003) used this protocol for half of each training session and Protocol 1 for the other half.

Clinical Benefits of Neurotherapy

In the case and controlled group studies, significant improvement has been reported in the following outcome measures: attention, cooperation and completion of academic tasks, intelligence, behavioral control, and reduction of hyperactivity. Evidence of such gains has been noted on standardized behavioral rating scales, tests of intelligence, CPTs, and qEEGs, as well as in the informal observations of parents, teachers, and therapists.

Three of the controlled group studies (Fuchs et al., 2003; Monastra et al., 2002; Rossiter & LaVaque, 1995) also involved comparisons with bona fide treatments for ADHD (i.e., stimulant medication). Initially, Rossiter and LaVaque (1995) conducted a study comparing the effects of NFT and stimulant medication. They reported significant improvement of attention and behavioral control in 23 children who received 3 to 5 EEG biofeedback sessions per week (20 sessions total). The children who had received NFT also demonstrated a level of performance on the Test of Variables of Attention (TOVA; Greenberg, 1994) and a level of functioning on the Behavioral Assessment System for Children (Reynolds & Kamphaus, 1994) that was equivalent to that demonstrated by 23 children treated with either methylphenidate or dextroamphetamine.

A similarly designed study was conducted by Fuchs et al. (2003), who treated 22 children with NFT and 12 children with Ritalin (average dose = 10 mg, three times daily; total daily dose range = 10–60 mg/day). NFT sessions were conducted three times per week (30–60 minutes) for a 12-week period. Again, children receiving NFT demonstrated a level of performance on the TOVA and on behavioral rating scales that was comparable to that associated with stimulant therapy.

Monastra et al. (2002) expanded this line of research by examining the effects of NFT in a study of 100 children, all of whom were treated with the stimulant medication Ritalin (average dose = 25 mg/day; typically administered as 10 mg after breakfast, 10 mg at lunchtime, and 5 mg after school; range = 15–45 mg/day for both groups). NFT sessions were conducted once per week (45–50 minutes). Treatment was continued until the patient demonstrated a degree of cortical activation on the qEEG measure that was within 1 standard deviation of the mean for age peers on the basis of normative data (Monastra et al., 1999) and could maintain this level of arousal for 45 minutes during three consecutive training sessions. All of the participants receiving NFT were able to achieve this target following training.

It is important to note that all of the participants who were treated with stimulant medication (including those who did not receive NFT) had their dose of medication adjusted at the beginning of treatment until qEEG theta:beta ratios at C_z were within the normal range according to the process developed by Monastra et al. (1999). Such a process requires a child to demonstrate "normal" levels of cortical arousal for four 90-second periods. In addition to careful initial titration of dose, interventions were provided at school and at home. An Individual Education Plan or 504 Accommodation Plan was developed for each child (in collaboration with his or her school district), and parent counseling was provided in classes and individual session, as described in Monastra (2005c).

One year after their initial evaluation, each of the participants were evaluated through a process that included standardized behavioral rating scales (i.e., the Attention Deficit Disorders Evaluation Scales or ADDES; McCarney, 2004), the TOVA, and the qEEG Scanning Process (Monastra et al., 1999). Patients were tested 1.5 to 2.0 hours postingestion of Ritalin. When tested within 2 hours of administration of Ritalin, no significant differences between the groups treated with stimulant alone or in combination with NFT were noted on behavioral, qEEG, or neuropsychological measures.

However, following this evaluation, a 1-week medication washout period was conducted for all participants. After 1 week, all participants were again evaluated using the ADDES, the TOVA, and the qEEG. Every child in the group who did not receive NFT relapsed on all of the dependent measures. In contrast, patients whose treatment included NFT demonstrated sustained improvement on the TOVA, qEEG, and school versions of the ADDES. A significant moderating effect was noted for parenting style. Those parents who were using the strategies taught in our class at least 50% of the time (systematic parenting style) reported improved behavioral control and attention at home. Those parents who did not apply class lessons (nonsystematic parenting style) continued to report excessive behavioral symptoms of inattention, impulsivity, and hyperactivity at home.

A long-term follow-up study, examining the endurance of clinical gains in the children who participated in the Monastra et al. (2002) study was also reported (Monastra & Monastra, 2004). In this study, 86 of the participants from the first study (43 members of each group) were reevaluated 6, 12, and 24 months after the conclusion of their 1st year of treatment. Evaluations were again conducted while taking stimulants and after a 1-week medication washout period.

The primary findings of this study were as follows:

1. There was no indication that stimulant medication caused an enduring change in any of the patients whose treatment did not include NFT. Although patients who had received stimulant medication demonstrated gains on all measures when tested on medication, none demonstrated maintenance of such gains when medications were withdrawn. In contrast, all of the members receiving NFT demonstrated maintenance of treatment gains at each follow-up period.

2. Thirty-four (80%) of the patients whose treatment included NFT were able to decrease the daily dose of stimulant by at least 50%. In contrast, none of the patients who did not receive EEG biofeedback was able to reduce dose. Instead, 85% needed to increase dose to maintain treatment gains.

3. Parents who rated themselves as nonsystematic reinforcers of appropriate behaviors at the conclusion of the 1st year of treatment varied in their eventual response to our parenting program. Parents whose children participated in NFT (but were initially nonsystematic in their parenting style) tended to return to the clinic for booster parenting sessions, eventually improving their style and their child's functioning at home.

Although the findings from the three studies involving direct comparisons with bona fide treatment provide support for the effectiveness of NFT, a valid critique of these studies is that each was an open trial, in which parents were able to select type of treatment (Barkley, 2003; Loo, 2003; Monastra, 2005a). In the absence of random assignment to group, such studies cannot be considered sufficient for a conclusion that NFT is an efficacious treatment.

Such criticism cannot be applied to two controlled group studies in which random assignment to group was included in the research design (Levesque et al., 2006; Linden et al., 1996). In the Linden et al. study (1996), 18 children who had been diagnosed with ADHD were randomly assigned to a waiting-list condition or NFT. None of the participants received pharmacological treatment for ADHD. Patients who received NFT received 40 training sessions (45 minutes each). As with the other controlled group studies, equivalence between the groups was noted on all dependent measures prior to initiating treatment. Following treatment, the children who received NFT demonstrated significant improvement on measures of intelligence and a reduction of symptoms of inattention on a standardized behavioral rating scale.

In the Levesque et al. (2006) study, 20 children were randomly assigned to receive NFT or were placed in a waiting-list control group (receiving no treatment). None of the children were treated pharmacologically. As in other studies, the dependent measures included standardized tests of memory (number sequence recall), attention, vigilance, behavioral control (impairment of visual accommodation), and the core symptoms of ADHD (Conners' Rating Scales; Conners, 2001). However, to assess whether the behavioral benefits of NFT were associated with evidence of improvement of neurological functioning, participants were evaluated via fMRI. The researchers were particularly interested in determining whether NFT resulted in changes in patterns of activation of the anterior cingulated gyrus, as measured by fMRI during completion of the Stroop Task (Stroop, 1935). Similar to the other controlled group studies, the findings of the Levesque et al. (2006) study revealed significant improvement in the group treated with NFT. Gains were noted on behavioral and neuropsychological measures of attention and behavioral control. Most important, significant changes in the activation of the right anterior cingulated gyrus were observed during completion of the Counting Stroop Task. Such findings are consistent with the emerging model of those structures involved in the mediation of attention and behavioral regulation and are supportive of the effectiveness of NFT.

Efficacy of Neurofeedback

On the basis of the publication of several randomized clinical trials (RCTs), as well as multiple controlled group studies using comparison with a bona fide treatment, NFT meets the initial requirement to be considered an effective treatment for ADHD using criteria published by the American Psychological Association (Chambless & Hollon, 1998) and the Association for Applied Psychophysiology & Biofeedback (LaVaque et al., 2002). In addition, Hirshberg et al. (2005) applied the guidelines for recommending evidence-based treatments developed by the American Academy of Child & Adolescent Psychiatry (AACAP; Greenhill et al., 2002) and concluded that NFT "meets AACAP criteria for 'Clinical Guidelines' for treatment of ADHD" (p. 12). Treatments meeting the requirement for Clinical Guidelines are those that apply approximately 75% of the time. Such practices "should always be considered by the clinician, but there are exceptions to their applications" (Hirshberg et al., 2005, p. 13).

At present, the exploration of strategies that can help patients learn to control cortical dysregulation is still at an early stage of development. Although at least 75% of participants in controlled group studies have demonstrated significant improvement in the core symptoms of ADHD, there are nonresponders who will need to be effectively treated (see Heywood & Beale, 2003). In addition, the controlled group studies conducted to date have evaluated the effects of NFT primarily in children and adolescents. Studies investigating effectiveness in adults are also needed.

A critical issue facing providers using NFT is the determination of type of protocol to use in the treatment of a specific patient. At present, there are three protocols that have been examined in controlled group studies. When choice of NFT protocol is determined by the presence or absence of cortical slowing during qEEG examination, improvement in response rates has been achieved (Monastra et al., 2002). Consequently, efforts to match type of NFT with type of dysregulation of cortical arousal appear to hold promise in our attempt to improve the response rates of NFT.

As neurophysiologists identify other types of qEEG abnormalities in patients diagnosed with ADHD, it seems likely that new protocols that yield clinical benefits in shorter training periods will emerge. In addition, at this time, several innovative approaches are being explored, including the training of slow cortical potentials (Heinrich, Gevensleben, Freisleder, Moll, & Rothenberger, 2004), hemoencephalography (Toomim & Toomim, 1999), and audiovisual entrainment (Siever, 2003). However, at present, the use of other types of training protocols would be considered to be experimental until there is empirical support from future RCTs.

Side Effects

Overall, a review of the results of the controlled group studies indicates that NFT has been consistently associated with significant improvement in the core symptoms of ADHD. However, both deBeus, Ball, deBeus, and Herrington (2003) and Monastra et al. (2005) have reported certain transitory side effects. These researchers reported that in children treated with both stimulant medication and NFT, increased irritability, moodiness, and hyperactivity may occur as the child begins to demonstrate improved self-regulation of cortical arousal. Such adverse effects typically respond to reduction in medication dose (rather than increase). In cases in which the primary residual symptoms are anxiety, irritability, or impaired anger control, antihypertensive medications (rather than stimulants) have proven helpful. Other side effects reported by Monastra et al. (2005) include headaches and dizziness. Such symptoms responded to brief resting periods (15–30 minutes) or the consumption of food.

Integration of Neurofeedback Into Clinical Practice

In our examination of 800 patients treated with NFT at our clinic (Monastra, 2005a), we found several factors that contributed to a parental or patient decision to initiate a trial of this type of treatment. The most common reason for a request for NFT was a patient's failure to respond to a series of at least two stimulant medications (68%). A secondary reason (noted in 22%) was the emergence of significant adverse side effects when taking stimulants (e.g., irritability, aggressive behavior, weight loss, severe and persistent headaches, insomnia). Approximately 10% of the parents who sought NFT for their child did so because of a family history of addiction, a fear that their child would become addicted, or other concerns about the safety of long-term use of stimulants.

As with any patient who seeks treatment for attention, impulsivity, and hyperactivity, a comprehensive evaluation (as described in chap. 4) is needed prior to initiating this type of treatment. Once screening for other medical conditions is completed, a multimodal treatment program is needed for patients selecting this type of treatment for the core symptoms of ADHD. As with stimulant medication, there is no compelling evidence that NFT effectively treats the wide range of functional impairments exhibited by patients with ADHD. In clinical practice, patients with ADHD will typically need a treatment plan that includes interventions at school and work (e.g., an Individual Education Plan or Accommodation Plan); life skills training; parent–child or marital counseling; and modifications of dietary, sleep, and exercise habits. Because our patients commonly exhibit difficulty in word fluency, reading comprehension, written expression, and other language-based skills, training in these areas could readily be included as part of a treatment session in which NFT was provided.

At our clinic, we approach the treatment of patients who receive NFT in the same manner that we approach those treated with pharmacological agents. Our first goal is to effectively treat the underlying dysregulation of cortical arousal and then address areas of residual functional impairment. To achieve rapid stabilization of symptoms (and reduce parental stress, improve family relationships, and reduce the patient's sense of failure at home and school), it is common for us to initially assist the patient's physician in determining a clinically effective dose of medication. Like a physician in an emergency room setting, we seek to stabilize the patient and then proceed with interventions to promote long-term functioning. Within such a framework, medications for ADHD provide immediate symptomatic relief; NFT promotes sustained improvement in functioning.

At this time, there seems little reason to deny patients the opportunity to benefit from both of these types of treatment. Although the cost for NFT varies regionally ($60–$150/session), the charge is consistent with that of other mental health services. This type of treatment is a covered benefit under most insurance programs if NFT is provided in combination with other interventions (e.g., parent counseling, individual and family therapy, cognitive behavior therapy, social skills training).

Practitioners interested in learning more about this type of treatment can contact the Association for Applied Psychophysiology & Biofeedback (see http://www.aapb.org) or the International Society for Neurofeedback and Research (see http://www.isnr.org). Certification standards for practitioners have been developed and are available through the Biofeedback Certification Institute of America (see http://www.bcia.org).

9

PROMOTING SCHOOL SUCCESS IN CHILDREN WITH ADHD

Children and teenagers with attention-deficit/hyperactivity disorder (ADHD) exhibit a wide range of academic and functional problems in school settings. As reviewed in chapter 1, these areas of concern encompass disorders of conduct, mood, and learning, as well as multiple types of social skill deficits. Without intervention, students with ADHD are at greater risk for academic failure, with 10% to 33% of students failing to graduate from high school (Barkley, 2006; Mannuzza, Klein, Bessler, Malloy, & LaPadula, 1993). College graduation rates indicate that adults without ADHD are 4 times more likely to attain a bachelor's degree than those with ADHD (Mannuzza et al., 1993).

Despite such high rates of academic failure, the existing scientific evidence indicates that school-related problems can be effectively addressed by school-based interventions, involving the coordinated efforts of parents, teachers, school mental health providers, the patient, and his or her physician and mental health specialist (see reviews by Hunter, 2004; Pfiffner, Barkley, & DuPaul, 2006; Robinson, 2004). However, a lack of intervention at the school level and the disconnection between care providers, educators, and parents have been cited as significant impediments to the effective treatment of chil-

161

dren with ADHD (National Institutes of Health, 1998), supporting the need to develop strategies for developing effective accommodation and intervention plans in the care of these patients.

In clinical practice, it is not uncommon for parents to seek counseling services for their children and teenagers who are struggling to complete school work, homework, and long-term assignments. It is also not unusual for them to request outpatient care for students who are exhibiting aggressive, defiant, or disruptive behaviors in class. However, among the lessons that we have learned over the past 2 decades, two principles are paramount.

First, without collaboration between the health care providers, the school district, the parent, and the student, little sustained improvement is likely. From my perspective, it makes little sense to engage in 1 hour of outpatient counseling on a weekly basis to address such problems. For behavioral change to occur, there needs to be instruction in desirable behavior, monitoring of performance, and systematic reinforcement of the child's actions. Without the collaboration between parents and teachers, monitoring and reinforcement efforts will be compromised.

Second, the complexity of any type of behavioral intervention program developed and implemented at school is inversely related to the adequacy of treatment for the medical and educational conditions that underlie a specific student's behavioral and functional problems. Although there are a variety of procedures that use tangible rewards, tokens, reprimands, and other response cost strategies (see review by Pfiffner et al., 2006), such strategies have been shown to fail to yield significant, sustained improvement in the functioning of patients with ADHD in the absence of effective medical care and appropriate levels of educational support (Multimodal Treatment Study of Children With ADHD Cooperative Group, 1999).

Proceeding from such a foundation, our clinic has investigated the types of interventions that were required to promote the successful functioning of students, once effective pharmacological treatment had been initiated and maintained. Three studies have been conducted over a 7-year period. In the first two studies, a total of 400 students were examined over a 5-year period to evaluate the effects of an Individual Education Plan (IEP) or 504 Plan on a variety of outcome measures, including number of disciplinary referrals per week, number of incomplete assignments per week, and overall academic average (Monastra, 2000). The results of the findings of these studies were then incorporated into the research design of a third study, a multimodal treatment project that examined the effects of stimulant medication, electroencephalographic biofeedback, and parent training in 100 students diagnosed with ADHD, in a context that included a program of academic support (Monastra, Monastra, & George, 2002).

The purpose of this chapter is to review the existing laws that protect the educational rights of students with ADHD, provide an overview of the types of interventions that are available in schools, and review the specific strategies that my research group found most beneficial to students during our three research programs. Consistent with the guiding principle of this book, the goal is to present a model of intervention that is economically feasible and could be implemented by practitioners in traditional clinical settings (i.e., individual or group practice, outpatient hospital clinics, or mental health centers).

EDUCATIONAL RIGHTS OF STUDENTS WITH ADHD

ADHD is recognized as a psychiatric disorder that entitles students to academic support and accommodations in school and work settings. One of the laws (Individuals With Disabilities Education Act [IDEA], most recently revised in 2004; see http://idea.ed.gov/) provides funding for students with ADHD (ages 3–21) who need special education services and related services. The other law (Section 504 of the Rehabilitation Act of 1973; see http://www.hhs.gov/ocr/504.pdf) provides "reasonable accommodations" to any U.S. citizen who has a physical or mental condition that substantially limits a major life activity (e.g., learning). A summary of the highlights of each of these laws follows.

Individuals With Disabilities Education Act

This federal law was developed so that students with disabilities could be afforded services to help them overcome the adverse effects of a variety of conditions, including learning disabilities, serious emotional problems, mental retardation, traumatic brain injury, vision or hearing impairments, physical disabilities, or other health problems (including ADHD). For a student with ADHD to qualify for supportive services under the IDEA, two important conditions must be met. First, the student must be diagnosed with ADHD by a person who is qualified to do so (e.g., a licensed psychologist or physician). Second, the ADHD symptoms must be shown to limit alertness to academic tasks and adversely affect educational performance.

Prior to recent revisions of the IDEA (e.g., 1998, 2004), a common misconception was that a child needed to be diagnosed with a specific learning disability to receive services. However, the IDEA supports the position that ADHD is a health impairment and students do not need to show evidence of a learning disability on standardized tests to qualify for services. Rather, the law requires that a school district complete a functional assessment of the student's school performance to determine the types of interventions that are needed.

Therefore, parents of students with ADHD no longer need to accept that their child, as many have said, "just needs to try harder and pay attention" because a school psychologist reported that the child's standardized test results indicated that the student did not have a learning disability. Quite often, a child diagnosed with ADHD is able to perform adequately on brief reading, spelling, or mathematical tests, administered on a one-to-one basis by a school psychologist in a low-distraction setting. However, when an examination of the child's functioning within the academic setting is conducted (using an assessment process such as a review of teacher comments on report cards or the Functional Assessment Checklist for Teachers [FACT]), evidence of the adverse effects of the child's ADHD becomes clear.

For instance, students with ADHD can be easily distracted by other children or activities in the room, in the hallways, or outside the window, thereby causing them to miss directions and instruction. Such a failure to attend could cause them to fail to hear that a test would be conducted tomorrow in math or that they would need to turn in a specific assignment on a targeted date. As a result, their grade in the subject would be significantly lowered, because of their inattention.

Another example is the common failure of students with ADHD to complete homework and turn in assignments to their teacher because of loss of attentional abilities and concentration in the late afternoon and early evening. For such students, their inability to sustain mental effort and complete homework causes them to receive zeros for their homework, again significantly lowering their report card grades. The IDEA mandates that school districts develop and follow a process to determine each area of functional impairment caused by the child's ADHD and to develop a comprehensive plan. Examples of the types of services that could be provided include the following:

- consultation between a special education teacher and a student's teacher to develop strategies that could promote the child's learning and functioning in class;
- consultation with a special education teacher, outside of the classroom (e.g., in a "resource room") to help with organizational problems and completion of homework;
- in-class assistance by a special education teacher to facilitate understanding of academic material in a specific class(es);
- in-class assistance by a classroom aide (under the supervision of a special education teacher), who could help the student remain on task;
- placement in a classroom with a lower student-to-teacher-to-aide ratio (e.g., 15:1:1; 12:1:1; 8:1:1) to permit more individualized instruction and pace of learning;
- individual and/or group counseling and participation in social skills groups to help the student develop improved behavioral and emotional control;
- participation in speech therapy, to improve word fluency and other expressive and receptive language functions;

- participation in occupational therapy, to improve coordination on tasks related to the writing process; and
- participation in physical therapy to improve balance and gross motor coordination needed for participation in exercise and athletic programs. In addition, some children with ADHD experience a calming effect from exercises that stimulate cerebellar functions (e.g., balance, rotational exercises).

Because students with ADHD commonly struggle to express their knowledge through handwritten response or experience difficulty sustaining attention while reading, a parent can also request that a district complete an assessment of the need for assistive technology. For example, at this time, there are computer software programs that can be used to read any printed text to a student (e.g., Read & Write, ReadPlease!, Kurzweil 3000). Once the text is entered into the child's computer (via disk, scanner, or download from the Internet), a text file is created. The child clicks on the file, and a copy of the homework page, article, book, and so on appears on the computer monitor. The child is prompted to inform the computer about his or her preferences about the voice that the computer will use to read to the student. The student also informs the computer about the desired speed of reading. Once this data is entered, these systems will then highlight the words for the student and read the text to them.

The advantages of such systems are readily apparent to students with ADHD. When I demonstrate such systems to them, they recognize that tasks that once seemed endless (e.g., reading a 20-page chapter) become manageable. Once they set the reading speed, they know when their task will be completed. A 20-page chapter could be completed in 30 to 40 minutes, rather than never. In addition, because the computer will correctly read any word, the student does not lose concentration or the meaning of texts because of gaps in their word recognition vocabulary.

Voice-recognition programs (e.g., Read & Write; Dragon Naturally-Speaking) can be used to simplify the writing process. Certain children with ADHD can take a long time to write homework responses. However, they can easily express their ideas verbally. For such children, use of computer programs that transcribe their spoken words into text can be quite helpful in reducing the emotional meltdowns that can occur at homework time. Children who are skilled at using word processors can be permitted to use laptop computers to type their homework.

Children who are prone to be distracted by the games on computers can use dedicated word processing tools such as AlphaSmart or DreamWriter. These systems are portable word processors that do not have any games to distract the child. A student can type on these devices and subsequently print out his or her homework on a printer. Information regarding such assistive technology can be found on multiple Web sites or through the local school district. I often direct parents and colleagues to the following Web site: http://www.upstatecommunications.com.

In addition to such services and tools, provisions of the federal No Child Left Behind Act (see http://www.ed.gov/nclb/landing.jhtml) require schools to provide academic support services to all students (regardless of the presence of a disability) in the areas of English and language arts, science, social studies, and mathematics. Each district must provide the services of a certified teacher for remediation in each of these areas to students at risk for academic failure in one of these core subject areas. Such remediation is to be provided in addition to daily instruction in each of these areas.

Section 504 of The Rehabilitation Act of 1973

The IDEA is intended to provide students with the assistance of special education teachers or other specialists (e.g., speech, occupational, or physical therapists) to help them overcome the impact of their attentional deficits on educational performance. However, not all students diagnosed with ADHD require the services of a special education teacher to overcome the adverse effects of impaired attention on educational performance. For those students, Section 504 of the Rehabilitation Act of 1973 can provide much needed modifications and accommodations.

Section 504 of the Rehabilitation Act of 1973 is intended to prevent discrimination against individuals with disabilities. This law requires that school districts provide reasonable accommodations to individuals diagnosed with a physical or mental condition that substantially limits a major life activity. Learning is defined as a major life activity. Therefore, a student who is diagnosed with a condition like ADHD may require modifications of the arrangement of the room, the manner in which lessons are presented, and the methods by which assignments and tests are given and completed. Accommodations can also be given to overcome the impact of symptoms of forgetfulness and disorganization on learning. A comprehensive listing of reasonable accommodations is provided in Exhibit 9.1. This list is derived from standards implemented on a national level and previously published (Monastra, 2005c) and is presented in a format that could be used to develop a 504 Plan.

Students who are referred to the 504 Committee are those who are not considered to be in need of special education services. Such students, however, are likely to benefit from being placed close to the source of instruction and from efforts by the teacher to ensure that the student has heard directions; has copied homework assignments accurately; has necessary materials needed for completion of homework; and is given access to tape recorders, word processors, or computers to learn and complete assignments. These students can also benefit from peer modeling, tutoring, and various interventions intended to improve motivation for task completion (e.g., praise, the development of a behavioral management program, daily or weekly parent–

teacher communication regarding completion of work and classroom behavior). In addition, as mandated by provisions of the No Child Left Behind Act, these students (like any student in danger of failing a course in mathematics, science, social studies, or English and language arts) are entitled to academic support services (i.e., remedial instruction), to be provided within their school day. As we discovered during the course of our clinical research (Monastra, 2000; Monastra et al., 2002), there are significant differences in the level of educational performance of students with ADHD who receive support and accommodations compared with those who do not. Moreover, we have noted that such differences persist despite the introduction of carefully titrated doses of medication for core ADHD symptoms.

PROCESS FOR ESTABLISHING A PROGRAM OF ACADEMIC SUPPORT AND ACCOMMODATION

A student diagnosed with ADHD who is demonstrating a level of educational performance that reflects the adverse effects of limited alertness is entitled to an evaluation by the Committee on Special Education (CSE). Such a referral can be made by a parent, teacher, school counselor, or administrator. Typically, this type of referral occurs after a period of time in which parents, teachers, and other members of the school's Child Study Team have collaborated and attempted to develop a formal or informal Instructional Support Plan. When such plans fail to address the factors causing the student's academic failure, referral to the CSE will be needed.

Despite the establishment of two federal laws that protect the educational rights of students with ADHD, there are multiple impediments to the development and implementation of an effective IEP or 504 Plan. As emphasized by Pfiffner et al. (2006) and the *National Institutes of Health (NIH) Consensus Statement on the Diagnosis and Treatment of Attention-Deficit/ Hyperactivity Disorder* (NIH, 1998), one of the primary impediments is the lack of basic knowledge among educators about the nature, causes, course, and treatments for ADHD. Another impediment is the reluctance of parents to have their child labeled, out of fear that their child will receive a substandard education. Finally, the lack of collaboration among teachers, parents, and health care providers and the resultant failure to create a therapeutic context in which relevant educational, motivational, and neurological factors are simultaneously being addressed in a cohesive manner combine to increase the likelihood of failure in school settings.

The therapeutic reality that needs to be created is one in which teachers understand and accept that ADHD is indeed a medical condition that impedes educational performance and that their role is to identify and create strategies that promote the development of those skills needed to succeed in school. In such a context, the role of the parent as a primary source of reinforcement is also recognized, and parents and teachers need to collaborate to

EXHIBIT 9.1
Accommodations Provided in Accordance With Section 504 of the Rehabilitation Act of 1973

Student's Name: _____ **Date of Birth:** _____
School District: _____ **Grade:** _____
Teacher: _____

Describe the nature of the handicapping condition: _____
_____
_____

Describe how the handicapping condition was determined: _____
_____
_____

Describe how the handicapping condition is affecting a major life activity: _____
_____
_____

On the basis of a review of this student's academic record, the school district has agreed that the following accommodations are reasonable in accordance with guidelines established by Section 504 of the Rehabilitation Act.

Physical Arrangement of the Room
_____ Student will be seated near the teacher.
_____ Student will be seated near a positive role model.
_____ Teacher will stand near the student when giving directions or presenting lessons.
_____ Student will be seated away from distracting stimuli (e.g., air conditioner, window, door).
_____ Teacher will increase the distance between the student's desk and those of classmates.

Lesson Presentation
_____ Pair students to check accuracy of work.
_____ Write key points on the board.
_____ Provide peer tutoring.
_____ Provide visual aides.
_____ Provide peer note taker.
_____ Provide written outline.
_____ Allow student to tape-record lessons.
_____ Have child review key points orally.
_____ Use computer-assisted instruction (software, Internet).
_____ Permit student to use word processing technology to take notes.
_____ Make sure directions are understood.
_____ Include a variety of activities during each lesson.
_____ Divide longer presentations into shorter segments.

Assignments and Worksheets
_____ Give extra time to complete tasks.
_____ Simplify complex directions.
_____ Hand out worksheets one at a time.
_____ Reduce the reading level of the assignments.
_____ Require fewer repetitions of practice work (e.g., writing spelling words).
_____ Reduce the number of homework assignments.
_____ Allow student to tape-record assignments or homework.
_____ Allow student to use typewriter, word processor, or computer to complete work.
_____ Provide structural guides for completing written assignments.

_____ Provide study skills training.
_____ Give frequent short quizzes and avoid long tests.
_____ Do not grade handwriting or spelling (unless during a spelling test).

Test Modifications
_____ Allow extra time to complete tests.
_____ Permit test to be taken in a low-distraction context.
_____ Permit use of assistive technology (e.g., tape recorder, computer, word processor, typewriter) to record answers.
_____ Read test items to the student.
_____ Read directions to the student; check to determine understanding of directions.
_____ Give exam orally.
_____ Give take-home tests.
_____ Use more objective questions (i.e., fewer essay responses).
_____ Give frequent short quizzes, not long exams.
_____ Allow breaks during testing.
_____ Allow periodic interaction with teacher or examiner to promote attention to task.

Organization
_____ Provide peer assistance with organizational skills.
_____ Assign homework buddy.
_____ Provide extra set of books at home.
_____ Send daily or weekly progress reports home, listing specific assignments that were not completed or returned and defining any behavioral concerns.
_____ Develop a reward system for classroom work and homework completion.
_____ Provide student with a homework assignment notebook.
_____ Check accuracy of daily assignment notebook.
_____ Prompt student regarding assignments and materials that need to be brought home.
_____ Prompt student in the morning to turn in completed homework.

Behavior
_____ Develop and implement a classroom behavior management system.
_____ Praise specific behaviors.
_____ Use privileges and rewards for specific behaviors.
_____ Make prudent use of negative consequences.
_____ Keep classroom rules simple and clear.
_____ Allow for short breaks between assignments.
_____ Use nonverbal cues to help student stay on task.
_____ Mark student's correct answers, not mistakes.
_____ Permit time out of seat for movement (e.g., run errands).
_____ Allow movement that does not distract others.
_____ Develop contracts with the student.
_____ Use time-out procedures.
_____ Ignore inappropriate behaviors not drastically outside classroom limits.

Participants (name and title)

_____   _____

_____   _____

Signature, Chairperson of the 504 Committee: _____

address the tendency of students with ADHD to avoid tasks requiring sustained mental effort. Finally, it is essential for parents and teachers to be supported by health care providers who seek to establish an effective treatment for the underlying neurological causes of a student's ADHD. Without adequate treatment for the neurological causes of ADHD in a specific student, no amount of intervention on the part of parents or teachers will be sufficient.

It is within such a collaborative context that an educational program can be developed for a student with ADHD. To initiate the process of evaluation for an IEP or 504 Plan, the school district's CSE chairperson needs to be informed that a student has been diagnosed with ADHD and be provided with documentation in support of such a diagnosis. Because many of the parents of students with ADHD have significant attentional and organizational problems, it is often helpful for the doctor who has made the diagnosis to assist the patient in writing a letter to the CSE chairperson (or the director of Special Education Services). At our clinic, we use the Request for Evaluation by the Committee on Special Education form provided in Exhibit 4.2 (see chap. 4, this volume). Because there are mandated time requirements for the completion of an evaluation by the CSE, parents or guardians would be well advised to send such a request via certified mail. Because of the high volume of mail received by a school district, the arrival of a certified letter alerts the district to the importance of the contents and ensures that the evaluation process will not be delayed.

Once the CSE chairperson receives such a certified letter, he or she will initiate an evaluation process. This evaluation will include assessment of the student's intelligence and reading, writing, and mathematical abilities. In addition, for students who are diagnosed with ADHD, the evaluation must include a functional assessment, to assess the degree of functional impairment in all areas related to the health condition. Because of the comprehensive nature of this evaluation process, a period of 60 days is commonly needed to complete the assessment.

After the assessment is completed, a meeting will be conducted. This meeting typically includes the parent or guardian of the student, the student (particularly at the junior and senior high school level), the CSE chairperson, a school psychologist, a special education teacher, at least one of the student's teachers, and another parent who has a child with a disability. At the CSE meeting (or 504 meeting), the results of testing of intelligence and core academic abilities are presented, as are a summary of the student's academic record. Information about the student's current progress in treatment for ADHD can also be provided, based on information from the physicians and mental health professionals caring for the patient. Finally, the results of the functional assessment (see FACT; chap. 7) are reviewed.

The initial task to be accomplished at the CSE meeting is to determine eligibility for services, support, and/or accommodations or modifications. For a student to be considered eligible under the IDEA, there must be evidence that the ADHD is limiting alertness and adversely affecting educational performance. For eligibility under Section 504, ADHD must be limiting learning. As a psychologist who has attended thousands of CSE and 504 meetings, I have heard these criteria to be misconstrued to mean that unless a child's performance on tests of academic skills is significantly suppressed relative to intelligence (i.e., falls at least 1.5 SD from expectations based on a test of intelligence), then the child is not demonstrating "adverse effects on educational performance." I have also heard a similar rationale used to justify denial of accommodations under Section 504, with the district asserting that the student's ADHD was not limiting learning because scores on tests of academic achievement were not sufficiently suppressed.

As has been clarified in recent revisions of the IDEA, the core principle of assessment is that it be comprehensive in nature and that all areas of functional impairment need to be carefully assessed. Scores on tests of intelligence or academic abilities cannot be used to deny eligibility if the qualifying condition is ADHD. Instead, evidence of how ADHD is limiting alertness and educational performance and demonstrations of learning must be reviewed and evaluated. Examples of how ADHD could adversely affect educational performance and/or limit demonstrations of learning in a specific student includes students who

- receive failing grades in a subject because they fail to *attend* to teacher instructions, record assignments, bring home materials, complete homework, return the assignment to school, and return it to the teacher;
- struggle to *sustain concentration* during class lectures, fail to take adequate notes, and do not study the correct information for a quiz or test;
- do not complete reading assignments, because of *lack of concentration* during the evening;
- are unable to *sustain concentration* while searching for information while reading and completing worksheets;
- are unable to *access working memory* to write answers during tests;
- are unable to retrieve information from memory because of *distractibility* in a class context;
- are unable to retrieve information needed for a test because of *slow processing speed* and time limitations;
- struggle to retrieve information and organize thoughts when writing paragraphs or short essays because of *slow processing speed* and word fluency problems;
- are unable to complete mathematical problems because of an *inability to retrieve* basic math facts;
- are *unable to focus* on class instruction because they are preoccupied with the teasing and insults that they have endured on the bus during transit to the school;
- are repeatedly removed from class instruction because of *impulsive, hyperactive, and disruptive behaviors*;

- are suspended from class instruction because of *inability to control impulsive aggressive physical behavior*; and
- are removed from instruction because of an *inability to regulate and control inappropriate verbal behavior*.

Each of these examples represents the types of impairments that require the development of a program of academic support and accommodation. By using a guide to conducting a functional assessment (such as the FACT), a district can obtain a comprehensive perspective of the multiple types of functional impairment evident in a specific student and develop an intervention and/or accommodation plan that targets each area of impairment, as mandated by the IDEA. However, as emphasized previously, the development of an IEP or 504 Plan without parental reinforcement and effective treatment for the neurological causes of a student's ADHD is not likely to yield optimal results.

For example, a district could develop a plan to provide daily or weekly progress notes of behavior and missing assignments to the student and parents. However, the student who has parents who do not monitor and reinforce completion of such work is not likely to improve the rate of task completion. A district could develop a plan to provide such progress notes, and parents could reinforce completion through a combination of incentives and response cost strategies (reviewed in chap. 10). However, without adequate treatment for the core ADHD symptoms, sustained improvement is not likely to be achieved.

Once the issue of eligibility for services under the IDEA or accommodations under Section 504 has been resolved, the committee needs to develop a comprehensive plan to address each area of functional impairment. For example, a student who is forgetful and disorganized will require monitoring and instruction in organizational skills. A student who has difficulty sustaining attention while reading may profit from instruction in focused reading exercises, the use of books on tape, or from the use of computer software that will read any text to the student. A student whose writing is illegible and who struggles to generate ideas in written form may benefit from instruction in writing skills, speech therapy to improve rate of word fluency, the use of a scribe, the use of a tape recorder to express ideas, the use of a word processor to type responses, or voice-recognition software that would transcribe spoken ideas into typewritten form.

On a similar note, a student who lacks retention of core mathematical facts (e.g., multiplication tables) could receive specialized instruction in mnemonic strategies to promote retention, use computer software programs to boost skills, and be provided with the accommodation of a calculator or multiplication chart to facilitate skill development. Depending on the school district, such instruction and monitoring may be provided by a special education teacher, through remedial instruction, or via computer software programs. A student who struggles to resolve conflict in a nonaggressive manner, who has limited conversational skills, or who is socially isolated may benefit from social skills training at school; speech–language therapy; and the guidance of a school counselor, social worker, or psychologist to promote involvement in peer activities at school.

Once the committee has reached an agreement on the plan of support and accommodation, a written version of the plan is prepared and distributed to the parent or guardian. This written version is typically not distributed to a student's teachers by the CSE chairperson. To ensure that the student's teachers are informed about the details of the plan, I encourage parents to provide copies of the IEP or 504 Plan to their child's teachers and arrange a follow-up meeting to review the plan. Such a meeting can be quite helpful in making sure that the plan is implemented. Because most plans are revised during the spring months, I also encourage parents to meet with the student's new team of teachers in the Fall, to ensure that the plan has been reviewed and will be implemented as written.

If the parents and CSE are not in agreement, there are several options available to the parents, including mediation and an impartial hearing. The option that I typically recommend is mediation. Unlike an impartial hearing, in which the school district and parents present their position to a hearing officer, who renders a binding decision, during mediation, parents (and their professional and legal representatives) and school officials (typically the CSE chairperson and the district's attorney) meet with a trained mediator. The role of the mediator is to promote a dialogue that leads to the resolution of areas of disagreement and the development of an acceptable plan.

Once a plan has been developed, reviewed with teachers, and implemented, current federal guidelines require that the plan be reviewed on an annual basis. However, should problems arise prior to the date for the annual review, a request for a meeting to revise a plan can be initiated at any time. This request should be made in writing to the CSE chairperson or the 504 Committee.

The rationale for requiring a review at least annually is based on both legal and scientific foundations. Both the IDEA and Section 504 specifically state that plans need to be reviewed and revised annually. In addition, evidence from several well-controlled studies examining the impact of comprehensive, school-based interventions (e.g., Conners et al., 2001; P. S. Jensen, Hinshaw, Swanson, et al., 2001; Shelton et al., 2000; Swanson et al., 2001) indicates that although children demonstrate improvements in terms of social skills and academic performance following such interventions, such gains do not appear to persist in the absence of carefully titrated pharmacological treatment, nor do they appear to generalize to new classroom contexts in the following years.

FUNCTIONAL ASSESSMENT VERSUS FUNCTIONAL BEHAVIORAL ASSESSMENT

Students who are diagnosed with ADHD are entitled to a comprehensive functional assessment to determine the impact of their limited alertness on educational performance. Such an assessment involves review of academic records, behavioral observation, completion of functional assessment checklists (e.g., the FACT), and assessment of academic and intellectual skills. This functional assessment needs to evaluate all areas potentially related to the health condition in question. Following completion of such an assessment, the CSE is in a better position to develop a comprehensive IEP to address each area of functional impairment caused by the health impairment ADHD.

However, among certain health care providers and educators, there appears to be confusion between such a comprehensive functional assessment and a functional behavioral assessment (FBA). In such educational contexts, a comprehensive functional assessment is not conducted and an FBA is initiated only if the student exhibits significant behavioral problems. Such an approach is in violation of the IDEA mandates.

The FBA is only one part of the evaluation process leading to the development of a comprehensive IEP. It is conducted to develop an effective treatment plan for specific symptomatic behaviors that are related to the reinforcement characteristics of specific educational contexts rather than caused by neurological or other medical factors. It does not compose the comprehensive type of assessment of functional impairment mandated by the IDEA. Rather, it is intended to address targeted behavioral or functional problems, which are caused by contextual factors.

The FBA was derived from the perspective that an undesirable behavior is the result of a combination of precipitating environmental stimuli, the occurrence of the undesirable behavior, and the absence of consistent reinforcement strategies following the occurrence of the behavior that could reduce or eliminate the frequency of the behavioral problem. In conducting the FBA, the therapist (or educational team) defines the behaviors to be eliminated, the environmental factors that appear to precipitate occurrence of the undesirable behaviors, and the environmental responses to the occurrence of the behavior. On the basis of such an analysis, the team develops a Behavioral Intervention Plan, which includes environmental consequences for the student's behavior (e.g., rewards such as time to engage in preferred tasks, response costs strategies such as loss of free time, punishments such as the assignment of additional work). Using such a perspective, therapists and educators have been able to address a wide variety of off-task and disruptive behaviors in children who do not have neuropsychiatric disorders such as ADHD. However, although such an approach has been quite useful in developing effective treatments for disorders that appear to be caused by contextual factors (e.g., oppositional defiant disorder), it does not provide a sufficient perspective for developing an intervention plan for patients with health conditions like ADHD. The following illustration may clarify this point:

> A teenager, with poorly controlled diabetes, exhibits lack of effort on tasks, irritability, and moodiness between 10:30 a.m. and 11:30 a.m. and between 1:15 p.m. and 2:45 p.m. An analysis of situational contexts determines that the behaviors occur during mathematics period and during social studies and English classes. Analysis of factors precipitating irritability and loss of effort determines that symptoms occur when the patient is required to do in-class assignments that require independent completion of worksheets or other writing tasks. The consequences of the behavior include removal from the classroom (i.e., disciplinary referrals) and avoidance of the school tasks (i.e., the student is able to avoid completion of the tasks). Because both consequences reinforce the continuation of the avoidance behaviors, an FBA would result in the development of a plan that includes the consequence "will make up any missing assignment and be assigned extra work."

In examining this case, it is important to realize that although the ability to engage in a behavior that results in the avoidance of an unpleasant task (completing schoolwork) would be considered reinforcing, medical factors appear highly relevant as well. If the patient is is experiencing fluctuating blood sugar levels due to dietary factors or the need to adjust medication, this type of behavioral intervention will have little impact. Instead, an intervention that calls for a medical evaluation and intervention for diabetes would appear highly relevant toward understanding both the medical and environmental factors contributing to symptom occurrence. Indeed, if the pattern of avoidance persisted following stabilization of blood sugar levels, the consequences determined in the FBA would make a great deal of sense.

A similar analysis could be conducted in a child diagnosed with ADHD who was being treated with a short-acting stimulant medication (e.g., Ritalin). If off-task behavior and irritability were being noted 3 to 4 hours postingestion and immediately following lunchtime dose, it would make far more sense to evaluate the adequacy of medication (using continuous performance test [CPT] and quantitative electroencephalographic [qEEG] data collected at off-task times) instead of developing a reward and response cost paradigm. Again, if symptoms persisted once the underlying medical conditions were addressed, then the development of such a plan would appear likely to succeed. Overall, in addressing residual functional problems in a student diagnosed with ADHD, assessment and treatment of the underlying neurological causes of ADHD need to occur prior to conducting and initiating a Behavioral Intervention Plan based on the FBA.

During the course of conducting two studies examining the role of the IEP and 504 Plans, certain key elements have emerged. In the initial study (Monastra, 2000), the effects of developing and implementing an IEP were examined in 400 students in Grades 1 through 12, who were diagnosed with ADHD on the basis of *Diagnostic and Statistical Manual of Mental Disorders* (4th ed.; *DSM–IV*; American Psychiatric Association, 1994) criteria and the assessment process described by Monastra et al. (1999). In addition to meeting *DSM–IV* criteria for ADHD, each of these students manifested evidence of cortical hypoarousal on qEEG examination and were being treated with stimulant medication. In each instance, dosage of medication was titrated until the student achieved scores consistent with age peers on both the qEEG and on visual and auditory CPTs (TOVA).

In the initial phase of the study ($N = 200$), Monastra (2000) examined the type of academic support and accommodation being provided to students diagnosed with ADHD who were being treated with an effective dose of stimulant medication (on the basis of qEEG and CPT data). This investigation revealed that only 18 of these students (9%) were receiving academic support via an IEP. In each case, students receiving support via an IEP had been diagnosed with a specific learning disability. Their program of support consisted of special education instruction (in a resource room; within a regular classroom context, or in a class setting with a lower student-to-teacher ratio), combined with testing modifications (extended time for tests; provision of a low-distraction testing context) and supervision of class and homework assignments. With such support, the 18 students with IEPs were functioning better on three critical dimensions: completion of assignments, frequency of disciplinary referrals, and overall grade point average.

On the basis of the results of this initial study, Monastra (2000) examined the impact of developing and implementing an IEP or 504 Plan for each of 200 students subsequently referred to our clinic and diagnosed with ADHD. Similar to our prior study, selection criteria were as follows: met *DSM–IV* criteria for a diagnosis of ADHD, exhibited cortical slowing on qEEG examination, scored in the impaired range (i.e., > 1.5 *SD* below age peers) on two CPTs, and did not have an IEP or 504 Plan prior to their participation in the study.

Following titration of medication dose (stimulants prescribed to all participants), a comprehensive evaluation was conducted by area school districts. Three dependent measures (disciplinary referrals per month; missing assignments per week; academic average) were monitored for the 10-week marking period prior to implementing the IEP or 504 Plan and for the 10-week marking period after the plan was implemented. Medication dosage was titrated prior to obtaining dependent measures pre- and postimplementation of the educational plan.

The results of this study illustrated the additional gains that can be achieved by implementation of a 504 Plan or IEP in the context of effective pharmacological treatment and active parental participation and reinforcement. On average, the number of missing assignments decreased from 9.00 per week to 0.61 per week, in both the ADHD, Predominately Inattentive Type, and ADHD, Combined Type, groups ($p < .01$). The average number of disciplinary referrals decreased from 1.41 per week to 0.39 per week (ADHD, Combined Type, group; $p < .05$). The number of disciplinary referrals for members of the ADHD, Predominately Inattentive Type, group remained negligible (0.09/week vs. 0.03/week). It is most significant to note that the overall grade point average for students in this study increased from 69.8 to 83.3. Again, it is important to stress that these gains occurred after pharmacological treatment for ADHD had been initiated, the dosage was titrated, and parents were supported and guided in the use of motivational strategies to increase educational performance and behavioral control in school.

Examination of the types of interventions needed to achieve these gains revealed several common themes. Among students in the primary grades, specialized instruction in reading, writing, or mathematics was required for 75% of students. Ninety-eight percent of these students required some type of monitoring to ensure that homework assignments were being recorded, completed, and returned. This was typically provided by daily parent–teacher correspondence, in which the child was rated for his or her classroom behavior (listening during instruction, completion of seat work, behavioral control in the classroom, behavioral control during transitions and unstructured period).

Consistent with well-established reinforcement principles, the student could earn privileges at school (e.g., time to engage in an enjoyable activity such as a computer game, read a high-interest book, or play with peers) as well as at home (e.g., time to engage in play activities immediately upon arrival at home). To address the tendency of children with ADHD to avoid tasks that require sustained mental effort, a child who did not complete seat work would be required to complete that task at home, as well as an additional task of similar type. The framework given to these children was that "if you play in school, instead of work, then you'll have to do extra work when you get home." Children in the primary grades quickly learned this principle. Although certain of the classroom teachers instituted variations of color charts and smiley-face programs (e.g., letting the child know how well he or she was performing during the day on the basis of the color of their chart or presence or absence of a smiley face), there was no indication that this approach resulted in increased compliance or task completion when compared with plans where a progress note was exchanged between parents and teachers at the end of the day.

Again, it is important to stress that these children were being treated with a carefully titrated dose of medication. Given the reinforcement of a simple behavioral program at home (and the provision of a pharmacologically effective dosage of stimulants), fewer than 10% of these students required the assistance of an aide. By the time these students reached the third grade, testing modifications (e.g., extended time to complete the test, permission to complete the test in a low-distraction context, use of a scribe to write answers) were being implemented for virtually all students (97%).

Among students in Grades 5 through 12, all of the students benefited from multiple types of support and accommodation. The primary types of intervention required were as follows: participation in a resource room class (one period/day) to help teach organizational skills and assist in the completion of homework and preparation for exams; weekly progress reports from teachers, indicating specific missing assignments; parental reinforcement of missing assignments (i.e., requiring that the student complete the missing assignment plus one extra assignment before being permitted to engage in recreational activities); participation in remedial or special education instruction in core context areas; testing accommodations; and the use of assistive technology to complete schoolwork (e.g., books on tape, word processors, calculators, voice-recognition software, computer software that could read text to the students). Because students at the middle and high school levels are typically afforded extended time to complete tests, extended time for homework was requested, because impairment of attention, concentration, working memory, and word fluency is not limited to times when tests are administered. Because of the positive response of students to these types of accommodations and support, IEPs and 504 Plans were developed for all participants in our subsequent study (Monastra et al., 2002). Similar levels of educational performance were noted in this subsequent study.

As noted in our studies, students with ADHD have significant difficulty concentrating and completing homework. When they advance into the high school grades, the demand for work increases significantly but the time available to complete it does not. However, unlike college students, who can take an additional dose of stimulant medication to help them sustain attention and concentration throughout the evening and compensate by waking at 9:00 a.m. or 10:00 a.m., high school students must typically wake at 6:00 a.m. Because stimulants interfere with sleep onset (if taken in the evening), high school students are unable to take an evening dose of medication.

Because of the need for additional time to complete homework and study, a student with ADHD would benefit by being treated like a college student, who is informed of upcoming assignments and quizzes in advance. I have often heard teachers comment that students with ADHD "need to be prepared for college." I agree. At the college level, professors inform their students of all assignments on the 1st day of class. The course syllabus is reviewed, which includes the types and deadlines of all assignments. Professors do not inform a student that a major test is coming in 4 days; the student knows well in advance so that he or she can prepare accordingly. Unfortunately, that is not the case in high school, where a student can discover on Monday that they will have two quizzes and two tests before the week is concluded (in addition to daily homework assignments).

Although it is unrealistic to propose that teachers in Grades 6 through 12 provide a course syllabus for a 10-week period, it is reasonable to request that they provide students with advance notice of upcoming assignments and tests. By providing such notice on the preceding Friday, students with ADHD can use some of their weekend time to complete certain assignments (e.g., vocabulary sheets, reading assignments, worksheets requiring definition of terms and concepts in science and social studies). Such an accommodation helps to create time during the week and weekend for studying and creates a foundation for improved organization at the college level.

As students proceed through the high school years, preparing them to accept support staff assistance at the collegiate level also appears to contribute to their success. It is common for teenagers with ADHD to resist the assistance of a resource room teacher or the monitoring of parents. As they head off to college, they are not inclined to avail themselves of the services provided by the Office for Students With Disabilities. Unfortunately, without such assistance, they are more likely to be placed on academic probation or to be dismissed from the university by the end of the 1st year.

As I review in the next chapter, there are multiple strategies that parents can use to overcome such resistance. The metaphor that we commonly use to help students is that most business owners, doctors, lawyers, and other professionals have a team of people who help them. The resource room teacher or college learning disorders specialist is similar to the office manager who helps a CEO stay organized and successful. Regardless of the size of a business, administrative assistants, who help with organization, are essential for success. Plumbers, carpenters, electricians, and others in the construction trades have an office staff to help them coordinate the scheduling of jobs and payment for work pending and completed. Doctors have numerous staff members to help with handling phone calls, finding and sorting files, completing insurance forms, transcribing reports, and performing a variety of accounting tasks so that the doctor can devote his or her time to what he or she enjoys most. Without such help, each of these businesses will fail. From my perspective, college students with ADHD are the CEOs of the business called "getting my degree." We simply ask students, "If the CEOs of every other business can accept that they cannot do everything by themselves, why can't you?"

Among the accommodations and assistive technology that seem most helpful to college students are the following: note takers during lectures and the availability of a learning center where the students can be assisted in understanding course content, completing essays and term papers, preparing for tests, and organizing their schedule. In addition, extended time for the completion of tests and provision of a low-distraction context can be quite helpful. Finally, the use of computer software that can read and write for students can greatly simplify the tasks of reading texts and journal articles for classes and transcribing the student's ideas for essay and term paper assignments. As described previously, such programs help students to better pace their completion of reading assignments and overcome reading decoding, reading comprehension, and writing problems.

Because of the significance of developing a plan of academic support for the college-bound student with ADHD, educators, guidance counselors, and mental health providers can play an important role in the selection process. By encouraging students and their parents to closely examine the types of accommodations and support services available at various colleges (e.g., by examining sources such as *Colleges for Students With Learning Disabilities* (2006), which are updated on an annual basis), counselors can guide students to examine and select programs that best fit their needs. A student who is well organized and has profited from a 504 Plan that provided little more than testing accommodations may fare well at a university with minimal support. However, another student who has needed the support and monitoring of parents and a resource room teacher to be successful is well advised to seek a setting that has a more comprehensive and structured program of support. An increasing number of colleges and universities maintain dormitory facilities specifically dedicated for the needs of students with disabilities and provide academic support within such facilities. Guiding parents and students to visit such programs seems an essential step in promoting a successful transition to college life for these students at risk.

IMPLICATIONS FOR CLINICAL PRACTICE

Because of the increased risk of academic failure in students with ADHD, the federal government has mandated that such students are entitled to academic support and accommodation. In addition, there is sufficient scientific evidence to support the value of such comprehensive psychoeducational interventions. Therefore, at this time, any provider who diagnoses ADHD in a student but does not take steps to ensure that the student is receiving an appropriate level of academic support is contributing to a process that denies these essential rights to their patients. From both a legal and clinical perspective, health care providers need to take an active role in ensuring the legal rights of their patients.

On the basis of findings that the beneficial effects of psychoeducational intervention are not sustained in the absence of effective treatment of the underlying neurological causes of ADHD, practitioners can promote their patients' academic success by routinely monitoring patient progress in the school setting. The requirement that a physician can prescribe only 1 month of medication at a time provides an opportunity for health care providers to receive a monthly update on patient level of functioning, so that medication effects can be assessed and treatment adjusted as needed. Sample forms to assist in such an assessment process are provided in Exhibits 6.1 and 6.2 (see chap. 6, this volume).

Finally, it is important to realize that teachers are accustomed to addressing classroom behavioral issues without support. They are highly resourceful individuals who will attempt to implement a wide range of interventions prior to asking for help. Such a process can take months before a teacher will initiate a request for assistance. To counter such tendencies, I encourage teachers to provide prescribing physicians with updates, particularly during months in which the student is clearly struggling to function effectively in their class. Such information from a teacher can result in the improvement of medical care for the child.

In children who are displaying significant functional problems but have not been evaluated or treated, I encourage teachers to ask parents for permission to write a note sharing their observations with the student's physician. I advise teachers not to comment about their opinions regarding possible diagnoses. Rather, I encourage them to inform parents that they are observing a degree of inattention, loss of concentration, and so on, that is unusual for their grade, and I allude to the fact that there are multiple explanations for such problems and that they would like to share these observations with the child's physician, who is in the best position to evaluate the possible causes of the child's problems. A letter from such a teacher to a physician can greatly facilitate the early identification of a condition like ADHD.

Over the years, I have come to develop a great appreciation and a tremendous respect for the efforts of teachers. I have also come to understand that without direct solicitation from a health care provider for a progress report, teachers will do the best they can and offer instruction in classroom contexts where several of their students will have behavioral or neuropsychiatric disorders that are not being effectively treated. During such time periods, the adverse effects of the child's untreated or poorly treated ADHD affect the acquisition of new skills and the self-esteem–boosting effects of successful school performance. By taking the time to solicit input from teachers on a monthly basis, practitioners can contribute to creating a context in which students with ADHD are able to benefit more fully from instruction, thereby enhancing their self-esteem.

10

COUNSELING PARENTS OF CHILDREN AND ADOLESCENTS WITH ADHD: THE NEUROEDUCATIONAL PARENT TRAINING PROGRAM

Children and teenagers diagnosed with attention-deficit/hyperactivity disorder (ADHD) display a wide range of functional impairments at home, as well as at school. With their parents, these patients exhibit more uncooperative and aggressive behaviors and are more forgetful, disorganized, inattentive, and impulsive than age peers (e.g., Barkley & Edelbrock, 1987; Cunningham & Barkley, 1979; DuPaul, McGoey, Eckert, & VanBrakle, 2001). Parents of such children tend to become more emotionally withdrawn and critical, attempting to control behavior through the use of a variety of response cost (e.g., loss of privileges) and punishment strategies, including verbal reprimands and corporal punishment (Cunningham & Barkley, 1979; DuPaul et al., 2001; Hinshaw et al., 2000; Monastra, Monastra, & George, 2002). However, as reviewed by Cunningham (2006) and Anastopoulos, Rhoads, and Farley (2006), there is little evidence that the nonsystematic application of various punishment or response cost paradigms is effective in improving cooperation, reducing disruptive and aggressive behaviors, and promoting social skills (e.g., eye contact, conversation, problem solving).

During the past 2 decades, a number of parenting programs for children with ADHD and other behavioral disorders have been developed and investigated, including Problem-Solving Communication Training (Robin & Foster, 1989), Behavior Management Training (Anastopoulos et al., 2006; Barkley, 1997), the Triple P-Positive Parenting Program (Sanders, 1999), the Community Parent Education Program (Cunningham, 2007; Cunningham, Bremner, & Boyle, 1995), the Intensive Social Skills Training Program (Pelham & Hoza, 1996), and the Neuroeducational Parent Training Program (NPTP; Monastra, 2005a, 2005c; Monastra et al., 2002).

Although there is considerable variation in the type of strategies taught in each of these parent training programs, there are several areas of overlap. In each of these programs, parents are taught to identify specific behavioral goals and to seek to reduce undesirable behaviors and increase more desirable ones through the systematic use of contingency management strategies including positive reinforcement, response cost, and/or time out. In addition, most of these approaches seek to provide some type of cognitive therapy intended to increase parental understanding about the causes of ADHD and the nature of effective treatments.

As reviewed by Chronis, Chacko, Fabiano, Wymbs, and Pellham (2004); Cunningham (2006); Robin (2006); and Anastopoulos et al. (2006), evidence of the positive impact of such treatments has also been reported in multiple studies. Most frequently, reduction in the degree of oppositionalism and aggression, as well as improved listening and conversational and problem-solving skills, have been observed. However, as reported by Anastopoulos et al. (2006), Monastra et al. (2002), and Monastra (2005a), there is considerable variability in the ability of parents to learn and implement such strategies in the daily care of their children. This variability of skill acquisition and the absence of long-term follow-up data make it difficult to derive conclusions about the efficacy of parent training alone. However, each of the listed types of parent training has been supported by the findings of at least one controlled group study.

In this chapter, the NPTP that was developed and researched at our clinic is presented. This program is one that can be easily adapted for use in solo or group practice, or in an outpatient clinic or a school setting. Sufficient detail is provided so that the principles taught in each of these classes can be applied in a variety of clinical settings. More detailed descriptions of each lesson are available in the book *Parenting Children With ADHD: 10 Lessons That Medicine Cannot Teach* (Monastra, 2005c) and in a DVD series documenting a 10-session parent class (Monastra, 2007).

THE NEUROEDUCATIONAL PARENT TRAINING PROGRAM

The NPTP has been administered in an outpatient clinical setting for the past 10 years. Similar to other types of parent training, it provides instruction in contingency management within a group context of adults who are raising children and teens diagnosed with ADHD. However, unlike other programs, the NPTP seeks to address those areas of functional impairment that persist after effective treatment(s) for the neurological causes of ADHD have been established. As such, the program is individualized for each participant in the group. In addition, recognizing that parents of children with ADHD are often overwhelmed by the complexity of behavioral charts, token economies, and other traditional behavioral approaches, the NPTP provides a more simplified approach to contingency management. Finally, by providing parents with a neurologically based understanding of the causes of their child's functional impairments, the NPTP seeks to help parents overcome residual feelings of guilt that can impede effort on parenting tasks.

Participants

Parents and guardians of children and teenagers who have been diagnosed with ADHD using *Diagnostic and Statistical Manual of Mental Disorders* (4th ed., text rev.; American Psychiatric Association, 2000) criteria, who have been thoroughly screened (and treated) for other relevant medical conditions, and who have been provided with effective treatment for the core symptoms of ADHD have successfully participated in our NPTP program. The program is composed of ten 90-minute sessions, conducted on a weekly basis by a licensed health care provider. Follow-up booster sessions are available as needed.

Because there is little evidence that children and teenagers with ADHD can learn and sustain new social skills in a context in which their core symptoms are not being effectively treated (Hinshaw et al., 2000), parental participation in such programs is not recommended until the child's core ADHD symptoms have been effectively treated. Premature participation in any type of parenting program can do little more than reduce a parent's belief that change is possible, rendering them much less likely to be responsive to instruction and ready to change (Prochaska, DiClemente, & Norcross, 1992).

This chapter provides a detailed description of the manner in which each class is taught. A handout, summarizing the core information taught in each class, is provided to participants in the class. This is done to help parents review information and to share with their spouse or partner, as typically only one parent will be able to attend (the other is busy with child care). Copies of these handouts are available through our clinic upon written request (see http://www.theADHDdoc.com). As described in Monastra

(2005c) and demonstrated in the video series by Monastra (2007), in each class there is a review of information presented in the previous class, instruction in a new skill, an opportunity to interact and practice skills, and the prescription of a homework assignment.

Several parent characteristics have differentiated clinical response to the NPTP (Monastra et al., 2002). Parents who schedule a time each week to meet and discuss their specific goals, teaching strategies, and child's progress report significantly better results. Such parents typically purchased a notebook; recorded these goals, strategies, and plans; and used some type of folder (to store the class handouts and track progress). On a similar note, Monastra et al. (2002) reported that parents who applied the instructional and reinforcement strategies taught in the NPTP at least 50% of the time reported significant gains in child functioning compared with those parents who were unsystematic in their reinforcement approach. Finally, those parents who decided to adopt a nonaggression policy for all members in the family reported significant reduction in the frequency of verbal and physical acts of aggression in the home (compared with parents who continued to use aggressive behavior as part of their parenting techniques).

The following sections are written in a style that is intended to provide clinicians with the instructional template used in actual class presentations. The participants in our programs have all been the guardians or parents of patients diagnosed with ADHD at our clinic. The fee for each class was $15. By providing a detailed presentation of class content, it is hoped that clinicians will find it easier to translate this presentation into clinical practice.

Class 1: The Causes of ADHD

In the first session, we begin to address several important misconceptions. First, many parents have begun to believe that they simply failed "Parenting 101." Second, there is a common belief that the lack of effective parenting caused their child's ADHD. Third, they feel that because of their previous failures, there is nothing that they can do to change their child's misbehavior or lack of attention. Following interventions to address parental guilt and sense of inadequacy, the therapist proceeds to a discussion of healthy dietary, eating, and sleeping patterns.

Class Content

1. Review the genetics and neuroscience of ADHD.
2. Present the importance of establishing an effective treatment for a child's core ADHD symptoms prior to beginning a parenting class.
3. Discuss the ways that the neurobiology of ADHD enhances performance in situations that are important, interesting, life-threatening, or fun.

4. Provide an opportunity for parents to address residual sources of guilt with a therapist who understands the genetic and neurological foundations of ADHD.

5. Review *Recommended Dietary Allowances* (Food and Nutrition Board of the National Academy of Sciences, 1989) regarding protein intake at breakfast and lunch, as well as healthy sleep and exercise habits.

Homework

Parents are requested to decide on a time during the week for a parent meeting. During this meeting, they are instructed to complete the Life Skills Questionnaire (LSQ): Child–Adolescent Form (see Exhibit 7.1, chap. 7, this volume). This format encourages the parents to complete a functional assessment of their child, which will serve as their focus as they proceed through the parenting program. Parents are also asked to monitor their child's eating, sleeping, and exercise patterns, as establishing healthy habits in these areas is beneficial for attention and behavioral control.

Class 2: Establishing Educational Support Plans for Children and Teens With ADHD

In clinical practice, the establishment of an appropriate plan of academic support is a critical element in the initial stages of treatment. I consider it to be secondary only to the initiation of effective treatment for the underlying neurological causes of ADHD and the establishment of healthy dietary, sleep, and exercise patterns. At our clinic, we have found that the degree of distress in the family is greatly reduced once these basic interventions have taken place. After the core symptoms of ADHD have been treated and the child has an effective educational support plan, the child and family can begin to focus on a broader spectrum of life skills development, through parent training and life skills training for the child.

Class Content

1. Collect LSQs.
2. Review parent progress in establishing a time for their parent meeting and discuss any impediments to initiating healthy dietary, sleep, and exercise programs.
3. Review the Individuals With Disabilities Education Act (see http://www.idea.ed.gov/) and Section 504 of the Rehabilitation Act of 1973 (see http://www.hhs.gov/ocr/504.pdf) and the process for initiating a request for a Committee on Special Education meeting.
4. Describe the Functional Assessment Checklist for Teachers (FACT; see Exhibit 7.3, chap. 7, this volume) and the impor-

tance of completing such an assessment in developing a comprehensive Individual Education Plan (IEP) or 504 Plan.

5. Review the kinds of accommodations that are helpful for students with ADHD.

6. Assist the parents in completing written requests to initiate and/or revise a plan of academic support, as needed.

Homework

The task for this week is for parents to request that each child's teacher complete the FACT. If the results of the FACT indicate that a child is functioning below expectations for his or her age, then the parents are requested to submit the letter (provided during class) that requests that an evaluation be conducted to either establish or revise an IEP or 504 Plan (as needed). They are also encouraged to continue to reinforce healthy dietary, sleeping, and exercise habits.

Class 3: Teaching New Skills to Children With ADHD

In this class, parents are taught an overview of the process for instructing and motivating children to learn new life skills. The development of any skill requires the physical capacity to perform the task, attention during the presentation of new skills, specific instruction in the desired behavior, and reinforcement of the desired behavior, as well as a cost for failing to perform the desired behavior. In addition, children and teens appear more likely to respond positively to instruction from a parent or teacher who they respect and who appears to respect and care about them.

Class Content

1. Review the results of the FACT; discuss the need for letters to request initiation or revision of a child's IEP or 504 Plan.

2. Review parent progress in establishing healthy dietary, exercise, and sleeping habits.

3. Present the steps for teaching a new skill to a child.
   (a) Select a skill that the child is physically and mentally able to learn;
   (b) instruct the child in a quiet, low distraction, low-conflict setting;
   (c) limit instruction to 1 minute, during which the parent presents the desired action and the time frame for performing the act; and
   (d) introduce reinforcers.
      (1) Time Stands Still: The child does not have parental permission to engage in any pleasurable activity until he or she performs the required behavior.

(2) Apologies and Amends: If the child resists performing the task and engages in other behaviors (e.g., watches TV anyway, yells at parents, becomes physically aggressive), the child will need to apologize to his or her parents, perform some type of act to indicate regret, and then complete the requested act before proceeding to enjoyable activities of his or her choice.

(e) Maintain a positive relationship with the child by engaging in recreational activities with him or her on a daily basis.

Homework

For the following week, parents are requested to perform the following tasks. First, spend at least 15 minutes per day with their child engaging in some type of enjoyable activity. During this period, the parents are instructed to not ask a question, give a direction, or correct their child. Instead, the time is to be spent having fun, whether it be playing a game, reading a book, preparing a snack, taking a hike, riding bikes, painting together, driving to the mall, or any other enjoyable activity.

Second, select six skills from the LSQ that they would like to establish during the parenting program. For each of the selected items, the parent is to attempt to determine what is interfering with skill development. Sometimes, the parent has selected a skill that is beyond the child's ability. More often, the parent only teaches in the middle of an emotional storm or has never actually shown the child what the parent wants done. Most often, the parents are using some type of big reward or punishment (an offer to take the child to a movie; grounding for the weekend) or are failing to apply any type of consequence for the child's actions, other than yelling. Parents are requested to record the results of their analysis and also record the kinds of activities that they are enjoying with their child each day.

Class 4: Motivational Strategies That Work

In this class, we examine the kinds of motivational strategies that parents have been using to teach their children new skills and introduce several new strategies that have emerged from our clinical research.

Class Content

1. Review parent journals, examining the impediments to their child's skill development.
2. Examine the limitations of mood management (i.e., setting limits only when angry or frustrated), the practical difficul-

ties of creating and maintaining home token programs or behavioral charts, the conflict associated with take aways (i.e., removing a privilege because of misbehavior), and the failure of children with ADHD to respond to large rewards (e.g., earning a trip to a vacation attraction).

3. Describe the following motivational strategies:

   (a) Dividing the day into four parts (before school, at school, before dinner, and after dinner): Parents are to decide on the tasks that the child is to perform during each of these periods.

   (b) Work-for-Play Rule: The child needs to complete the required tasks for a specific period to be permitted the reward of permission to engage in pleasurable activities of his or her choice. It is this freedom to be involved in activities of his or her choosing that is the primary reward used in this parenting program. If the child fails to complete the required tasks for a specific time period, he or she is not permitted to engage in reward activities until he or she has done so.

   (c) Time Stands Still: This is a nonconfrontational approach for addressing defiance and oppositionalism. If a child refuses to perform the required task, the parent informs him or her that his or her life is "on hold" and the child does not have permission to engage in any pleasurable activity until he or she completes the assigned task. The parent is instructed not to attempt to physically coerce or restrain the child, rather to simply encourage the child to comply to avoid the need to apologize and make up for his or her misbehavior.

   (d) Apologies and Amends: As humans, we all make mistakes. When we do, we need to apologize and offer to perform an action that indicates that we are sorry. In this parenting program, an effort is made to teach social reciprocity through this strategy. If a child says or does something that is hurtful, he or she is required to apologize and perform a task that communicates regret before engaging in pleasurable activities.

   (e) The Parent–Child Nonaggression Pact: Parents are encouraged to experiment with the notion that "it's not okay for any member of a family to yell, scream, strike, criticize, or threaten another member of the family." For the remainder of the parenting program, we invite parents to establish the following rule: If any family member acts in an aggressive way (including mom and dad), he or she will apologize and offer to do some type of act to show he or she is sorry. This strategy is used to model nonaggression in the home and reinforce the value of apologizing and making amends in our relationships with others.

Homework

Parents are requested to decide on the types of tasks to be performed by their child during each time period of the day. They are also requested to experiment with the types of motivational strategies taught during the class and record any problems in implementation in their journal. We continue to encourage 15 minutes of recreational time each day with their child and to stress the importance of healthy dietary, sleep, and exercise patterns. We also encourage them to begin holding family meetings (with their children) after their weekly parent planning session and to initiate these meetings with a discussion of the Parent–Child Nonaggression Pact.

Class 5: Problems of Emotional Control

This class represents a shift from general instruction to specific applications. By this time in our program, children are beginning to respond to a combination of improved dietary, sleep, and exercise habits. Their school districts have developed or revised IEP or 504 Plans, so school is becoming less stressful. They are being treated with medications that have been titrated to optimize response. They are enjoying daily fun time with their parents. Although home life is not perfect, parents have begun to see movement on specific goals and have noted that their children are beginning to respond to the motivational strategies taught in our program.

Despite these positive changes, there are a variety of problems that continue to trouble parents. For some, the concerns center on issues of emotional control (e.g., loss of temper, statements suggestive of depression, anxiety). For others, issues of impulsivity, disorganization, social skills deficits, and impairment of problem-solving skills are the primary concerns. During the next four classes, we focus on each of these areas.

Class Content

1. Review parent progress in implementing motivational strategies.
2. Present the types of emotional control problems demonstrated by children and adolescents with ADHD (e.g., outbursts of anger, excessive worry, depressive reactions).
3. Discuss the types of medications used to treat emotional control problems (e.g., antihypertensives, antidepressants).
4. Provide instruction in anger management skills (e.g., systematic deep breathing, rational "self-talk" designed to help the

patient identify "What do you want . . . what can you do to make it happen when frustrated?") and practice these skills in session.

5. Discuss calming activities (exercising, participating in physical activities of a nonaggressive nature, listening to music, journaling, drawing, playing music).

6. Present the essentials of desensitization, the value of facing fears, and the importance of a child's participation in activities that matter to peers; being good at activities that count for a child's age contributes to a sense of self-esteem and confidence that can lessen anxiety and depressed mood.

7. Review ways to teach children effective ways to communicate frustration and disappointment.

Homework

For this class, we request that parents review goals from the LSQ that are related to emotional control and develop a plan that incorporates strategies taught in this class. Again, we encourage parents to record their plan and their child's progress in their journal so that we can brainstorm ways to improve their teaching approach in our next class.

Class 6: Problems of Impulse Control

Although medications help to reduce the frequency of impulsive behaviors, children with ADHD will continue to act in thoughtless ways in a variety of situations. In this class, we ask parents to consider ways that they could help their children learn to control impulsivity.

Class Content

1. Review journal records of the prior week and troubleshoot parenting strategies that do not appear successful.

2. Assist parents in defining the types of impulsive behaviors that continue to be exhibited by their children.

3. Review the steps for eliminating an impulsive behavior: inform the child about the impulsive behavior in a nonstressful, nonconflictual teaching moment; inform the child what the desired behavior is in the situation in which he or she is acting impulsively; review the motivational strategies that will be used to promote the reduction of the impulsive behavior (typically Apologies and Amends).

4. Practice these steps with parents, using examples of impulsivity described in this class, role-playing in the class as needed.

Homework

Parents are requested to select one type of impulsive behavior to be addressed during the week. As with other types of skill development, we encourage them to initiate instruction during a family meeting, being brief and specific in their instruction and making sure to mention the motivational strategies that they will use to teach impulse control.

Class 7: Problems of Organization and Responsibility

One of the most common complaints that we hear from parents is about the disorganization and irresponsibility of their children. Parents tell us that their children can't keep track of anything. Their clothes are strewn all over the place. These parents have essentially become their child's brain, keeping track of everything, including the location of books, papers, favorite shirts, swimsuit, sneakers, toys, and so on. The parents have to remind their children over and over and over again about the basics, ranging from brushing teeth and changing clothes to taking a shower and actually using soap. In this class, we begin to review those organizational problems that have persisted despite previous interventions and to guide parents in ways to improve completion of essential organizational tasks.

Class Content

1. Review parent journals and troubleshoot efforts to improve impulse control, as well as other previously taught lessons.
2. Discuss organizational issues, emphasizing the need to organize personal possessions, family possessions, and time (appointments, schedules).
3. Define parental goals regarding organization of the child's possessions, the child's role in organizing family possessions, and the child's schedule.
4. Review the importance of instructing the child in organization, establishing a time line for completing tasks and the use of previously presented motivational strategies to ensure compliance.

Homework

Parents are requested to define at least one organizational goal, present this task during a family meeting, and use motivational strategies taught in our class to promote compliance.

Class 8: Teaching Problem-Solving Skills to Preteens and Teenagers

One of the most important lessons that we teach children is how to resolve a conflict with another person, particularly when the conflict prevents the child from obtaining some desired goal. In this class, we teach parents a relatively simple strategy for solving interpersonal problems. The basic principle is that when people say "no" to a request, typically they do so because they either need something or are afraid of something. We teach parents to help children to identify what needs or fears are blocking them from getting what they want, resist the urge to argue or criticize, and seek to find ways to address these fears, so that they can get what they want.

Class Content

1. Review parent progress in teaching organization.
2. Describe the steps for effective problem solving.
3. Identify the fears or needs of the person saying "no."
4. Brainstorm ways to address each fear or need.
5. Develop a plan to address these issues so that you can get what you want.
6. Practice and role-play problem solving with parents.

Homework

Parents are requested to teach this problem-solving strategy during their family meeting time and to use it at least once during the week.

Class 9: Helping Your Child Succeed With Peers

In the earlier classes, we discussed a variety of strategies to help children with ADHD succeed at home. In this class, we focus on helping kids with ADHD find success in peer relationships.

Class Content

1. Review parent progress in teaching problem-solving skills.
2. Present strategies for promoting increased success with peers.
3. Take steps to ensure that the child is involved in school-based activities each season of the year. It does not matter if the activity involves sports, music, drama, art, or community service. The key element is that the activity occurs at school, with classmates, and involves performing some type of action that is observed by others (desensitizing them to fear of failure). For children who are too young to participate in such activities at school, exposing them to the types of activities that will be available to them at the middle and high school levels is helpful.
4. Help the child socialize with classmates outside of school.
5. Because children with ADHD often do not know the names and phone numbers of classmates, parents often can help by

finding out such information while working on bake sales, and other school activities and fund raisers.

6. Teach conversational skills to the child, because patients with ADHD often will either speak excessively or not say anything in social settings.

7. Instruct the child in strategies for responding to teasing (i.e., acknowledge the truth of what is said, do not look sad or mad, remain calm, cheerfully oblivious, and maintain an unbothered "whatever" look, that says, "I'm not scared of you, I mean you no harm, but I don't want to play the teasing game").

Homework

Encourage parents to review the strategies presented in the class, and initiate at least one in the coming week.

Class 10: Promoting Self-Care in Parents of Children With ADHD

In the last class of the parenting program, we focus on identifying ways that parents can maintain the level of energy needed to effectively parent children with ADHD for the 2 decades (or so) of childhood. We provide a description of four strategies that can boost the spirits of parents during the toughest days and nights.

Class Content

1. Review the results of parental efforts to improve their child's peer relationships.

2. Describe four self-care strategies.

   (a) Engage in three pleasurable activities each day (e.g., picking enjoyable foods to eat, music to listen to, a television program to watch, a book or other reading material; making a phone call to a friend or family member).

   (b) Establish healthy dietary, sleep, and exercise patterns.

   (c) Set some type of goal or dream and begin to pursue it. In our class, we give a list of sentence stems to promote the process of goal setting, for instance, "If I weren't so old, I'd . . ."; "If I weren't so afraid, I'd . . ."; "Even though it's silly, I'd like to . . ."; "There's nothing like . . ."; "I really would like it if me and my dad, mom, brother, sister, or spouse and I could . . ."; "I always wanted to teach my child to . . ."; "I always wanted to learn to . . . ."

   (d) Set aside part of 1 day each week to enjoy the company of your spouse or loved one; if possible, get away for an overnight vacation each season.

At the conclusion of the program, we invite parents to remain in contact, as needed, to address residual areas of difficulty. Participation in a support group (e.g., Children and Adults With Attention Deficit/Hyperactivity Disorder [CHADD]) is also recommended.

IMPLICATIONS FOR CLINICAL PRACTICE

Structured clinical programs for promoting more effective parenting strategies to address a variety of residual functional problems in children and adolescents with ADHD have been developed for use in clinical practice and have demonstrated at least short-term benefits. However, because children will encounter new social problems as they proceed through the various developmental stages and risk relapse, strategies for follow-up counseling for parents are needed. A challenge for practitioners is to develop parenting programs that provide both instruction and systematic follow-up as there is evidence that clinical gains may dissipate within 24 months without such care.

To address such needs, innovative programs that provide such follow-up have begun to emerge, including the Parent-to-Parent networks being encouraged by CHADD (see http://www.chadd.org). Similar support networks can also be coordinated by practitioners who provide care to a substantial number of families including a member diagnosed with ADHD. Other strategies for providing follow-up care include the development of Internet blogs; computer networking facilitated by free Internet telephone carriers, such as Skype (see http://www.skype.com), which would permit parents to listen to guidance provided by experts in the field; and weekly mental health segments on local news programs. For the gains noted in parenting programs to be sustained, ongoing support is needed.

11

SOCIAL SKILLS TRAINING FOR CHILDREN AND TEENS WITH ADHD: THE NEUROEDUCATIONAL LIFE SKILLS PROGRAM

As reviewed in chapter 1, children with attention-deficit/hyperactivity disorder (ADHD) display a wide range of functional problems that persist even after effective pharmacological treatment has been initiated and maintained. At our clinic, and other specialized ADHD treatment centers, social skills programs for patients with ADHD have been developed to address such areas of functional impairment. There is initial evidence that children and adolescents can learn certain skills through reinforced practice (Frankel, Myatt, Cantwell, & Feinberg, 1997; Hinshaw et al., 2000; Monastra, Monastra, & George, 2002; Pelham & Hoza, 1996; Pfiffner & McBurnett, 1997) and that such training appears particularly effective when a combination of patient social skills training and parent training is provided in the context of effective treatment of the underlying neurological factors responsible for symptom onset and maintenance (Arnold et al., 2004; P. S. Jensen, Hinshaw, Swanson, et al., 2001). However, it is unclear how enduring these training

197

effects may be, as there is evidence that the superiority of combined pharmacological and behavioral treatments (vs. intensive medication management) dissipates within 24 months (Multimodal Treatment Study of Children With ADHD Cooperative Group, 2004).

On the basis of earlier studies (Barkley, Edwards, Laneri, Fletcher, & Metevia, 2001; Frankel et al., 1997; Monastra et al., 2002; Pelham & Hoza, 1996), several areas of intervention appeared critical to include in an instructional program for children and adolescents with ADHD. Initially, presentation of those self-care skills (e.g., eating, sleeping, exercise habits) that are the foundation of attention and behavioral control needed to be reviewed. In addition, the low self-confidence, impaired conflict resolution skills, deficient conversational skills, inadequate mood regulation, and disorganization exhibited by our patients also required intervention. Given the need to facilitate generalization of skills to home and other settings, systematic involvement of parents also seemed necessary, as reported by Cousins and Weiss (1993); Pfiffner and McBurnett (1997); and Tutty, Gephart, and Wurzbacher (2003).

Consequently, we developed a life skills program that includes a pretreatment session with the patient and a parent to review the nature of ADHD, the rationale for our life skills program, and the kinds of skills that they wanted to develop. We incorporated a 10-session instructional group for children and parents, with an additional five sessions to practice skills that appeared more difficult to master (e.g., conversation, emotional control, problem solving). We also provide follow-up skill training sessions for children and parents, as needed.

An essential component of our program is that instruction is provided in a context that includes the patient and at least one parent. We have found that such a format helps to keep the students on task, ensures that parents are informed about the content of each session, provides an opportunity for parents and children to practice skills in an educational setting with guidance, enables parents and children to team up to compete in group activities, facilitates completion of homework assignments, and sets the stage for socialization with class members outside of the clinic setting.

An additional requirement for participation in our life skills program is that the child's core ADHD symptoms are being effectively treated. Children who are unable to remain seated, attend during instruction, and remain in control over impulsive behavior are unlikely to profit from classes until these symptoms are addressed. On a similar note, including such a child in the class setting is likely to disrupt instruction, limiting the acquisition of new skills by members. Consequently, we delay involving students in our life skills program until they are able to attend, sit still, and not interrupt, hence are more likely to profit from instruction.

PRETREATMENT ORIENTATION SESSION

During this meeting, the child and his or her parent(s) receive an overview of the life skills program. The initial focus emphasizes helping the child understand the purpose of the classes and what occurs during meetings. The following presentation illustrates one example of how this orientation is provided by a therapist.

Katie, your mom and dad have told me that you are having a hard time at school. Kids are teasing you, you don't have too many friends, and it's starting to bug you. I want to help you out. I'd like you to think about signing up for a class that we have for kids to help them with these kinds of problems. Let me give you an idea of what our classes are like.

Have your parents ever taken you to a swim class? [Most kids say, "yes"]. They did it because they wanted you to learn how to survive in the water. You'd go to the class, hang out with other kids and their parents, and the teacher would teach you some very important skills. At our clinic, we have a different kind of class. It's a class that will teach you how to succeed on the land, in your everyday life. We call it a "Life Skills Class."

The idea of grown-ups teaching kids how to survive is not a new one. A long time ago, before we had television, DVDs, video games, and computers, families and their neighbors would sit together in the evening and talk about what happened that day. The kids would run around and play games for awhile. But after it started to get dark, people would sit by the fire and tell stories. Sometimes, the stories were funny; sometimes the stories were scary; and sometimes the stories were meant to teach kids valuable life lessons.

Parents and the older members of the community would talk about where to go to catch the biggest fish. They'd teach kids what kinds of plants were good to eat and what kinds were poisonous. They'd teach kids what kinds of animals were friendly and what kinds were dangerous. They'd teach kids how to grow vegetables, make bread, sew clothes, and build a home. Just as important, they'd teach kids how to get along with their neighbors, solve problems peacefully, and become a kind and caring member of their community.

Our class is similar to those meetings. Each time we get together, we'll share a meal and talk about your week. The kids decide what we're eating, so it's usually pretty good stuff. After we eat, we'll teach the class one lesson that should help each kid live a better life. We'll teach you about the foods that help us to be able to concentrate better, and how sleep and exercise are important too. We'll teach you how to calm down when you get frustrated and how to negotiate to get what you want in life, without hurting other people. If you have a hard time having conversations with other kids, or are getting teased a lot, we'll share some tips with you. We'll talk about ways you can become more confident.

After we teach the lesson, you and your mom or dad will practice with the other kids. Then we'll have a kind of game in which you and your parent will compete with other families. The winner wins some cash! After the game, everybody heads home and, we hope, practices what we taught. Oftentimes, kids make some pretty good friends in the class and start hanging out together. So it is a pretty good deal. What do you think?

At that point, the child and his or her parents will typically have a variety of questions. Usually, the first questions include "What do we eat?" and "How much money can you win?" However, some of the kids will be hesitant to participate in such a group. Rather than trying to convince them, I will simply reflect on the kinds of problems that are happening and offer our help, letting them know that we are here to help them feel better and succeed in life. If the child wants to visit a class or two before deciding to join, that's fine. If the child wants to try to handle a particular situation on his or her own for a month or 2, that's fine: "We'll get together in a couple months and see how it's going. If the problems have gone away, great! If not, we're here to help."

THE NEUROEDUCATIONAL LIFE SKILLS PROGRAM FOR CHILDREN AND TEENAGERS

This program is conducted in 15 weekly classes. Each class lasts about 75 minutes. Children in Grades 3 through 11 have participated. At least one of their parents must attend and participate each week. We limit the group to no more than 8 children and parent teams: We group children as follows—primary: children in Grades 3, 4, and 5 (depending on interests); intermediate: children in Grades 5, 6, 7, and 8 (depending on interests); secondary: children in Grades 8, 9, 10, and 11.

Fifth- and eighth-grade students are placed with peers who have similar interest patterns. Some fifth graders have interests more consistent with older students; some, with younger ones. The same holds true for our eighth graders. As described previously, the session includes a meal (e.g., chicken nuggets, fries, and vegetables with fruit drink; pizza with fruit drink; tacos with fruit drink; roast beef sandwiches with curly fries and fruit drink) while we review the previous week's homework. After the meal and review, the instructor presents a brief lesson (15–20 minutes). The students then practice the lesson with their parent(s) and other students in the class. Finally, we play a game that is related to the day's lesson, and one child–parent team wins $10. This gives children practice each week in handling the frustration of losing and how to be a gracious winner. A homework assignment is given each week.

Over the years, we have experimented with different types of lessons. After 2 decades, we have developed a core curriculum of the following 10 lessons. A brief description of each class lesson, the practice exercise(s), and games used follows. As with our parenting program, a handout, summarizing the day's lesson, is provided to each student and his or her parents. Copies of these handouts can be provided upon written request (see http://www.theADHDdoc.com).

Because some lessons are more difficult to learn than others, we do not proceed to the next lesson until either each child has demonstrated mastery of the skill or the parent and child report that the patient is actively practicing the skill at home and in school settings. As a result, we may continue to review and practice a specific skill for several classes. In school districts that have adopted our program, the class may continue for a semester or the entire school year.

SESSION SUMMARIES

To facilitate the development of life skills programs in outpatient clinical settings, the following sections provide the instructional templates used in our class presentation. The participants in our programs are patients diagnosed with ADHD, who attend classes with at least one parent or guardian. The fee for each class is $20.

Class 1. Ya Gotta Eat, Ya Gotta Sleep, and Ya Gotta Get Some Exercise if You Want To Succeed in Life

Lesson: Part A

In this portion of the class, children are taught what kinds of foods help us to concentrate better in the morning and afternoon. We teach children how to estimate the protein content of various common foods and how much protein should be eaten at breakfast and lunch according to the *Recommended Dietary Allowances* published by the Food and Nutrition Board of the National Academy of Sciences (1989, approximately 10 g for primary grades; 15–20 g for intermediate grades; 20–30 g for junior and senior high school).

Practice: Part A

We play a game in session called "Test Your Food IQ." We present 15 different food pairs and ask kids and their parents to decide which of the two foods has more protein. The child–parent score from this task is tallied and will be combined with another task later in the session to determine who wins the cash reward.

Lesson: Part B

Children are next taught about the importance of getting 30 minutes of exercise each day. Because some of our children are pretty sedentary and others are involved in activities only two to three times per week, we demonstrate four basic exercises that are relatively easy to perform by anyone yet require the effort of multiple muscle groups.

Practice: Part B

There are four exercises that we practice with the kids and their parents:

1. *Easy push-up.* Kneel down (on hands and knees). Place your hands about 6 to 9 inches in front of your shoulders. Lean forward, touch your chin on the ground, lean back. Repeat 10 to 15 times.
2. *The plank.* Lie on your back. Place your arms in front of you, elbows bent. Now push off with your toes and forearms, rising up and holding your body flat, sort of like a platform or the plank of a boat. Hold the position for a count of 5. Repeat 10 to 15 times.
3. *Superman or Superwoman.* Lie on your back. Extend your hands as far as you can reach and point your toes straight back, extending them as far as you can. Hold the position for a count of 5. Repeat 10 to 15 times.
4. *Wall squat.* Place your back against the frame of a door or against a wall. Extend your arms straight out. Slide down the wall, bending your knees until you are nearly in a seated position. Hold the position for a count of 5. Repeat 10 to 15 times.

Part C

The last part of instruction is a review of the minimum requirements of sleep. For younger children, we recommend 10 hours of sleep; for teens, 8 to 9 hours minimum.

Challenge Game

In today's session, each child–parent pair teams up for a game of table-top basketball (or other table-top sports games, in keeping with the exercise theme). Each team tries to make as many baskets as they can in 1 minute. The total number of baskets is added to the total from the Food IQ game. The winning team gets a check for $10, after thanking the other kids for a good game. The other kids offer some words of congratulations.

Homework

This week, the children are asked to keep track of how many days they meet sleep, diet, and exercise guidelines. We provide them with a list of the protein content of a variety of foods that are commonly eaten by children, as well as the *Recommended Dietary Allowances* (Food and Nutrition Board of the National Academy of Sciences, 1989). We recommend that parents incorporate these requirements as part of how their child earns his or her free play periods.

Class 2. Calm Down! Breathe

Lesson

In this class, students are taught the value of breathing in maintaining emotional control. We demonstrate that yelling, whining, and screaming are ways that infants and toddlers use to get their way. We refer to statements such as "that's not fair" as what 3-year-olds say when they can't get what they want. We teach our students that everyone else needs to learn how to breathe when upset, calm down, and say nothing until they have the answer to two questions: (a) What do you want, and (b) what can you do to make it happen?

During our instruction, we stress the power of breathing, emphasizing that breathing is more powerful than anger, fear, and sadness. We teach that when a person is in a situation in which they experience a rush of anger (e.g., due to frustration), fear (e.g., due to an anxiety-provoking situation), or sadness (e.g., due to an awareness of a potential loss), the feeling of anger, fear, or sadness will dissipate if they can reestablish a calm, natural, deep breathing pattern. Once breathing is reestablished, a person can identify what they want, as well as strategies to make it happen.

Practice

During our practice phase, we demonstrate that breathing stops and becomes very shallow when people get angry, scared, or sad. Heart rate increases and a person starts to feel uncomfortable. However, if a person starts to bring more air to their brain (by breathing more deeply with each breath), then the brain wakes up, and the person starts to calm down and is able to figure out how to get what they want. We practice a type of counting breathing exercise in which we start with a breath while mentally counting to 1, hold the breath for a 3 count, and then release. Then we all take a breath, while mentally counting to 2, hold the breath for a 3 count, and then release. We continue this process until we can take in a breath (while mentally counting to 10), hold the breath for a 3 count, and release.

Challenge Game

In this class, each parent–child team takes turn taking a deep breath and holding it until they can't hold it any longer. We time the parent and the child and total their time. Best total score wins $10!

Homework

We ask the children to practice this breathing exercise once per day. Parents are to include this practice as one of their child's tasks each day.

Class 3. Increasing Self-Confidence: Part 1

Lesson

In this class, we review two sources of self-confidence. The first is getting good at something that counts to kids your age. The second is facing fears.

Practice

During the class, each child–parent pair develops two lists, one of the skills that matter to other kids; the other, the child's fear list. We use the prompt "If I weren't so afraid, I'd _____" to trigger the fear list.

Challenge Game

After the children complete the lists, we ask them to circle one fear that they think that no one would guess and give the instructor the sheets. The instructor then selects 15 fears and asks the children to guess who wrote that specific fear. Winner is the one who guesses the most correctly.

Homework

Children are instructed to pick at least one skill that they want to get good at and one fear that they want to face. Again, home practice of this skill is part of each child's daily responsibility, to be reinforced using strategies reviewed in chapter 10.

Class 4. Increasing Self-Confidence: Part 2

Lesson

In this class, we teach children that self-confidence is also increased by making and keeping friends. We teach two basic rules: Rule 1 is that everyone is interested in something, and Rule 2 is that most everyone likes to talk about their interests. Because most children with ADHD don't really pay close attention to what other people like, we begin by focusing on learning the interests of others.

Practice

To help kids begin to learn about the interests of others, we ask the children to look closely at the other kids in the room. We give each child a sheet of paper and write down his or her guess as to one interest that each other kid has. Afterward, we ask the kids to read their guesses aloud and to indicate the reasons for their guesses (e.g., the logo on the child's shirt, a comment the other kid made). We tally the number of correct guesses.

Challenge Game

For this game, we ask each child–parent team to complete a list of questions about the interests of each other. The questions include simple items such as their favorite food, TV show, and room in the house and what they like to do for fun. More personal items (e.g., what makes the other person angry, sad, or proud) are also included. We tally the number of matches and add it to the score from the peer guessing game. The winner gets $10.

Homework

At dinner time, each child is requested to bring up one topic that he or she thinks their mom, dad, sister, or brother would like to discuss.

Class 5. Even Conversations Can Be Fun!

Lesson

Most children with ADHD have a lot of interests and like to be active. This works out great during those preschool and early childhood years, when laughing and running around and playing games are what counts. However, as children get older, the ability to have a conversation and show enthusiasm about the interests of others (as well as themselves) becomes as important. In this class, we teach children several tips for having good conversations:

> *Tip 1:* Before you leave home each day, think about a couple of topics that you can bring up in a conversation at school. It could be something you played the night before; it could be something that happened at home; or it could be something you watched on TV. Try to have three stories that you could bring up.
>
> *Tip 2:* Learn about the interests of other kids in school. Play detective, listen, and learn. Then take the time to bring up something related to their interests. The best kinds of conversations are when you are talking about something of interest to you and the other person.
>
> *Tip 3:* Be a minute minder. Try to learn what a minute feels like and try not to speak for longer than a minute before you ask the other person some version of "What do you think?"
>
> *Tip 4:* Show some enthusiasm. If you are not enthused about what you are talking about, how could anyone else be?

Practice

In this part of the session, we pair students with each other and practice having 3-minute conversations. We have parents work as coaches, helping kids to watch the 1-minute rule described in Tip 3, and help the flow of conversation from the interests of one kid to the interests of another.

Challenge Game

We randomly pair the kids up for a 3-minute conversation. The other kids rate the team (1–10) for how well they took turns in sharing interests, minded the 1-minute rule, and showed enthusiasm. Each member of the team with the highest rating wins $10.

Homework

This week, the children are requested to have one conversation per day with a member of their family in which they talk about one interest and also discuss an interest of the other person.

Class 6. Ignoring Teasing Will Not Make It Go Away

Lesson

In this class, we discuss why kids tease each other and strategies for dealing with this common problem. We talk about a simple fact: Teasing is a pathetic way that some kids use to feel good about themselves. Although everyone will get teased, the kids who are targeted are the ones who lack confidence and a way of showing the bullies "I'm not afraid of you; I mean you no harm, but I'm not interested in playing the teasing game."

Practice

During this session, we ask the kids to tell us the most common teases in their school. We then demonstrate a look that shows "you don't scare me" and words that express "I don't waste my time on the teasing game." The first step is helping kids practice their "you don't scare me" look in response to teasing. Everyone has their version of the look. So we take turns teasing each other and practicing "the look." Mirrors and video cameras can be used to help provide feedback to the students. Then we review brief statements that say "I'm not interested in the teasing game": could be a "whatever," could be "I think teasing is a waste of time," could be agreeing with the tease (e.g., "Sure, I'm overweight . . . and your point is?").

Sometimes kids express concerns about another student being physically violent toward them in school. In that type of situation, talking does little good. We instruct children, if hit, kicked, pushed into a locker, and so on, to turn toward the attacker, and in a loud, attention-drawing voice, say some version of "there must be something seriously wrong with you to act like that" and immediately go to the building principal or disciplinary office. Kids who act in a violent way need treatment, and it makes no sense for parents, teachers, or administrators to act like it's a normal part of life. It's not!

Challenge Game

For this class, we make a teasing comment to the entire class. Each child is given a paper and pencil to write down as many things as he or she can think of to say in 5 minutes. Students receive no credit if they write a teasing or aggressive comeback.

Homework

Practice responding to potential or actual forms of "teasing" with parents.

Class 7. Sometimes Making Faces Can Be A Good Idea

Lesson

In this class, we emphasize the importance of facial expressions in establishing friendships. We discuss how showing a face that says "I care about you and what you're saying" can help establish and keep friendships. Just as when we practiced the "I am not afraid; I mean you no harm" look, we practice "I care about you, I'm interested" actions in this class. Among the behaviors we review are the following: look at people when they talk, smile or nod when you like or agree with what is said, give a puzzled look when confused, and say something that shows interest (e.g., ask a question, request more information).

Practice

In this session, we work with parent–child pairs first. We ask the parent to begin a conversation and have the child practice his or her "I care" face. Next, we practice making an "I'm interested" or "I'm confused" look or statement. Last, we pair the children up for conversations. As in the previous class, mirrors and video cameras can be helpful.

Challenge Game

During the pairing of children for conversations, we ask the other kids to rate the facial expressions of each other during conversations. We ask kids to rate (1–10) how well other kids' faces show "I'm interested" or "I'm confused."

Homework

Children are asked to practice their "I care" faces during conversations with their parents.

Class 8. Getting What You Want In Life Without Getting Into Trouble

Lesson

In this class, we review the essentials of problem solving. We teach children that when someone says "no" to them, there are two primary reasons getting in the way: (a) The other person (mom, dad, friend, etc.) is afraid of something or (b) the other person needs something.

Getting what you want requires a person to find out what the other person needs and/or fears and figure out a way to address those issues. Once those issues are addressed, the child can typically get what he or she wants.

Practice

During this class, we practice the three components of problem solving:

- determining the other person's fear;
- determining the other person's need; and
- generating ideas to address those needs and fears while getting what the student wants.

We typically generate several scenarios in which a child is told "no" and ask students to generate lists of possible fears and needs. We then conduct a practice activity with their parent in which they ask for something they truly want but their parent must say "no." We coach the child in discovering needs and fears and developing a solution to get what they want.

Challenge Game

We present a typical scenario in which a child is told "no." The students are given a paper and pencil and asked to write down as many needs and fears as they can generate in a 5-minute period. The winner is the student who generates the most.

Class 9. Organization Is Not A Four-Letter Word

Lesson

In this class, we review the basics of organization: Everyone needs to develop a system for organizing their stuff and responsibilities. In addition, we introduce the concept that organization is not just about taking care of what is important to others. It is also about planning to achieve personal goals and dreams.

Practice

During the class, we pair students and parents to determine where books, papers, clothes, toys, food, and dishes are to go and the time frame for accomplishing these tasks. We also talk about how each student prefers to keep track of their schedule (e.g., dry marker board in their room). Finally, we ask them to write down one dream or goal they have. We'll develop an action plan for their dream during the next session.

Challenge Game

Because the lesson is centered on pick up, we typically play a pick-up game. Being a psychologist, I have the Lafayette Pegboard available. However, there are lots of other types of puzzle boards that could be used. The student who completes the puzzle in the shortest time wins.

Homework

This week, the assignment is to establish a place for stuff and a way to keep track of important dates. A time frame for maintaining organization is also recommended.

Class 10. Anyone Can Have A Dream: Successful People Make Dreams Come True

Lesson

In this class, we teach children that with planning, many things that we want and many activities we'd like to try can happen. We also stress that it is not getting stuff that counts, it is the process of pursuing what we want that seems to be beneficial. People who believe that they are free to pursue personal goals typically feel better than those who do not have that belief. Determining goals and planning ways to make our goals happen is another habit that builds self-confidence and life satisfaction.

Practice

We provide students with a list of sentence stems to generate possible goals, including "I always wanted my dad to _____"; "I think it would be neat if my mom and I could _____"; "I'd like to be able to do with my Grandpa or Grandma _____"; "I really wish that my brother or sister and I could _____"; "I think it would be great to have a friend who would _____"; "I really wish that I were better at _____"; "I'd love to have enough money to be able to _____"; and "I always wanted to go to _____." Once the list is completed, we ask the students to pick one goal and write down the roadblocks and ways to overcome them. Finally, we ask the parent–child pair to develop a game plan to make their goal happen.

Challenge Game

We end the class series the same way we began, with a game of table-top basketball.

Homework

Put the game plan into action.

Follow-Up Consultations

After the conclusion of the 15-week program, we have attempted to provide follow-up classes on a bimonthly and monthly basis. However, attendance is typically quite low for such classes. The most common reason given by parents is the absence of any significant crisis in the child's life and the positive, short-term benefits of the program. During our follow-up phone consultations, we have found that most of the children continue to demonstrate improved dietary, exercise, and sleeping habits. On a similar note, the majority of our patients have begun to participate in activities of interest to peers (which conflicts with attendance at our follow-up classes) and are using the problem-solving techniques taught in our class. The most common issues presented in our follow-up sessions center on issues of emotional control, struggles to handle teasing, and difficulty in generating ideas for conversation. Therefore, in our follow-up classes, we often practice these skills. We have been particularly interested in examining the response of children to a variety of word fluency and working memory tasks (e.g., games such as Outburst and Scattergories, word fluency challenges in which students are asked to generate words beginning with a particular letter or within a specific category or both). However, at this time, our research is in a preliminary phase with respect to the impact of such practice on fluency and working memory during conversations (Monastra & Carlson-Gotz, 2006).

IMPLICATIONS FOR CLINICAL PRACTICE

At present, there are multiple models for promoting the development of social, or life, skills. The models that appear to hold the greatest promise integrate parent training and skills classes for children and provide instruction in a context that includes effective pharmacological treatment of the core symptoms of ADHD. However, there are insufficient data regarding ways to optimize the learning process and enhance generalization to a broader range of social environments.

The program developed and used at our clinic represents one approach for promoting such skills in multiple social contexts. In contrast with previous programs, it does not require multiple therapists, counselors, or aides. Instead, parents serve as "assistant teachers" to help teach skills and promote generalization to other settings. As a result, the Neuroeducational Life Skills Program (NLSP) is more easily provided in a wide range of clinical settings. Although there is initial indication that this type of instructional format may optimize transfer of skills (Frankel et al., 1997), additional research examining programs such as the NLSP are needed. By providing practitioners with a detailed description for conducting the NLSP, it is hoped that traditional counseling sessions for children and parents can shift to a more skill-building approach and that systematic clinical studies examining this model can be conducted.

12

SPECIAL ISSUES IN THE TREATMENT OF ADULTS WITH ADHD

Between 30% and 70% of individuals diagnosed with attention-deficit/ hyperactivity disorder (ADHD) during childhood will continue to exhibit moderate to severe levels of inattentive, hyperactive, and impulsive symptoms as adults (Barkley, Fischer, Smallish, & Fletcher, 2003; Mannuzza, Klein, Bessler, Malloy, & LaPadula, 1993, 1998; Rasmussen & Gillberg, 2001; M. Weiss & Hechtman, 1993). Of these patients, approximately 75% will also present symptoms of other psychiatric disorders, including major depressive disorder, anxiety disorders, personality disorders (e.g., antisocial, passive–aggressive, borderline, histrionic), conduct disorders, and psychoactive substance abuse and/or dependence disorders. Significant functional impairment persists in academic, occupational, and social contexts in the vast majority of these patients.

Because of the multiple types of psychiatric and functional problems exhibited by adults presenting for an evaluation, access to information from a variety of sources is essential in establishing a differential diagnosis. However, obtaining such information is not as easily achieved in adults as it is with children. Adults with ADHD do not routinely arrive for evaluation sessions accompanied by a parent or spouse, nor do they typically bring reports from their teachers or supervisors. Instead, they arrive alone, reporting a range of symptoms that meets diagnostic criteria for multiple psychiatric disorders (Barkley, 2002; Barkley, Murphy, & Kwasnik, 1996b; Murphy, Barkley, & Bush, 2002). In addition, these individuals display difficulties in word finding, memory, and organization of speech, which further impedes efforts to determine a differential diagnosis based on self-report. In such a context, accurate assessment and effective treatment can be compromised.

In this chapter, strategies for the assessment and treatment of adults with ADHD are reviewed. In contrast to the extensive literature with children and adolescents, the clinical research on the assessment and treatment of adults with ADHD is limited. However, despite these limitations, certain patterns have emerged from the existing literature, which can begin to guide clinical practice.

ASSESSMENT OF ADULTS WITH ADHD

The *Diagnostic and Statistical Manual of Mental Disorders* (4th ed., text rev.; *DSM–IV–TR*; American Psychiatric Association, 2000) makes no differentiation between adults and children with respect to the criteria for a diagnosis of ADHD. The diagnosis requires evidence of six of nine symptoms of inattention, six of nine symptoms of hyperactivity and impulsivity, or both. A childhood onset of symptoms, combined with evidence of a degree of symptomatology that is developmentally atypical and clear indication of significant functional impairment remain the cornerstones of the diagnosis. Finally, the diagnosis requires that these symptoms cannot be better accounted for by another psychiatric or medical disorder.

Practice guidelines, offered by Roy-Byrne et al. (1997); Murphy and Gordon (2006); Silver (2000); and Wender, Wolf, and Wasserstein (2001) suggest the use of a comprehensive semistructured clinical interview and the completion of rating scales in the assessment of adults. Although such sources of information can contribute to the assessment process, it is important for clinicians to realize that ratings of the presence and severity of core ADHD symptoms are greatly affected by the source of information. Adults who were diagnosed as children have been shown to report an extraordinarily low rate of symptom retention (e.g., 3%–5%: Barkley et al., 2003; 4%, 8%: Mannuzza et al., 1993 and 1998, respectively). In addition, previously diagnosed adults tend to report significantly lower impairment ratings than parent raters (Barkley, 2006; M. Fisher, 1997; Silver, 2000), although the opposite pattern has also been noted (Murphy & Gordon, 2006).

The high rate of discrepancies among the responses of multiple informants (Murphy & Gordon, 2006) further complicates the clinical interpretation of rating scales. Although Murphy and Gordon (2006) noted that "assessing the credibility of each source is crucial" (p. 440), there are no empirically founded guidelines for such a credibility check in clinical practice. Without incorporating other types of information (e.g., review of academic records from childhood, the results of a targeted medical evaluation assessing conditions known to impair attention and concentration in adults, analysis of performance on continuous performance tests [CPTs] and quantitative electroencephalographs [qEEGs]), the determination of ADHD in an adult based solely on the behavioral report from the patient should be considered provisional at best, pending the results of a more comprehensive assessment.

Investigations of the diagnostic accuracy of several commonly used rating scales—Conners' Adult ADHD Rating Scales (CAARS; Conners, Erhardt, & Sparrow, 1999), Attention Deficit Scales for Adults (ADSA; Triolo & Murphy, 1996), and the Wender Adult Questionnaire Childhood Characteristics Scale (AQCCS; Wender, 1985)—support the need for such caution. Although these scales appear sensitive to the presence of ADHD in adults (accurately identifying 65%–92% in studies reviewed by McCann and Roy-Byrne, 2004), they yield a potentially dangerously high rate of false positives among individuals without ADHD. For example, McCann, Scheele, Ward, and Roy-Byrne (2000) reported a 43% false positive rate for non-ADHD patients using the AQCCS. Their subsequent review of the literature indicated that between 36% and 67% of non-ADHD patients are falsely identified with ADHD according to behavioral rating scales such as the AQCCS, the CAARS, and the ADSA.

The high degree of discrepancy among informants, combined with the unacceptably high rate of false positives, poses a significant risk for patients who are screened for ADHD by practitioners who rely on such data to confirm a diagnosis of ADHD. As noted by McCann and Roy-Byrne (2004), "the implications of false positives in ADHD screening and diagnosis are potentially serious" and "self-report measures are very poor indicators of an ADHD diagnosis and are likely to produce an unacceptably high number of misdiagnoses" (p. 182).

In contrast, studies examining the diagnostic accuracy of both CPTs and qEEG procedures have yielded significantly higher rates of test sensitivity (see review in chap. 4). In addition, the false positive rate of qEEG screening measures is less than 10%. The high sensitivity and specificity of neuropsychological and neurophysiological measures support the use of such techniques, particularly in the assessment of patients whose clinical history is unclear (because of impairment of patient recall; lack of information from multiple informants; discrepancies among the ratings of multiple sources).

Therefore, similar to our conclusion regarding the process of assessment for children and adolescents, the evaluation of adults presenting for an evaluation of symptoms of inattention, impulsivity, and hyperactivity needs to be far more comprehensive than a clinical interview with the patient and the administration of behavioral rating scales, particularly when such data are provided by informants whose executive functions are suspect. As reviewed in chapter 3 (this volume), and emphasized by Braverman (1995, 2003) and Murphy and Gordon (2006), adults are at risk to develop numerous types of medical conditions that can produce symptoms of inattention, hyperactivity, and impulsivity, including thyroid disorders, diabetes, hypoglycemia, perimenopause, hormonal deficiencies, and heart and lung disease, in addition to the aging process. The assessment of such medical conditions is likewise essential in the evaluation of adults for ADHD.

To address *DSM–IV–TR* criteria for a diagnosis of ADHD, the assessment strategies described in the next section have proven to be helpful in our assessment of adults at our clinic.

Clinical History

In addition to conducting a comprehensive clinical interview with adult patients, conducting interviews with biological parents or childhood caretakers of patients to review early childhood symptoms can yield information that is essential to the diagnostic process. Although parents who are older may have difficulty completing a retrospective ADHD symptom checklist for their 30-, 40-, or 50-year-old son or daughter, they are often able to recall details of the patient's childhood medical, educational, and social histories that are relevant for a diagnosis of ADHD. It is not uncommon for a parent to recall that he or she took his or her child to a specialist because of concerns about the child's hearing or vision, even though the parent failed to report any significant attentional problems on the ADHD checklist.

On a similar note, it is not uncommon for the parents of our adult patients to recall that they had to "stay on top of their child" and "make sure their child did their homework every night" or that it took their child "all night long" to complete homework, beginning in middle school. Similar recollections about the use of private tutors, the need for summer school, delayed entry into kindergarten, retention in the primary grades, involvement in special education programs, or other indications of impaired school functioning can be quite helpful in the determination of age of symptom onset. In addition to information about functional problems, parental reports can also provide a great deal of information about potentially relevant medical conditions that contribute to attentional problems. It is rare that an adult patient is aware of his or her early childhood medical history, yet such information is highly relevant for determining the causes of symptom manifestation in childhood.

Review of Academic Records

Evidence of symptom manifestation during early childhood can also be obtained from a review of school records. However, most adults with ADHD are unsure where their academic records are stored. To facilitate the retrieval of such information, clinicians can assist the patient in contacting schools from their office, faxing necessary signatures to expedite the process. Practitioners may be surprised to learn that school districts archive student educational records in both electronic and paper formats. Even in the most abbreviated of such records, evidence of impairment is apparent when level of academic performance is substantially less than anticipated on the basis of estimated level of intelligence (which is also contained in such records).

Review of Medical History

Most patients have maintained a relationship with a primary physician during their adulthood. Clinicians can learn much about the presence of relevant medical conditions from directly examining the physician records of their patients. Because of the organizational problems of adult patients, practitioners can assist in this process by providing their patients with medical release forms and faxing or mailing them from their office.

Review of Pharmacy Records

Because it is often difficult to read the clinical notes from physicians, a review of the pharmacy records of an adult patient can also be informative. At minimum, it is often helpful to obtain a listing of medications taken during the past 5 years from the patient's pharmacist. Again, because of the impairment of working memory found in patients with ADHD, such records can provide a wealth of information about the patient's current medical status.

Consultation With Spouse, Family Members, and Other Significant Individuals

In addition to input from parents, interviews with others who have frequent contact with the patient can provide information regarding types of symptoms and areas of functional impairment. Such information is essential in the development of a comprehensive treatment plan.

Administration of Continuous Performance Tests

To help clarify diagnostic issues, it is quite useful to obtain an objective measure of capacity for attention, concentration, and behavioral control. Such measures are helpful both during the initial assessment phase and as an indicator of treatment response. Both visual and auditory tests can be helpful. We have found that individuals with a primary convergence insufficiency disorder score in the impaired range on the visual test but exhibit no such impairment on the auditory one. The converse has held true for those individuals with a primary central auditory processing disorder.

Quantitative Electroencephalographic Examination

On the basis of neuroscience findings that support the perspective that ADHD is associated with dysregulation of cortical arousal, a qEEG evaluation can also contribute to the assessment process. Although evidence of cortical hypoarousal or hyperarousal is not specific for ADHD (other medical conditions can also cause such dysregulation), abnormal findings on qEEG examination alert the practitioner to the high likelihood that the patient's impairment is due to some type of medical disorder, providing impetus for a thorough medical evaluation. Both the multichannel qEEG and the qEEG scanning process developed and investigated by Monastra and his colleagues (Monastra, Lubar, & Linden, 2001; Monastra et al., 1999) can provide information that is useful to identify patterns of cortical dysregulation.

Medical Evaluation

Patients who meet *DSM–IV–TR* criteria for a diagnosis of ADHD must be evaluated by their physician to rule out other medical conditions that can cause symptoms of inattention, impulsivity, and hyperactivity. As presented in chapter 4, such an evaluation includes (at minimum) the following conditions: anemia; thyroid disorders; hypoglycemia; allergies; cardiac and respiratory disorders; deficiencies of zinc, magnesium, and vitamin B; hormone deficiencies; the effects of perimenopause and menopause; illegal psychoactive use; and the adverse effects of current medications on attention and concentration.

TREATMENT OF ADULTS WITH ADHD

Pharmacological Treatments

Adults with ADHD report multiple types of psychiatric symptoms and functional impairment during clinical interview (Murphy & Barkley, 1996; Span, Earleywine, & Strybel, 2002; Wender et al., 2001). Commonly reported psychiatric symptoms include chronic depression, generalized anxiety, impaired anger control, conduct disorder, and substance abuse or dependence. Functional impairment can include forgetfulness, disorganization, distractibility, procrastination, poor listening skills, and aggressive behavior, together with reports of significant marital and parenting problems, lack of friendships, and a history of employment problems. Without a comprehensive assessment, such patients can be mistakenly treated for any of these psychiatric disorders.

However, when *DSM–IV–TR* criteria are used and a comprehensive assessment is conducted, adults with ADHD can be reliably and accurately diagnosed and treated. Similar to approaches for children and adolescents, pharmacological treatments are the most commonly provided. At present, there is evidence of the effectiveness of several different types of medications, including stimulants (e.g., methylphenidate, pemoline, Dexedrine, and mixed amphetamine salts), antidepressants (e.g., buproprion, desipramine), and the norepinephrine-specific reuptake inhibitor (NSRI) atomoxetine (see reviews by Maidmert, 2003; Prince, Wilens, Spencer, & Biederman, 2006; Wilens, 2003; Wilens, Spencer, & Biederman, 2002). Response rates have varied in studies, ranging from 33% to 70% of patients improved. On the basis of such response rates, the FDA has approved methylphenidate, mixed amphetamine salts, and atomoxetine for the treatment of ADHD in adults.

In reviewing medication efficacy studies, it appears that issues of insufficient dose, the process used to determine ADHD, and the degree of comorbidity have, in all likelihood, suppressed the response rate in studies conducted to date. In clinical settings that conduct a comprehensive assessment and provide treatment of relevant medical conditions; counseling to improve dietary, exercise, and sleep habits; and titration of dose on the basis of therapeutic effect (as determined through CPT, qEEG, and self-report measures), improved medication response rates seem likely. In adults, dosages of methylphenidate ranging up to 30 milligrams, three to four times daily, and amphetamine ranging up to 15 to 20 milligrams, three to four times daily, have been reported to be well tolerated and clinically necessary to achieve optimal effects (Prince et al., 2006). However, because of potential adverse effects on cardiovascular functions, monitoring of cardiac symptoms is advised, particularly in the treatment of adults, when stimulants are prescribed.

The NSRI atomoxetine has also been approved for the treatment of adults with ADHD. Like the stimulants, atomoxetine has been associated with improvement in approximately 50% to 70% of patients. The average daily dose ranged from 60 to 120 milligrams in the two studies (Michelson et al., 2001; Spencer, Biederman, Wilens, & Faraone, 1998). In these studies, the most common dose was 90 milligrams per day, administered in two daily doses ranging from 30 to 60 milligrams. However, several side effects merit consideration in clinical practice. First, although rare, there is an increased risk for jaundice, which should be monitored. Second, slight increase in heart rate and blood pressure have also been noted, hence caution is advised in treating adults with hypertension as well as ADHD. Third, there are reports of interactive effects when atomoxetine is prescribed with antidepressants such as fluoxetine and paroxetine, leading Prince et al. (2006) to advise reduction in dose of atomoxetine when combined pharmacotherapy is used. Finally, at our clinic we have repeatedly noted patient reports of a sedative effect of atomoxetine, particularly when administered in the morning, as well as insomnia when taken too close to bedtime. On the basis of such reports, use of a lower morning dose and administration of a larger dose in the afternoon or early evening has been initiated, with reduction of these side effects described by our patients.

Antidepressant medications, such as buproprion, desipramine, and venlafaxine, have been evaluated in the treatment of adults with ADHD. Although these medications have not been approved by the Food and Drug Administration (FDA) for the treatment of this disorder, we have found that the majority of the adult patients evaluated at our clinic report a history of prior or current treatment with such antidepressant medications. This is not surprising, given the demoralization that occurs during a lifetime of untreated or insufficiently treated ADHD. Reviews of studies have found that, similar to stimulant therapy and atomoxetine, the effectiveness of antidepressants indicates a response rate ranging from approximately 50% to 75% (Prince et al., 2006).

Clinically effective doses of buproprion (sustained or extended-release preparations) have been identified via gradual titration from 100 to 150 milligrams to approximately 400 to 450 milligrams per day. With desipramine, daily doses ranging from 50 to 250 milligrams have been needed, with most patients requiring approximately 150 milligrams per day. Venlafaxine, administered in doses ranging from 75 to 150 milligrams per day, has also proven effective. However, significant side effects warrant caution in the use of these medications. Buproprion has been associated with increased risk for seizures, as well as insomnia and irritability. Desipramine has been associated with increased risk for cardiac disorders. Venlafaxine has also been associated with increased risk for hypertension, as well as nausea and gastrointestinal distress. Consequently, such medications, although potentially beneficial, remain a second-line treatment for ADHD in adults, as cardiovascular and gastrointestinal disorders are common in adults and are likely to be exacerbated by these medications.

Antihypertensive medications, such as guanfacine and propranolol, have also been examined in controlled group studies with adults (Mattes, 1986; Taylor & Russo, 2001). In both studies, significant positive response was noted in the majority of patients. The mean dose of propranolol needed to achieve clinical effects was 528.0 milligrams. The average dose of guanfacine needed to yield significant clinical effects was quite low (1.1 mg) yet was sufficient. Although well tolerated, the risk for cardiovascular symptoms, particularly hypertensive rebound if medications are discontinued abruptly, is cause for caution in using such medications.

Given the research available at this time, the following medication strategies appear to be empirically supported:

1. When an adult has been determined to meet *DSM–IV–TR* criteria for ADHD, and other relevant medical conditions have

been ruled out, a clinical trial of a stimulant medication merits consideration, particularly in patients who demonstrate cortical hypoarousal on qEEG examination.

2. In patients who present with comorbid anxiety or depression, as well as ADHD, stimulant medications remain the medication of first choice, as it is unlikely that the patient will be able to effectively profit from cognitive or other types of psychological treatment without improved attention and concentration.

3. Titration of dose should proceed until evidence of positive response is noted on CPT and/or qEEG measures, as well as in patient report (i.e., scores are within the nonclinical range).

4. Antidepressants, antihypertensives, and NSRIs merit consideration as second-line treatments for ADHD, particularly in patients who cannot tolerate stimulant side effects. Antihypertensives appear particularly helpful in treating anxiety and anger outbursts that commonly are noted in adults with ADHD.

Psychological Treatments for ADHD in Adults

Several types of psychological treatment have emerged as potentially beneficial for the treatment of adults with ADHD, including electroencephalographic (EEG) biofeedback, cognitive behavior therapy (CBT), parent counseling, marital therapy, and social skills training through individualized coaching. Although the research support for these types of treatments is far less extensive than for pharmacological treatments, the research conducted to date is generally supportive of these approaches.

Electroencephalographic Biofeedback (Neurotherapy)

This type of treatment, reviewed in detail in chapter 8 (this volume), has been associated with a level of improvement in core ADHD symptoms that is comparable to pharmacological treatments, with approximately 75% of participants in studies demonstrating positive response with minimal adverse effects (J. F. Lubar, 2003; Monastra, 2005a; Riccio & French, 2004). Although primarily examined as a treatment for ADHD in children and adolescents, two studies (Rossiter & LaVaque, 1995; Monastra, Monastra, & George, 2002) have indicated that significant improvement has occurred in young adults as well. Because this type of treatment has not been associated with any type of adverse effect on cardiovascular, respiratory, or gastrointestinal functions and has yielded a level of benefit similar to both stimulant and nonstimulant medications, a clinical trial of this type of treatment merits consideration, particularly for adults with comorbid medical conditions that could be exacerbated by pharmacological treatment.

Cognitive Behavior Therapy

Recently, several controlled group studies have appeared in the scientific literature describing the beneficial effects of CBT when provided in combination with pharmacological treatment for adults diagnosed with ADHD (Rostain & Ramsay, 2006; Safren et al., 2005). In the Safren et al. (2005) study, patients were randomly assigned to a medication or combined medication-plus-CBT treatment protocol. Safren et al. indicated that patients treated with the combined approach reported fewer ADHD symptoms, less anxiety, and less depression. Assessments performed by an independent evaluator also revealed fewer ADHD symptoms, less anxiety, and less depression. Rostain and Ramsay (2006) likewise reported significant improvement on measures of ADHD, depression, anxiety, and level of social functioning in the group treated with a combination of pharmacotherapy and CBT. However, this was an open trial, without a comparison group.

Consistent with the model presented in this book, Safren (2006) recommended that in the treatment of adults with ADHD, medical evaluation and stabilization be completed first. Following such medical treatment, provision of psychological treatments (e.g., CBT) may provide additional beneficial effects on comorbid symptoms and social functioning. The treatment models proposed by Rostain and Ramsay (2006) and Safren (2006) represent a foundation for future research in this area.

Parent Counseling

Adults with ADHD have significant difficulty in child rearing and have profited from participation in classes such as those described in chapter 10. As reviewed in that chapter, significant gains in the functioning of children have been reported following parental participation in such programs. In clinical practice, the participation of adults with ADHD in parenting classes seems beneficial for multiple reasons. First, adults with this disorder are able to profit from this type of instruction and are able to reduce the level of family stress, teach essential skills to their children, and facilitate the development of healthy family relationships. Second, adults with ADHD who participate in such classes begin to experience improved self-esteem as they address multiple kinds of family problems that previously appeared insurmountable.

In our clinical practice, we have found that adults with ADHD report greater benefit from participation in this type of counseling when they are being effectively treated for their ADHD. Although coparenting with a spouse who does not have ADHD can lead to improved child functioning, parenting strategies are more consistently implemented when the adult with ADHD is being treated. Without such treatment, these parents begin to feel overwhelmed and increasingly guilty and "stupid" as they attempt to initiate changes in their family structure. In such instances, we provide support and assistance through the evaluation process, emphasizing that, like their children, they will be able to succeed as parents when they are being effectively treated.

Marital Therapy

Adults with ADHD display a wide range of problems in their marital relationships, including loss of attention, impaired verbal and nonverbal communication, deficits in organization and problem solving, procrastination, failure to fulfill commitments, and lack of emotional control (Betchen, 2003; Eakin et al., 2004; Murphy, 2006; Robbins, 2005; Robin & Payson, 2002). Although at present there is an absence of controlled group studies that support the efficacy of any specific approach to marital therapy with adults with ADHD, observational and single-case studies have been reported that may provide some guidance to practitioners who seek to promote improved marital functioning.

Common across current treatment models is the position that couple counseling efforts that ignore the reality of ADHD will fail to yield beneficial results and that a multimodal approach is essential for optimal outcomes (Betchen, 2003; Halverstadt, 1998; Nadeau, 1996; Robbins, 2005; L. Weiss, 1997). Each of these clinicians suggests a treatment approach for couples that incorporates medical evaluation and treatment, education of both partners on the nature of ADHD, behavioral interventions (to promote improved trust, intimacy), cognitive restructuring, communication and social skills training, and consultation with an ADHD coach. Although multiple case studies are presented by each of these authors, to date there is no controlled group study that evaluates the individual and combined effects of these treatment components.

At our clinic, we have begun to explore the effects of a program that incorporates several of these components. Paralleling our life skills program for children and teenagers, we have developed a program for adults with ADHD and their spouses. The 10-class program (with follow-up) provides the opportunity for adults with ADHD and their spouses to meet other couples and participate in a structured program intended to provide education regarding ADHD; improve the dietary, sleep, and exercise habits of both partners; promote improved self-esteem; enhance verbal and nonverbal communication; develop problem-solving skills; and address the organizational issues that so many of our patients experience. As in our life skills program for children and teenagers, a Couple's Meeting Time is encouraged for couples to review their goals as well as strategies to achieve them. However, because of the attentional and organizational problems of adults with ADHD, we recommend daily meetings rather than weekly ones.

Consistent with the impressions of other clinicians, this type of treatment proceeds from the evaluation of the adult patient and the establishment of an effective treatment for the patient's core ADHD symptoms. During this process, the results of the evaluation are reviewed with the patient's partner, and the nature of ADHD is discussed. Once an effective treatment for the patient's ADHD is established, we conduct three initial counseling sessions. These preparatory meetings are intended to review the class format and to provide the couple with several initial strategies that they can use during the initial months of treatment.

The first intervention requires the patient and partner to respond to the following question: "How could your spouse show you that he or she loves you?" For instance, a spouse may devote an extraordinary amount of time on household chores, inside or outdoors. However, that might not translate to "I love you" to his or her spouse. A spouse may work hard to generate income for the family, as a way of showing love. However, that might not mean "love" to his or her spouse.

In our first preparatory session with the couple, we ask each person to generate a list of ways that their spouse could express love in a way that mattered to them. Most adults enjoy this type of activity. After we compile a list of at least 10 loving acts, we encourage each spouse to share their list (aloud) and then give the list to their partner. The homework assignment is a simple one: Each day, do at least two things that spell love to your partner.

During the second preparatory session, we provide an overview of problem solving. Most adults with ADHD have difficulty engaging in extended conversations. Consequently, we seek to simplify this task with respect to problem solving. Consistent with the approach to problem solving that is presented during our life skills program classes, we teach couples that the key to resolving conflict is to identify the fears and needs of the other person. Once they identify the needs and/or fears, they can proceed to generate possible solutions that address these concerns and then moved toward reaching a decision.

During our third preparatory session, we seek to identify those hurtful actions that have occurred during the years of marriage but have not yet been forgiven. Such unforgiven acts can sabotage treatment progress. Therefore, we ask our patients and their spouses to develop a list of such events so that we can guide them in the process of obtaining forgiveness. Following these preparatory sessions, we invite adult patients and their spouses to participate in our life skills program for adults. If they are uncomfortable with participation in such a group, we provide the instruction in an individual format.

At this time, we have conducted case studies of patients who have completed this program. However, like other counseling programs for couples in which one spouse has ADHD, we have not completed a controlled group study. To date, a review of the literature reveals that a similar program for adult patients with ADHD (without spousal participation) has yielded improvement on core ADHD symptoms, the Symptom Checklist–90–R (Derogatis, 1992), and the Beck Depression Inventory (Beck, Ward, &

Mendelson, 1961; Hesslinger et al., 2002). However, this too was a pilot case study involving 8 patients. Clearly more research is required to develop effective programs for couples including a partner with ADHD. Given the apparent need for such services, there is little doubt that such research will be forthcoming.

Adult Coaching

Another type of treatment for adults with ADHD that has generated considerable interest but has minimal empirical support is consultation with a coach to assist patients in developing life skills. The concept of "coaching," as an adjunctive treatment for adults with ADHD, was initially presented by Hallowell (1995). In his discussion of multiple-case vignettes, Hallowell presented the concept of a "performance coach," who could be available on a much more frequent basis than a therapist. Such a person would ideally offer practical guidance and support, as needed, to help the patient with ADHD accomplish a variety of life tasks (e.g., organizing paperwork, cleaning the home, paying bills, managing finances, developing a tracking system for keeping appointments, managing time, setting and achieving personal goals).

Since the appearance of Hallowell's (1995) article, professional associations for coaching have emerged, numerous books on coaching have been written, and training opportunities have been developed (see detailed description by Ratey, 2002). However, as noted by Goldstein (2005) and Murphy (2006), controlled group studies examining the efficacy of coaching are absent. My impression is that given the interest and need to explore strategies for skill development in this population, research in this approach will emerge in the coming years, providing additional guidance to practitioners interested in providing such a service.

Interventions in the Workplace

As noted previously, ADHD is a condition that qualifies an individual for reasonable accommodations in work settings. Unfortunately, adults with ADHD are often unaware of such legal protection, and without informing their employers, they place themselves in jeopardy of losing their jobs. Far too often, adults with ADHD are terminated from their employment because of late arrival for work, disorganization, failure to meet deadlines, difficulty listening to and following directions, and other functional problems. In fact, one of the more common reasons that adults seek evaluation for ADHD is poor work performance (Murphy et al., 2002).

Similar to other types of interventions, consideration of accommodations in the workplace follows the establishment of an effective treatment program for the core symptoms of ADHD. Once such an intervention program is implemented, a functional assessment can be conducted, similar to the type used in school settings. For some adults with ADHD, the primary functional problem is attendance issues. Others struggle with time management or have difficulty listening to directions or organizing and completing writing tasks.

Because of the significant repercussions of failing to arrive on time, organizing the day, prioritizing responsibilities, listening to directions, recording assigned tasks, completing writing tasks, returning work materials to designated storage areas, and so on, treatment targeting the functional impairments of ADHD is an essential component of care for adults with ADHD. Assessment strategies, such as the Life Skills Questionnaire: Adult Form (see Exhibit 7.2, chap. 7, this volume), can be helpful in identifying specific concerns. Counseling sessions for adults with ADHD are far more likely to focus on such issues than those of trauma and neglect. It is within this context that coaching services may prove to be most helpful.

In addition to functionally targeted counseling sessions, adults with ADHD can profit from assistive technology. There are a variety of electronic devices that can facilitate the completion of tasks in work settings. Personal computers contain programs that are often helpful in maintaining addresses and contact numbers and noting appointments on a calendar. Cell phones have numerous options that make communication easier and more instantaneous, enabling adults with ADHD to make contact when they become aware of the need, rather than wait until they are at a land phone. Electronic banking services can enable adults with ADHD to remain current on bills, thereby protecting them from the fees charged to delinquent and late accounts.

Several computer software programs have also proven to be quite helpful to adults with ADHD. Programs such as Read & Write, ReadPlease!, and Kurzweil 3000 read any computer-scanned or electronic text file. These programs prompt the patient to select voice type and reading speed and then read aloud the text to the patient (while highlighting each word). This type of program performs three essential functions: It provides auditory and visual input, overcomes any reading decoding problems, and sets a time frame for completing a reading task.

Another type of program translates the spoken word into written form. Although some patients with ADHD are able to use word processing software to complete writing assignments, other patients lack keyboarding skills. Those patients have found that speaking into a computer microphone facilitates the expression of their ideas. Programs such as Dragon NaturallySpeaking and the Read & Write system work well for such students. Once the patient completes a tutorial program, the computer transcribes their spoken word into text displayed on the computer monitor.

IMPLICATIONS FOR CLINICAL PRACTICE

At present, there are several emerging nonpharmacological therapies for adults with ADHD. Some treatments, such as EEG biofeedback, target core ADHD symptoms. Other interventions, such as parent counseling, marital therapy, and coaching, target specific areas of functional impairment. Technological advances in computer science provide additional tools that can be used by patients to complete essential life tasks, such as reading, writing, and organization of time and work. Although there is clearly a need for additional controlled group studies examining the effects of these treatments with adults, it is evident that there is considerable public interest in these types of services.

Clinicians interested in providing such services are encouraged to design research studies examining the effects of these treatments. The development of simple research designs incorporating random assignment and wait-list or standard-care controls can be readily incorporated in clinical settings in which the effects of additional treatment components are being evaluated. For example, a clinic that currently offers pharmacological treatments and "supportive" counseling services could design and conduct a study in which its standard program of care is compared with an "enhanced" program that provides EEG biofeedback, CBT, parent counseling, marital therapy, or coaching, using one of the models. Although such research designs would not provide conclusive evidence of efficacy, they would contribute to the development of empirically based programs to guide clinical practice. Such a foundation is largely missing in the treatment of adults at this time.

13

UNCOMMON SOLUTIONS TO COMMON CLINICAL PROBLEMS

Throughout this book, an effort has been made to illustrate how comprehensive, integrative care can be provided at the individual- or group-practice level. However, in clinical practice, patients do not always respond to first-line treatments. In this chapter, strategies for helping patients overcome their symptoms when initial treatment approaches fail are presented. It is hoped that such a presentation will provide guidance for practitioners, based on my experience in treating thousands of patients with attention-deficit/hyperactivity disorder (ADHD) over the past 2 decades.

CASE ILLUSTRATION 1:
FAILURE TO RESPOND TO MULTIPLE STIMULANTS

A 10-year-old boy was referred by his pediatrician after failing to respond to methylphenidate-based and amphetamine-based stimulants. He was initially diagnosed with ADHD at age 6 years and was treated with Ritalin, 5 milligrams, three times daily. Response was positive for several weeks. However, the patient gradually became more hyperactive at home and school, and increased levels of irritability and aggressiveness were noted at home.

The physician decided to increase dose of medication to 10 milligrams upon waking and at noon, continuing the 5-milligram dose after school. Again, reduction in hyperactivity was noted at school but irritability continued at home. The after-school dose was then increased to 10 milligrams. The patient became more irritable in the evening and displayed sleep-onset insomnia.

Medication was next changed to 10 milligrams of Adderall XR in the morning and 5 milligrams of Adderall after school. The patient continued to exhibit irritability at home and school, and there was no change in degree of hyperactivity. Dose was increased to 20 milligrams of Adderall XR in the morning and 10 milligrams of Adderall after school. The patient had an incident at school in which he became aggressive in the class after his teacher told him to remain in his seat. He overturned his desk in the classroom, yelling that he was going to kill his teacher. He was suspended from school, pending evaluation and treatment by a psychologist or psychiatrist.

Assessment Results

ADHD Symptoms

Eight of nine symptoms of inattention and nine of nine symptoms of hyperactivity and impulsivity were reported. Onset was at age 4. There was functional impairment at home and school. Rating scale data (Attention Deficit Disorders Evaluation Scales [ADDES]; McCarney, 2004) indicated a frequency of ADHD symptoms that was greater than 99% of peers (Home and School Versions), despite treatment with stimulant medication.

Continuous Performance Tests

Test of Variables of Attention (TOVA) standard scores were impaired on the visual and auditory tests. Degree of impairment was greater than 99% of peers, with atypically high numbers of errors of omission and commission and marked variability noted. No significant improvement occurred when the visual test was repeated 2 hours postingestion of a 20-milligram dose of Adderall XR. Although frequency of commission errors decreased (standard scores = 64), standard scores for inattention and variability remained less than 40.

Quantitative Electroencephalography

The Attention Index (AI) obtained when the patient was tested without medication was 7.92 (3.0 SD above the mean for age peers). When evaluated 2 hours postingestion of medication, the AI was 6.03. Although improvement was noted, the degree of cortical slowing remained greater than 98% of age peers.

Medical

Physician evaluation of relevant medical conditions failed to identify any other physical causes of the child's symptoms.

Diet

The patient ate cereal for breakfast; snack foods for lunch (e.g., French fries with juice; ice cream sandwich and water).

Exercise

The patient was active on several sports teams during the week and was exercising on a daily basis.

Sleep

The patient was unable to fall asleep until nearly midnight, thereby obtaining approximately 6.5 hours of sleep per night.

Clinical Impression

The patient met *Diagnostic and Statistical Manual of Mental Disorders* (4th ed., text rev.; *DSM–IV–TR*; American Psychiatric Association, 2000) criteria for a diagnosis of ADHD and exhibited cortical slowing on quantitative electroencephalographic (qEEG) examination. Such patients routinely respond to stimulants. However, dietary and sleeping habits were not sufficient to sustain attention and it had not been determined (via continuous performance test [CPT] or qEEG) whether lower doses of stimulant could be effective in a context of adequate sleep and dietary patterns.

Treatment Plan

The treatment plan was as follows:

1. Establish dietary habits that provide 15 to 20 grams of protein at breakfast and lunch.
2. Establish sleeping patterns that ensure at least 9 hours of sleep each night, and use a melatonin supplement if needed.
3. Evaluate response to 5 milligrams of Adderall XR via CPT and qEEG, and behavioral reports of parents and teachers. If CPT and qEEG are within age expectations, maintain 5 milligrams of Adderall XR. If not, increase dose by 5 milligrams, until normal scores are obtained.

Treatment Response

After nutritional counseling was provided, and desirable foods were identified for breakfast and lunch, the patient was able to maintain levels in the *Recommended Dietary Allowances* (Food and Nutrition Board of the National Academy of Sciences, 1989) for protein intake at breakfast and lunch. Sleep-onset insomnia persisted, but use of a melatonin supplement (2 mg; administered 1.5 hours before bedtime) addressed this symptom. Melatonin was administered for a 3-week period before it was discontinued.

Evaluation of medication response revealed insufficient response to the 5.0-milligram dose. The patient was able to successfully complete both auditory and visual forms of the TOVA 2 hours after treatment with 10 milligrams of Adderall XR. However, afternoon evaluation (conducted at 4:30 p.m.) revealed declining benefits at that time on qEEG measure. A 5.0-milligram dose of Adderall was administered immediately after school (3:30 p.m.), which boosted attention but resulted in sleep-onset insomnia. A 2.5-milligram dose of Adderall was introduced after school, with positive response on the qEEG and CPT and no adverse effects evident on sleep. This case illustrates a commonly seen pattern of poor response to increased dosage of medication when insufficient dietary and sleep patterns are not addressed in a patient who exhibits cortical slowing on qEEG, in the absence of other medical conditions.

CASE ILLUSTRATION 2: ADHD IN COMBINATION WITH ANXIETY AND SOCIAL SKILL DEFICITS

A 9-year-old boy was referred by his parents because of multiple presenting problems. At school, he was unable to remain seated, attend to instruction, and complete written assignments. He was highly reactive to changes in school schedule and had become agitated, refusing to comply with directions from a substitute teacher. He had run out of the classroom and struck his principal when he attempted to restrain the child. This resulted in the child being suspended from school, prompting a consultation at our clinic.

At home, this child exhibited multiple symptoms of anxiety and inattention. He avoided certain rooms of the house (e.g., basement, his bedroom) and slept with his parents. He consumed a greatly restricted range of foods (i.e., macaroni and cheese, cereal, hot dogs, chips, and ice cream) and became highly agitated if forced to eat any other types of foods. He did not visit with friends and was not involved in any group social activities at the time of the consultation. His parents reported that they had tried to involve him in T-ball, soccer, and basketball but their son refused to go to practice. He was quite fascinated by Construx and Legos and would spend his days constructing new designs. He also enjoyed playing video games and collected Yu-Gi-Oh! cards. His conversations centered on descriptions of his latest conquest in video games or the power or attack points of his cards. Although interested in sharing his interests with others, he lacked any sense of social or emotional reciprocity.

Prior treatment had included a school evaluation, which determined delays in fine motor coordination but no evidence of a specific learning disability. Occupational therapy had been provided by his school district, with improvement noted on a variety of measures but not on handwriting. Outpatient psychotherapy had been provided for 6 months. The treatment consisted of play therapy with the child and parent counseling. No positive response was reported. Although the parents had discussed their concerns with their son's pediatrician, pharmacological treatment had not been initiated.

Assessment Results

ADHD Symptoms

Seven of nine symptoms of inattention were reported, and two of nine symptoms of impulsivity were acknowledged. Onset was age 3 years. Functional impairment was noted at home and school. Rating scale data (ADDES) indicated a frequency of ADHD symptoms that was greater than 95% of peers at home and at school. In addition to ADHD, this patient met *DSM–IV–TR* criteria for Asperger's Disorder and a Generalized Anxiety Disorder.

Continuous Performance Tests

TOVA standard scores were impaired on the visual and auditory tests. Degree of impairment was greater than 98% of peers, with an atypically high number of errors of commission, slow rate of decision making, and marked variability of response rate noted.

Quantitative Electroencephalography

The AI was 6.48 (2.5 *SD* above the mean for age peers).

Medical

Environmental allergies were being treated symptomatically with antihistamines. No screening had been conducted. Otherwise, prior medical evaluations had not identified any other relevant medical concerns.

Diet

The patient's diet was highly restricted. He ate cereal for breakfast; yogurt for lunch; macaroni and cheese, or a hot dog and French fries, for dinner. He avoided drinking milk, preferring water.

Exercise

The patient was quite sedentary.

Sleep

The patient was unable to fall asleep alone. He waited until his parents went to bed and then crawled into bed with them, attaining approximately 7 hours of sleep per night.

Clinical Impression

The patient met *DSM–IV–TR* criteria for diagnoses of ADHD, Predominately Inattentive Type; Asperger's Disorder; and a Generalized Anxiety Disorder, and qEEG examination revealed cortical slowing, a neurophysiological indicator associated with positive response to stimulant medication. However, prior medical evaluation had not been comprehensive. Allergies were suspected; dietary insufficiencies seemed likely. Sleeping habits were not sufficient to support attentional functions. Therefore, prior to initiating treatment for DSM–IV–TR diagnoses, thorough medical evaluation and treatment for relevant medical concerns seemed required.

Treatment Plan

The treatment plan was as follows:

1. Refer for medical evaluation to assess other relevant medical concerns, particularly allergies and nutritionally related deficiencies. Establish sleeping patterns that ensure at least 9 hours of sleep each night. Use a melatonin supplement if needed.
2. Once relevant medical concerns are addressed, reevaluate attentional abilities via qEEG and CPT. If impairment persists, initiate a clinical trial of a sustained-release stimulant medication (e.g., Focalin XR).
3. Titrate dose until normal scores are obtained on CPT and qEEG. A clinical trial of electroencephalographic (EEG) biofeedback could be considered, on the basis of parent and patient interest.
4. If significant levels of anxiety are evident, despite stimulant therapy, initiate a trial of an antihypertensive medication (guanfacine).
5. Refer the child to his district's Committee on Special Education (CSE) to develop an Individual Education Plan (IEP) or 504 Plan, with particular emphasis placed on improving communication and social skills, and develop a behavioral intervention plan.
6. Encourage parental participation in parenting classes and patient participation in our life skills program.

Treatment Response

Medical evaluation determined specific allergies to foods including corn, eggs, and wheat, as well as pollens such as dust, mold, and animal dander. Anemia was also diagnosed. Treatment consisted of initiation of an elimination diet and treatment with Zyrtec (for airborne allergens). Consultation with a nutritionist was initiated to assist in establishing a dietary plan based on the *Recommended Dietary Allowances* (Food and Nutrition Board of the National Academy of Sciences, 1989) for daily intake, and each of the members of the family began a program of at least 30 minutes of exercise per day (typically performed with their child). Following improved diet, the patient no longer exhibited symptoms of anemia. Sleeping patterns likewise improved, following initiation of a behavioral treatment plan to gradually desensitize the patient to sleeping alone. However, anxiety, social skill deficits, and attentional problems persisted.

The qEEG and CPT results continued to reveal significant impairment of attention and cortical arousal. Focalin XR was initiated (5 mg) and titrated to 15 milligrams before scores on the qEEG and CPT were within normal limits. Following establishment of an effective dose of stimulant, significant improvement in attention, quality of handwriting, and completion of seat work and homework was noted. However, significant anxiety and social skills deficits persisted.

A clinical trial of guanfacine was introduced to address symptoms of anxiety. Dosage was initiated at 2 milligrams at bedtime and titrated to 3 milligrams (1 mg in the morning; 2 mg at bedtime). Reduction in the patient's tendency to worry excessively and improved ability to tolerate change in routine were noted. However, lack of involvement in peer activities persisted. Conversation continued to lack a sense of "connection" with the interests of others.

Consequently, the patient was referred for participation in our life skills program and consultation with the child's speech therapist was conducted, to encourage the practice of such communication skills in speech therapy. His parents established the family rule that he needed to be involved in at least one activity with peers on a season-to-season basis, reinforcing this rule with strategies taught to them in our parenting program. The patient became involved in a science–adventure type of club at school and enrolled in a karate program. His parents facilitated the process of learning the names of other children and guided their son in ways to invite other children over to their house. He continued to practice conversational skills in speech therapy, at home, and in our life skills program, with positive response.

Because of parental concerns about the potential adverse effects of long-term use of stimulant medication, this student also participated in EEG biofeedback. He required 35 sessions of this type of treatment before he met criteria for "graduation" (i.e., AI within normal limits for a 45-minute period while completing schoolwork; no evidence of impairment on the CPT). As a result of this type of treatment, medication dose was reduced to Methylin (5 mg) as needed to help sustain concentration while completing homework. Guanfacine was reduced to 2 milligrams (h.s.) after 18 months.

This case illustrates the importance of a careful medical evaluation; the positive effects of stimulant therapy even when symptoms of anxiety and other comorbid conditions (e.g., Asperger's disorder) are present; the role of nonstimulant medications in addressing comorbid symptoms, the process for implementing a multimodal treatment plan; targeting specific areas of functional impairment; and the beneficial effects of EEG biofeedback.

CASE ILLUSTRATION 3: TREATMENT-RESISTANT ADHD

An 11-year-old girl was referred by her parents following 4 years of nonsuccessful pharmacological treatment for ADHD. This patient was initially evaluated by a psychologist in the second grade, because of delays in the development of reading and writing skills. On the basis of a review of clinical history, academic records, completion of behavioral rating scales (both ADHD specific and broad spectrum), and testing of intelligence and core academic skills, the child was diagnosed with ADHD, as well as specific learning disabilities in reading and written expression. An IEP was developed at her school, which included specialized instruction in these core areas, testing accommodations, and classroom modifications. Clinical trials of Ritalin-LA, Metadate CD, Adderall XR, and Strattera had yielded minimal response and significant adverse effects were reported.

At the time of our evaluation, the child had begun to display disruptive behavior in the classroom. She would talk to classmates, interrupt instruction, and fail to complete in-class and homework assignments. As a result, she was in danger of having to repeat the fifth grade. Her parents also observed frequent off-task behavior and were frustrated over the amount of time and the degree of assistance needed to help their daughter complete homework tasks. They also were becoming increasingly concerned about their daughter's defiance and loss of temper at home. Because they were unsure whether retention was best for their daughter, they decided to seek a consultation at our clinic.

Assessment Results

ADHD Symptoms

Eight of nine symptoms of inattention and three of nine symptoms of hyperactivity and impulsivity were reported. Onset was at age 6. Functional impairment was noted at home and school. Rating scale data (ADDES) indicated a frequency of symptoms that was greater than 96% of age peers (Home and School) despite current treatment with Adderall XR (20 mg).

Continuous Performance Tests

TOVA standard scores were significantly impaired on the Visual Form but not on the Auditory Form. The patient exhibited a significant number of errors of omission and commission, performing more poorly than 99.9% of age peers on the Visual Test. Her performance on the Auditory Form of the TOVA was above average. No significant improvement was noted on the Visual Form of the TOVA when administered 2 hours postingestion of Adderall XR.

Quantitative Electroencephalography

The AI obtained when the patient was tested without use of stimulant was 2.89. When the qEEG was conducted 2.5 hours postingestion of Adderall XR, no significant change was noted (AI = 3.12). Both scores are within 1.0 standard deviation of the mean for age peers. Observation of the girl during the qEEG examination revealed excessive eyeblinking during testing and a tendency to place reading materials close to her face.

Medical

Physician evaluation of relevant medical conditions had been conducted prior to initiation of medication. No other physical causes of her attentional problem had been identified. Routine visual examinations for acuity had indicated no impairment.

Diet

The patient typically ate yogurt, cereal, and a glass of milk for breakfast and had a balanced school lunch.

Exercise

The patient actively participated in athletic activities on a daily basis. She had a group of friends with whom she played on a consistent basis.

Sleep

No evidence of sleep disturbance was reported. The girl was able to obtain between 9 and 10 hours of sleep nightly.

Clinical Impression

The patient met *DSM–IV–TR* criteria for a diagnosis of ADHD, Predominately Inattentive Type. However, her excessive eyeblink, her positioning of reading materials close to her eyes, her age-appropriate performance on an auditory test of attention, and her "normal" qEEG increased the likelihood that a visual problem was contributing to her performance problems at school.

Treatment Plan

The treatment plan was as follows:

1. Obtain an evaluation from an optometrist or ophthalmologist who can conduct a comprehensive examination of visual tracking and convergence.
2. If convergence insufficiency (CI) is identified, reassess attentional abilities after treatment of visual problems is completed.

3. If no CI is identified, initiate treatment with a nonstimulant medication, systematically evaluating dose, and consider assistive technology to help with reading and writing tasks (e.g., Read & Write).
4. Provide follow-up parent counseling and family counseling, if needed after Steps 1 through 3 are completed.

Treatment Response

Evaluation by an optometrist revealed significant CI. Bifocals were prescribed and visual training was initiated. With this intervention, the patient reported that she could focus while reading. Her level of educational performance improved dramatically. At home, her parents purchased a Read & Write system, so that their daughter could proceed more quickly through reading assignments and dictate her responses. Speed and quality of homework completion improved. Her parents participated in our parenting program, and began applying strategies taught in these classes to address motivational issues. Reevaluation of attention via the Visual Form of the TOVA revealed a level of performance consistent with age peers, when tested while wearing bifocals.

Year-end academic evaluation at her school revealed significant gains on test of reading, although residual mild impairment of writing skills was noted. Her district changed her support program to a 504 Plan, providing extended time for tests and permission to use assistive technology. No further treatment was required. This case illustrates the importance of thoroughly assessing visual impairment, particularly in students who present with a combination of inattention and delays in reading and writing skills.

CASE ILLUSTRATION 4: TREATING ADHD WHEN LEARNING DISABILITIES ARE FORGOTTEN

A 15-year-old boy was referred for evaluation by his probation officer. He was diagnosed with learning disabilities in reading, mathematics, and written expression during the primary grades and was provided with an IEP. By the end of the fifth grade, his scores on achievement tests were within 1.0 standard deviations for his grade. Although his primary classroom teacher was concerned about his lack of organization and his difficulty attending during class instruction, the patient was declassified at the end of the fifth grade.

His mother reported that without assistance, he failed every class in the sixth and seventh grades, primarily because of a lack of completion of homework and poor performance on tests. He was required to attend summer school both years. By the eighth grade, he was routinely skipping classes and was truant from school. He refused to do seat work, walked out of classes, and failed to complete homework assignments. His parents met with his teachers repeatedly and verbally requested that their son be reevaluated. However, the perspective of the school district was that his problems were, as they said, "motivational" and that "he needed to take responsibility for his actions."

He began staying overnight at friends' homes and would not respect curfew. Because of his behavioral problems and truancy, his parents sought an evaluation with a licensed psychologist. The patient was diagnosed with oppositional defiant disorder and dysthymia. Treatment consisted of parent counseling, individual therapy, and family therapy, without significant improvement. A clinical trial of Zoloft (prescribed by his pediatrician) was unsuccessful. Because of the lack of response to treatment, his parents sought the assistance of the probation department. Their son was determined to be a Person in Need of Supervision and assigned a probation officer. To determine the causes for his educational and behavioral problems, the probation department referred this patient to our clinic.

Assessment Results

ADHD Symptoms

Nine of nine symptoms of inattention and eight of nine symptoms of hyperactivity and impulsivity were reported. Onset was at age 7 years. Functional impairment was noted at home and school. ADDES scores were indicative of a markedly atypical frequency at home (exceeding 99% of peers). However, high school teacher ratings indicated a degree of inattentive and hyperactive symptoms that was less than 85% of age peers.

Teacher ratings consistently indicated that the patient did not attend during class or complete assignments. However, their perspective (shared in handwritten comments on the rating form) was that the patient was "unmotivated" and "lazy."

Continuous Performance Tests

TOVA standard scores were impaired on both the Visual Form and the Auditory Form. Degree of impairment was greater than 99% on both tests, with impairment noted on subscales assessing accuracy, impulse control, and consistency of decision-making speed.

Quantitative Electroencephalography

The AI obtained during the evaluation was 5.84. This ratio represented a degree of cortical slowing greater than 99% of age peers (> 3.0 SD).

Medical

The patient had not been evaluated for other relevant medical conditions by his physician.

Diet

The patient skipped breakfast and ate pizza with a cola for lunch.

Exercise

Although the patient had been a good athlete and participated in competitive youth leagues, he withdrew from such activities during middle school. When home, he spent most of his time in his room, playing video games or instant messaging his friends.

Sleep

The patient was unable to fall asleep before 12:30 a.m. He obtained approximately 6 hours of sleep each night.

Clinical Impression

The patient met *DSM–IV–TR* criteria for a diagnosis of ADHD, Combined Type, as well as Oppositional Defiant Disorder. The qEEG findings revealed cortical hypoarousal, a pattern noted in students who typically respond to stimulant therapy. However, dietary and sleep problems required intervention prior to stimulant treatment, and evaluation of other relevant medical factors (including the possibility of illegal psychoactive substance usage) was needed.

Treatment Plan

The treatment plan was as follows:

1. Obtain a comprehensive medical evaluation to rule out relevant medical conditions.
2. Provide nutritional counseling to ensure that the patient is consuming amounts of protein at breakfast and lunch as outlined in *Recommended Dietary Allowances* (Food and Nutrition Board of the National Academy of Sciences, 1989).
3. Treat any identified medical condition. Reassess attentional abilities following such treatment. Initiate a clinical trial of stimulant medication if attentional problems are evident on TOVA and qEEG. Titrate dosage until TOVA and qEEG results are within the "normal" range.
4. Inform CSE that the patient had been diagnosed with ADHD. Request evaluation of academic abilities, completion of a functional assessment, and a functional behavioral assessment to develop a comprehensive IEP.
5. Provide follow-up parent counseling, family therapy, and social skills training, as needed.

Treatment Response

Medical examination revealed anemia and illegal psychoactive substance use (i.e., cannabis). Nutritional intervention targeting improvement of protein content at breakfast and lunch improved anemia. Melatonin (2 mg) was provided at 9:00 p.m., resulting in sleep onset between 10:30 and 11:00 p.m. Stimulant medication (Adderall XR) was initiated at the 10-milligram dose and titrated to 20 milligrams. The qEEG and TOVA findings subsequent to administration of 20 milligrams of Adderall XR revealed a level of cortical arousal and performance consistent with age peers. Because of reoccurring outbursts of anger, the antihypertensive medication clonidine was prescribed (0.1 mg at bedtime; 0.05 mg in the morning). Random drug screening for psychoactives, counseling at our clinic and from the probation officer (emphasizing the legal ramifications of continued positive screens), resumption of involvement in at least one school-based activity each season, closer monitoring of patient social activities by his parents, and prohibition of overnight visits at friends' homes led to discontinuation of marijuana use.

At school, the CSE evaluation indicated that the patient was a student of above-average intelligence (Full-Scale Intelligence Quotient [FSIQ] = 115). However, a specific learning disability in written expression was identified. An IEP was developed that included daily consultation with a special education teacher, the use of assistive technology, advance notice of assignments (on Friday), weekly progress reports (listing missing assignments), systematic application of consequences (as outlined in our parenting program), and testing modifications (e.g., extended time, permission to record answers via keyboard or orally through voice-recognition software or a scribe, permission to seek clarification of the meaning of exam questions). This intervention resulted in a 22-point improvement in overall average.

With regard to social interaction, the patient was encouraged to identify school-based activities for involvement. His guidance counselor was quite helpful in supporting this intervention, meeting with the patient and assisting him in making the necessary contacts with coaches. The patient tried out for the lacrosse team in the spring, and made the team. His social network expanded to include members of this team. He participated in our life skills program for teenagers and exhibited improvements primarily in conflict resolution and problem-solving skills. Subsequently, clonidine was gradually discontinued. The active treatment phase was concluded after 9 months, with follow-up care provided as needed.

This case illustrates the importance of recognizing the likelihood that a previously diagnosed learning disability will not just go away and that a substantial percentage of adolescents presenting with oppositionalism, truancy, and poor academic performance are likely to have undiagnosed ADHD as well. By addressing the underlying learning and attentional disorders (as well as relevant medical, nutritional, and sleep problems), prognosis is significantly increased.

CASE ILLUSTRATION 5: THE DEPRESSED AND/OR ANXIOUS ADULT WITH ADHD

A 48-year-old woman sought evaluation at our clinic after being informed by her employer that she would be terminated from her clerical position within 30 days because of poor job performance (unless substantial improvement was noted). The woman indicated that she was chronically late for work, was highly disorganized with managing paperwork, and would lose completed work projects. She typically stayed late at work to try to, in her words, "catch up"; however, she was "overwhelmed." She indicated that this had been a problem for her in clerical positions prior to, as she said, the "child-birth and child-rearing years" and that she had been terminated from several positions in her early 20s. She had returned to clerical work approximately 6 months ago and felt like the same problems were "happening all over again."

The patient described a lifelong pattern of impaired attention, concentration, and performance. As a child, she had difficulty comprehending while reading and struggled to, as she said, "put her ideas down on paper." She reported that she "wore glasses for a couple of months" as a little girl, but they did not help, so she stopped using them. Although she was never evaluated for a specific learning disability, she did indicate that her parents had her tutored in reading and hired a teacher to help her during exam time and when she had term papers. Despite this assistance, she described herself as a "marginal" student. Review of report cards confirmed this appraisal. She graduated from high school with an overall average of 71, requiring summer school to pass courses in English, social studies, and science. She attended college briefly but was unable to complete course requirements. Because she was an outgoing and personable young woman, she sought positions as a receptionist. She enjoyed the interaction with customers; however, she was overwhelmed by the paperwork.

As a wife and mother, the patient also felt overwhelmed. Although she described her relationships with her husband and children as "close and loving," she indicated that her "house was a disaster" and that she frequently lost important papers, failed to pay bills on time, and forgot important appointments for herself and her children. In contrast, her spouse was "super organized," which made her feel like she was "inept" and "an idiot."

Throughout adulthood, she had compared herself with her spouse and with "other moms" and could not understand why she "couldn't do the simplest of tasks." Over the years, she reported an increased sense of shame and social withdrawal. Depression was diagnosed by her physician approximately

10 years prior to her consultation at our clinic. For the past decade, she was treated with a variety of antidepressants (e.g., Wellbutrin, Effexor, Prozac, Paxil), without positive response. At the time she was seen at our clinic, she was obese and described herself as "depressed and anxious all the time," and unsure how to "get better."

Assessment Results

ADHD Symptoms

Nine of nine symptoms of inattention and one of nine symptoms of hyperactivity–impulsivity were reported by the patient. Her mother also completed a rating form and described seven of nine symptoms of inattention, with an onset during the "primary grades." Functional impairment was reported at home, school, and work. Rating scale data indicated a frequency of inattentive symptoms that was greater than 98% of age peers, according to patient and spouse report.

Continuous Performance Tests

The patient demonstrated significant disparity in level of performance between the Visual and Auditory Forms of the TOVA. On the Visual Form, she made numerous errors of omission and commission and exhibited marked variability of response. Level of performance was poorer than 99% of age peers. On the Auditory Form, her level of accuracy was improved to within the 50th percentile. However, her rate of response and consistency of decision-making speed was poorer than 96% of peers.

Quantitative Electroencephalography

The patient's AI was 4.98, which is more than 3.00 standard deviations above age peers. Observations during testing revealed a slow rate of reading and writing and impaired comprehension.

Medical

The patient had undergone a comprehensive medical evaluation prior to our consultation. Aside from obesity and elevated cholesterol and triglyceride levels, no significant medical problems were evident. Perimenopausal symptoms were absent.

Diet

The patient typically drank 2 cups of coffee for breakfast. Lunch consisted of yogurt or a salad. However, after work she "ate constantly."

Exercise

The patient did not exercise.

Sleep

The patient was unable to fall asleep until 1:00 a.m. Snoring was reported by her husband. The patient reported that she woke at least two or three times per night. She finally woke in the morning at 6:00 a.m., achieving less than 5 hours of sleep per night.

Clinical Impression

The patient met *DSM–IV–TR* criteria for a diagnosis of ADHD, Predominately Inattentive Type, as well as Major Depressive Disorder (on the basis of comprehensive clinical interview and assessment). She exhibited cortical slowing on qEEG examination, which is commonly noted in patients with ADHD who respond to stimulant therapy. However, her dietary, exercise, and sleeping habits were insufficient to support attention during the workday. In addition, there were concerns about possible visual and reading problems, and spousal and patient reports were suggestive of apnea.

Treatment Plan

The treatment plan was as follows:

1. Refer for evaluation of vision (acuity; CI).
2. Refer for evaluation for sleep apnea.
3. Establish dietary patterns that provide 20 grams of protein at breakfast and lunch.
4. Establish a program to provide at least 30 minutes per day of exercise.
5. Initiate a clinical trial of stimulant medication (pending results of medical evaluations); titrate dose until scores on TOVA and qEEG indicate age-appropriate levels of attention and cortical arousal.
6. Assess for reading and writing disorders and consider assistive technology.
7. Share evaluation results with employer and develop accommodation plan if needed.
8. Provide follow-up coaching and marital, parenting, and family counseling as needed.

Treatment Response

The results of the visual examination revealed that the patient had significant oculomotor impairment and needed bifocal lenses, which were prescribed with positive response. Evaluation by a sleep disorders clinic revealed sleep apnea and a continuous positive accuracy pressure (CPAP) machine was prescribed for use at home. In addition, dietary modifications and an exercise program were recommended by the physician at the sleep disorders clinic, and consultations with a nutritionist and fitness expert were arranged. The patient was able to collaborate effectively with these individuals, used the CPAP devices, and reported improved energy and mood during the day and better sleeping habits at night.

Following stabilization of sleeping and eating patterns, attentional abilities were reassessed. Although improvement was noted on both the TOVA and qEEG, significant impairment persisted. A clinical trial of Focalin XR was initiated (5 mg) and titrated to 15 milligrams. Additional gains in attention and cortical arousal were noted. To rule out possible learning disabilities, intellectual and academic testing was then conducted. Results indicated above-average intelligence (FSIQ = 118); however, specific learning disabilities in reading decoding and comprehension, as well as written expression, were identified.

Because of these disabilities, instruction was provided in the use of assistive technology programs (e.g., Read & Write), and her employer was informed of the benefits of these programs. Her employer agreed to install these programs in the computer system at her office, with positive response. However, the patient realized that she would always feel like she was, as she stated, "paddling upstream" in a clerical position. We administered the Strong Interest Inventory (2006) to assess career paths more consistent with her abilities, identifying positions in real estate and sales as careers of high interest. The patient subsequently enrolled in a real estate class, used assistive technology to help her with reading assignments, passed her certification class, and was hired as a realtor.

At home, disorganization remained an issue. She was referred to a professional organizer, who met with her at her home and systematically worked with her to organize her papers, finances, and household items. Parent counseling was provided at our clinic, as were several marital therapy sessions directed at improving problem-solving skills. The active phase of treatment lasted approximately 12 months, with periodic follow-up counseling provided as needed.

This case illustrates the importance of comprehensive medical, as well as psychological, intervention to address the multiple factors that can impede the functioning of adults with undiagnosed ADHD. In addition, it highlights the value of a thorough clinical interview process that includes contact with the parents and spouse of adult patients and direct examination of academic records. With such information, the use of stimulant medications can be far more appropriate and effective than can antidepressants in the treatment of an ostensibly depressed or anxious adult, whose symptoms were associated with undiagnosed ADHD.

CONCLUSION

In clinical practice, health care providers encounter numerous problems that require innovative solutions. In this book, a framework for creating such solutions through the comprehensive assessment and treatment of patients with ADHD is presented. This model emphasizes the identification of the specific medical causes of symptoms of inattention, impulsivity, and hyperactivity in a specific patient; the importance of diet, exercise, and sleep for attention and concentration; the value of incorporating neuropsychological and neurophysiological measures in the assessment of patients and in the selection of pharmacological treatments; the need for a comprehensive functional evaluation after effective medical interventions have been initiated; and the perspective that multimodal intervention should be considered part of the treatment plan for every patient with ADHD, not just those treated at specialty clinics. As illustrated throughout this book, clinical solutions derived from such a model of patient care, although uncommon, may hold the key to unlocking the potential of patients with ADHD.

ADDITIONAL RESOURCES

Clinicians seeking to provide effective care for their patients with attention-deficit/hyperactivity disorder (ADHD) may find the following resources to be helpful.

NATIONAL SUPPORT GROUPS FOR CHILDREN AND ADULTS WITH ADHD

Children and Adults With ADHD

Children and Adults With ADHD (CHADD) provides essential information regarding ways to understand and treat ADHD. Through local chapters, patients and their families can meet others with this condition and share information and develop friendships that can be invaluable in the recovery process. CHADD publishes a very informative magazine (*Attention*), which is available to members. Visit http://www.chadd.org.

Attention Deficit Disorder Association

Another excellent support organization for individuals with ADHD and their families is the Attention Deficit Disorder Association, which also publishes a useful and informative newsletter. Visit http://www.add.org.

RESOURCES PROVIDING RESEARCH PAPERS, SUMMARIES, AND REVIEWS ON ADHD

National Institute of Mental Health: http://www.nimh.nih.gov/
    healthinformation/adhdmenu.cfm
National Resource Center for ADHD: http://www.help4ADHD.org
ADDitude magazine: http://www.additudemag.com
Attention Research Update: http://www.helpforadd.com
The ADHD Report: 1-800-365-7006

INTERNATIONALLY RECOGNIZED SPECIALISTS IN ADHD

Daniel Amen: http://www.amenclinic.com
Russell Barkley: http://www.russellbarkley.org
Sam Goldstein: http://www.samgoldstein.com
Ned Hallowell: http://www.drhallowell.com
Vincent Monastra: http://www.theADHDdoc.com
John Ratey: http://www.johnratey.com

PRACTITIONER DIRECTORIES

Professionals Specializing in ADHD

Children and Adults With ADHD: http://www.chadd.org
ADD Professionals: http://health.groups.yahoo.com/group/ADDprofessionals

Biofeedback Providers

Association for Applied Psychophysiology & Biofeedback: http://
    www.aapb.org
International Society for Neurofeedback & Research: http://www.isnr.org
Biofeedback Certification Institute of America: http://www.bcia.org

Coaches

ADD Coach Academy: http://www.addcoachacademy.com
American Coaching Association: http://www.americoach.org

Professional Organizers

National Association for Professional Organizers: http://www.napo.net

PRODUCTS AND SOFTWARE FOR PATIENTS WITH ADHD

Products to Aid in Organization: http://www.myADDstore.com
Assistive Technology Resources: http://www.upstatecommunications.com

REFERENCES

Achenbach, T. M., & Edelbrock, C. S. (1983). *Manual for the Child Behavior Profile and Revised Child Behavior Checklist.* Burlington, VT: Authors.

Achenbach, T. M., McConaughy, S. H., & Howell, C. T. (1987). Child/adolescent behavioral and emotional problems: Implications of cross-informant correlations for situational specificity. *Psychological Bulletin, 101,* 213–232.

Adesman, A. R., Altshuler, L., Lipkin, P., & Walco, G. (1990). Otitis media in children with learning disabilities and in children with attention deficit disorder with hyperactivity. *Pediatrics, 85*(3, Pt. 2), 442–446.

Akhondzadeh, S., Mohammadi, M.-R., & Khademi, M. (2004). Zinc sulfate as an adjunct to methylphenidate for the treatment of attention deficit hyperactivity disorder in children: A double blind and randomized trial. *BMC Psychiatry, 4,* 9–15.

Aman, M. G., Mitchell, E. A., & Turbott, S. H. (1987). The effects of essential fatty acid supplementation by Efamol in hyperactive children. *Journal of Abnormal Child Psychology, 15,* 75–90.

Amara, S. G., & Kuhar, M. J. (1993). Neurotransmitter transporters: Recent progress. *Annual Review of Neuroscience, 16,* 73–93.

Ambroggio, J. D., & Jensen, P. S. (2002). Behavioral and medication treatment for ADHD—Comparisons and combinations. In P. S. Jensen & J. R. Cooper (Eds.), *Attention deficit hyperactivity disorder: State of the science—best practices* (pp. 14-1–14-14). Kingston, NJ: Civic Research Institute.

American Academy of Child & Adolescent Psychiatry. (1997). Practice parameters for the assessment and treatment of children, adolescents, and adults with attention-deficit/hyperactivity disorder. *Journal of the American Academy of Child & Adolescent Psychiatry, 36*(Suppl. 10), 85–121.

American Academy of Pediatrics. (2000). Clinical practice guidelines: Diagnosis and evaluation of the child with attention-deficit/hyperactivity disorder. *Pediatrics, 105,* 1158–1170.

American Psychiatric Association. (1994). *Diagnostic and statistical manual of mental disorders* (4th ed.). Washington, DC: Author.

American Psychiatric Association. (2000). *Diagnostic and statistical manual of mental disorders* (4th ed., text rev.). Washington, DC: Author.

American Speech–Language–Hearing Association Task Force on Central Auditory Processing Consensus Development. (1996). Central auditory processing: Current status of research and implications for clinical practice. *American Journal of Audiology, 5,* 41–54.

Anastopoulos, A. D., Rhoads, L. H., & Farley, S. E. (2006). Counseling and training parents. In R. A. Barkley (Ed.), *Attention-deficit hyperactivity disorder: A handbook for diagnosis and treatment* (pp. 453–479). New York: Guilford Press.

249

Anderson, J. C., Williams, S., McGee, R., & Silva, P. A. (1987). *DSM–III* disorders in preadolescent children: Prevalence in a large sample from the general population. *Archives of General Psychiatry, 44*, 69–76.

Angold, A., Erkanli, A., Egger, H. L., & Costello, E. J. (2000). Stimulant treatment for children: A community perspective. *Journal of the American Academy of Child & Adolescent Psychiatry, 39*, 975–984.

Anokhin, A. P., Vedeniapin, A. B., Sirevaag, E. J., Bauer, L. O., & O'Connor, S. J. (2000). The P300 is reduced in smokers. *Psychopharmacology, 149*, 409–413.

Appel, S. J., Szanton, V. L., & Rapaport, H. G. (1961). Survey of allergy in a pediatric population. *Pennsylvania Medical Journal, 64*, 621–625.

Arbeiter, H. J. (1967). How prevalent is allergy among United States school children? A survey of findings in the Munster (Indiana) school system. *Clinical Pediatrics, 6*, 140–142.

Arcos-Burgos, M., Castellanos, F. X., Lopera, F., Pineda, D., Palacio, J. D., Rapoport, J. L., et al. (2003). Genome-wide scan in multigenerational and extended pedigrees segregating ADHD from a genetic isolate. *American Journal of Human Genetics, 73*, 476–481.

Arnold, L. E. (2002). Treatment alternatives for attention deficit hyperactivity disorder. In P. S. Jensen & J. R. Cooper (Eds.), *Attention deficit hyperactivity disorder: State of the science—best practices* (pp. 13-2–13-29). Kingston, NJ: Civic Research Institute.

Arnold, L. E., Chuang, S., Davies, M., Abikoff, H. B., Conners, C. K., Elliott, G. R., et al. (2004). Nine months of multicomponent behavioral treatment for ADHD and effectiveness of MTA fading procedures. *Journal of Abnormal Child Psychology, 32*, 39–51.

Arnold, L. E., Clark, D. L., Sachs, L. A., Jakim, S., & Smithies, C. (1985). Vestibular and visual rotational stimulation as treatment for attention deficit and hyperactivity. *American Journal of Occupational Therapy, 39*, 84–91.

Arnold, L. E., Pinkham, S. M., & Votolato, N. (2000). Does zinc moderate essential fatty acid and amphetamine treatment of attention-deficit/hyperactivity disorder? *Journal of Child and Adolescent Psychopharmacology, 10*, 111–117.

Arnsten, A. F., Steere, J. C., & Hunt, R. D. (1996). The contribution of alpha-2-noradrenergic mechanisms to prefrontal cortical cognitive functions. *Archives of General Psychiatry, 53*, 448–455.

Aronen, E. T., Paavonen, E. J., Fjallberg, M., Soininen, M., & Torronen, J. (2000). Sleep and psychiatric symptoms in school-age children. *Journal of the American Academy of Child & Adolescent Psychiatry, 39*, 502–508.

Ashkenazi, R., Ben-Shachar, D., & Youdim, M. B. H. (1982). Nutritional iron and dopamine binding sites in rat brain. *Pharmacology Biochemistry and Behavior, 7*, 43–37.

August, G. J., Realmuto, G. M., MacDonald, A. W., Nugent, S. M., & Crosby, R. (1996). Prevalence of ADHD and comorbid disorders among elementary school children screened for disruptive behavior. *Journal of Abnormal Child Psychology, 24*, 571–595.

August, G. J., Stewart, M. A., & Holmes, C. S. (1983). A four-year follow-up of hyperactive boys with and without conduct disorder. *British Journal of Psychiatry, 143*, 192–198.

Ayres, A. J. (1979). *Sensory integration and the child.* Los Angeles: Western Psychological Services.

Ayres, A. J. (1989). *Sensory integration and praxis tests.* Los Angeles: Western Psychological Services.

Bakker, S. C., van der Meulen, E. M., Buitelaar, J. K., Sandkuijl, LA., Pauls, D. L., & Monsuur, A. J. (2003). A whole genome scan in 164 Dutch sib pairs with attention-deficit hyperactivity disorder: Suggestive evidence for linkage on chromosomes 7p and 15q. *American Journal of Human Genetics, 72*, 1251–1260.

Baloh, R., Sturm, R., Green, B., & Gleser, G. (1975). Neuropsychological effects of chronic asymptomatic lead absorption. *Archives of Neurology, 32*, 326–330.

Barkley, R. A. (1997). Behavioral inhibition, sustained attention, and executive functions: Constructing a unifying theory of ADHD. *Psychological Bulletin, 121*, 65–94.

Barkley, R. A. (2002). ADHD: Long-term course, adult outcome, and comorbid disorders. In P. S. Jensen & J. R. Cooper (Eds.), *Attention deficit hyperactivity disorder: State of the science—best practices* (pp. 4-1–4-12). Kingston, NJ: Civic Research Institute.

Barkley, R. A. (2003). Editorial comment. *The ADHD Report, 11*(3), 7.

Barkley, R. A. (2006). *Attention-deficit hyperactivity disorder: A handbook for diagnosis and treatment.* New York: Guilford Press.

Barkley, R. A., & Edelbrock, C. S. (1987). Assessing situational variation in children's problem behaviors: The Home and School Situations Questionnaires. In R. J. Prinz (Ed.), *Advances in behavioral assessment of children and families* (Vol. 3, pp. 157–176). Greenwich, CT: JAI Press.

Barkley, R. A., Edwards, G., Laneri, M., Fletcher, K., & Metevia, L. (2001). The efficacy of problem-solving communication training alone, behavior management training alone, and their combination for parent–adolescent conflict in teenagers with ADHD and ODD. *Journal of Consulting and Clinical Psychology, 69*, 926–941.

Barkley, R. A., Fischer, M., Edelbrock, C. S., & Smallish, L. (1990). The adolescent outcome of hyperactive children diagnosed by research criteria: I. An 8-year prospective follow-up study. *Journal of the American Academy of Child & Adolescent Psychiatry, 29*, 546–557.

Barkley, R. A., Fischer, M., Smallish, L., & Fletcher, K. (2003). Does the treatment of attention-deficit/hyperactivity disorder with stimulants contribute to drug use/abuse? A 13-year prospective study. *Pediatrics, 111*, 97–109.

Barkley, R. A., Guevremont, D. C., Anastopoulos, A. D., DuPaul, G. J., & Shelton, T. L. (1993). Driving-related risks and outcomes of attention deficit hyperactivity disorder in adolescents and young adults: A 3- to 5-year follow-up survey. *Pediatrics, 92*, 212–218.

Barkley, R. A., & Murphy, K. R. (2006). *Attention-deficit hyperactivity disorder: A clinical workbook* (3rd ed.). New York: Blackwell.

Barkley, R. A., Murphy, K. R., & Kwasnik, D. (1996a). Motor vehicle driving competencies and risks in teens and young adults with ADHD. *Pediatrics, 98,* 1089–1095.

Barkley, R. A., Murphy, K. R., & Kwasnik, D. (1996b). Psychological adjustment and adaptive impairments in young adults with ADHD. *Journal of Attention Disorders, 1,* 41–54.

Barry, R. J., Clarke, A. R., & Johnstone, S. J. (2003). A review of electrophysiology in attention-deficit/hyperactivity disorder: I. Qualitative and quantitative electroencephalography. *Clinical Neurophysiology, 114,* 171–183.

Barry, R. J., Johnstone, S. J., & Clarke, A. R. (2003). A review of electrophysiology in attention-deficit/hyperactivity disorder: II. Event-related potentials. *Clinical Neurophysiology, 114,* 184–198.

Bashore, T. R. (1989). Age, physical fitness, and mental processing speed. *Annual Review of Gerontology and Geriatrics, 9,* 120–144.

Baumgaertel, A., Wolraich, M. L., & Dietrich, M. (1995). Comparison of diagnostic criteria for attention deficit disorders in a German elementary school sample. *Journal of the American Academy of Child & Adolescent Psychiatry, 34,* 629–638.

Beck, A. T., Ward, C., & Mendelson, M. (1961). Beck Depression Inventory. *Archives of General Psychiatry, 4,* 561–571.

Beelmann, A., Pfingsten, U., & Losel, F. (1994). Effects of training social competence in children: A meta-analysis of recent evaluation studies. *Journal of Clinical Child Psychology, 23,* 260–271.

Beeson, P. B., McDermott, W., & Wyngaarden, J. B. (1979). *Cecil textbook of medicine.* Philadelphia: W. B. Saunders.

Bekaroglu, M., Aslan, Y., Gedik, Y., Deger, O., Mocan, H., Erduran, E., & Karahan, C. (1996). Relationships between serum free fatty acids and zinc, and attention deficit hyperactivity disorder: A research note. *Journal of Child Psychology and Psychiatry, 37,* 225–227.

Belenky, G., Wesensten, N. J., Thorne, D. R., Thomas, M. L., Sing, H. C., Redmond, D. P., et al. (2003). Patterns of performance degradation and restoration during sleep restriction and subsequent recovery: A sleep dose-response study. *Journal of Sleep Research, 12,* 1–12.

Benloucif, S., Orbeta, L., Ortiz, R., Janssen, I., Finkel, S. I., Bleiberg, J., & Zee, P. C. (2004). Morning or evening activity improves neuropsychological performance and subjective sleep quality in older adults. *Sleep, 27,* 1542–1551.

Benton, A. L. (1973). La medición de afección del afasia [The measurement of aphasic disorders]. In A. C. Valesquez (Ed.), *Aspectos patologicos del language* (pp. 17–29). Lima, Peru: Centro Neuropsicologico.

Benton, D., & Sargent, J. (1992). Breakfast, blood glucose, and memory. *Biological Psychiatry, 33,* 207.

Betchen, S. J. (2003). Suggestions for improving intimacy in couples in which one partner has attention-deficit/hyperactivity disorder. *Journal of Sex and Marital Therapy, 29,* 103–124.

Bhatara, V., Clark, D. L., Arnold, L. E., Gunsett, R., & Smeltzer, D. J. (1981). Hyperkinesis treated by vestibular stimulation: An exploratory study. *Biological Psychiatry, 16,* 269–279.

Bhatia, M. S., Nigam, V. R., Bohra, N., & Malik, S. K. (1991). Attention deficit disorder with hyperactivity among pediatric outpatients. *Journal of Child Psychology and Psychiatry, 32,* 297–306.

Biederman, J., Faraone, S. V., Keenan, K., Benjamin, J., Krifcher, B., Moore, C., et al. (1992). Further evidence for family-genetic risk factors in attention deficit hyperactivity disorder: Patterns of comorbidity in probands and relatives in psychiatrically and pediatrically referred samples. *Archives of General Psychiatry, 49,* 728–738.

Biederman, J., Faraone, S. V., Mick, E., Spencer, T., Wilens, T., Kiely, K., et al. (1995). High risk for attention deficit hyperactivity disorder among children of parents with childhood onset of the disorder: A pilot study. *American Journal of Psychiatry, 152,* 431–435.

Biederman, J., Faraone, S. V., Milberger, S., Guite, J., Mick, E., Chen, L., et al. (1996). A prospective 4-year follow-up study of attention-deficit hyperactivity and related disorders. *Archives of General Psychiatry, 53,* 437–446.

Biederman, J., Keenan, K., & Faraone, S. V. (1990). Parent-based diagnosis of attention deficit disorder predicts a diagnosis based on teacher report. *Journal of the American Academy of Child & Adolescent Psychiatry, 33,* 842–848.

Biederman, J., & Spencer, T. J. (2002). Nonstimulant treatments for ADHD. In P. S. Jensen & J. R. Cooper (Eds.), *Attention deficit hyperactivity disorder: State of the science—best practices* (pp. 11-1–11-16). Kingston, NJ: Civic Research Institute.

Biederman, J., Wilens, T. E., Mick, E., Faraone, S. V., & Spencer, T. J. (1998). Does attention-deficit hyperactivity disorder impact the developmental course of drug and alcohol abuse and dependence? *Biological Psychiatry, 44,* 269–273.

Biederman, J., Wilens, T. E., Mick, E., Faraone, S. V., Weber, W., Curtis, S., et al. (1997). Is ADHD a risk factor for psychoactive substance use disorders? Findings from a four-year prospective follow-up. *Journal of the American Academy of Child & Adolescent Psychiatry, 36,* 21–29.

Biederman, J., Wilens, T. E., Mick, E., Milberger, S., Spencer, T. J., & Faraone, S. V. (1995). Psychoactive substance use disorders in adults with attention deficit hyperactivity disorder (ADHD): Effects of ADHD and psychiatric comorbidity. *American Journal of Psychiatry, 152,* 1652–1658.

Biederman, J., Wilens, T. E., Mick, E., Spencer, T. J., & Faraone, S. V. (1999). Pharmacotherapy of attention-deficit/hyperactivity disorder reduces risk for substance abuse disorder. *Pediatrics, 104,* e20.

Biggins, C. A., MacKay, S., Clark, W., & Fein, G. (1997). Event-related potential evidence for frontal cortex effects of chronic cocaine dependence. *Biological Psychiatry, 42*, 472–485.

Bilici, M., Yildirim, F., Kandil, S., Bekaroglu, M., Yildirmis, S., Deger, O., et al. (2003). Double-blind, placebo-controlled study of zinc sulfate in the treatment of attention deficit hyperactivity disorder. *Progress in Neuro-Psychopharmacology & Biological Psychiatry, 28*, 181–190.

Binnie, C. D. (1994). Cognitive impairment—Is it inevitable? *Seizure, 3*(Suppl. A), 17–21.

Birbaumer, N., Elbert, T., Canavan, A., & Rockstroh, B. (1990). Slow potentials of the cerebral cortex and behavior. *Physiology Review, 70*, 1–41.

Bird, H. R. (2002). The diagnostic classification, epidemiology, and cross-cultural validity of ADHD. In P. S. Jensen & J. R. Cooper (Eds.), *Attention deficit hyperactivity disorder: State of the science—best practices* (pp. 2-1–2-12). Kingston, NJ: Civic Research Institute.

Blissitt, P. A. (2001). Sleep, memory, and learning. *Journal of Neuroscience Nursing, 33*, 208–215.

Bobb, A. J., Castellanos, F. X., Addington, A. M., & Rapoport, J. L. (2005). Molecular genetic studies of ADHD: 1991–2004. *American Journal of Medical Genetics: Part B. Neuropsychiatric Genetics, 132*, 109–124.

Boller, R., & Vignolo, L. A. (1966). Latent sensory aphasia in hemisphere-damaged patients: An experimental study with the Token Test. *Brain, 89*, 815–831.

Bor, W., Sanders, M. R., & Markie-Dadds, C. (2002). The effects of the Triple P-Positive Parenting Program on preschool children with co-occurring disruptive behavior and attentional/hyperactive difficulties. *Journal of Abnormal Child Psychology, 30*, 571–587.

Boris, M., & Mandel, F. S. (1994). Foods and additives are common causes of the attention deficit hyperactive disorder in children. *Annals of Allergy, 72*, 462–468.

Borkowski, J. G., Benton, A. L., & Spreen, O. (1967). Word fluency and brain damage. *Neuropsychologia, 5*, 135–140.

Borkowski, W. J., Ellington, R. J., & Sverdrup, E. K. (1992). Effect of sleep deprivation on the EEG of learning-impaired children with absence seizures. *Clinical Electroencephalography, 23*, 62–64.

Borsting, E., Rouse, M., & Chu, R. (2005). Measuring ADHD behaviors in children with symptomatic accommodative dysfunction or convergence insufficiency: A preliminary study. *Optometry, 76*, 588–592.

Botting, N., Powls, A., Cooke, R. W. I., & Marlow, N. (1997). Attention deficit hyperactivity disorders and other psychiatric outcomes in very low birthweight children at 12 years. *Journal of Child Psychology and Psychiatry, 18*, 931–941.

Boutros, N., Fristad, M., & Abdollohian, A. (1998). The fourteen and six positive spikes and attention-deficit hyperactivity disorder. *Biological Psychiatry, 44*, 298–301.

Bradley, J. D., & Golden, C. J. (2001). Biological contributions to the presentation and understanding of attention-deficit hyperactivity disorder: A review. *Clinical Psychology Reviews, 21*, 907–929.

Braverman, E. (1995). *PATH wellness manual.* Skillman, NJ: Publications for Achieving Total Health.

Braverman, E. (2003). *The healing nutrients within: Facts, findings, and new research on amino acids.* North Bergen, NJ: Basic Health Publications.

Breakey, J. (1997). The role of diet and behaviour in children. *Journal of Paediatrics and Child Health, 33*, 190–194.

Bresnahan, S. M., & Barry, R. J. (2002). Specificity of quantitative EEG analysis in adults with attention deficit hyperactivity disorder. *Psychiatry Research, 112*, 133–144.

Bresnahan, S. M., Barry, R. J., Clarke, A. R., & Johnstone, S. J. (2006). Quantitative EEG analysis in dexamphetamine-responsive adults with attention-deficit/hyperactivity disorder. *Psychiatry Research, 141*, 151–159.

Breton, J., Bergeron, L., Valla, J. P., Berthiaume, C., Gauder, N., Lambert, J., et al. (1999). Quebec children mental health survey: Prevalence of *DSM–III–R* mental health disorders. *Journal of Child Psychology and Psychiatry, 40*, 375–384.

Brown, T. E. (2004). Atomoxetine and stimulants in combination for treatment of attention deficit hyperactivity disorder: Four case reports. *Journal of Child and Adolescent Psychopharmacology, 14*, 129–136.

Buckley, R. H., & Metcalfe, D. (1982) Food allergy. *Journal of the American Medical Association, 248*, 2627–2631.

Cantwell, D. P., & Baker, L. (1989). Stability and natural history of *DSM–III* childhood diagnoses. *Journal of the American Academy of Child & Adolescent Psychiatry, 28*, 691–700.

Cantwell, D. P., Swanson, J. M., & Connor, D. F. (1997). Adverse response to clonidine. *Journal of the American Academy of Child & Adolescent Psychiatry, 36*, 539–544.

Carskadon, M. A., Cavallo, A., & Rosekind, M. R. (1989). Sleepiness and nap sleep following a morning dose of clonidine. *Sleep, 12*, 338–344.

Carskadon, M. A., & Dement, W. C. (1981). Cumulative effects of sleep restriction on daytime sleepiness. *Psychophysiology, 18*, 107–113.

Carter, C. M., Urbanowicz, M., Hemsley, R., Mantilla, L., Strobel, S., Graham, P. J., & Taylor, E. (1993). Effects of a few food diets in attention deficit disorder. *Archives of Disease in Childhood, 69*, 564–568.

Castellanos, F. X., Giedd, J. N., Marsh, W. L., Hamburger, S. D., Vaituzios, A. C., Dickstein, D. P., et al. (1996). Quantitative brain magnetic resonance imaging in attention-deficit hyperactivity disorder. *Archives of General Psychiatry, 53*, 607–616.

Centers for Disease Control and Prevention. (2006). *Epilepsy.* Atlanta, GA: Author.

Centers for Disease Control and Prevention. (2007, February 9). Prevalence of autism spectrum disorders—Autism and Developmental Disabilities Monitoring

Network, 14 sites, United States, 2002. *Morbidity and Mortality Weekly Report Surveillance Summaries, 56,* 12–28.

Cermak, S. A. (1991). Somatodyspraxia. In A. G. Fisher, E. A. Murray, & A. C. Bundy (Eds.), *Sensory integration: Theory and practice* (pp. 137–170). Philadelphia: F. A. Davis.

Chabot, R. J., di Michele, F., & Prichep, L. (2005). The role of quantitative electroencephalography in child and adolescent psychiatric disorders. *Child and Adolescent Psychiatric Clinics of North America, 14,* 21–53.

Chabot, R. J., di Michele, F., Prichep, L., & John, E. R. (2001). The clinical role of computerized EEG in the evaluation and treatment of learning and attention disorders in children and adolescents. *Journal of Neuropsychiatry and Clinical Neuroscience, 13,* 171–186.

Chabot, R. J., Merkin, H., Wood, L. M., Davenport, T. L., & Serfontein, G. (1996). Sensitivity and specificity of QEEG in children with attention deficit or specific developmental learning disorders. *Clinical Electroencephalography, 27,* 26–34.

Chabot, R. J., Orgill, A. A., Crawford, G., Harris, M. J., & Serfontein, G. (1999). Behavioral and electrophysiological predictors of treatment response to stimulants in children with attention disorders. *Journal of Child Neurology, 14,* 343–351.

Chambless, D. L., & Hollon, S. D. (1998). Defining empirically supported therapies. *Journal of Consulting and Clinical Psychology, 66,* 7–18.

Chan, E., Hopkins, M. R., Perrin, J. M., Herrerias, C., & Homer, C. J. (2005). Diagnostic practices for attention deficit hyperactivity disorder: A national survey of primary care physicians. *Ambulatory Pediatrics, 5,* 201–208.

Chan, Y.-P. M., Swanson, J. M., Soldin, S. S., Thiessen, J. J., Macleod, S. M., & Logan, W. (1983). Methylphenidate hydrochloride given with or before breakfast: II. Effects on plasma concentration of methylphenidate and ritalinic acid. *Pediatrics, 72,* 56–59.

Chermak, G. D., Hall, J. W., & Musiek, F. E. (1999). Differential diagnosis and management of central auditory processing disorder and attention deficit hyperactivity disorder. *Journal of the American Academy of Audiology, 10,* 289–303.

Chermak, G. D., & Musiek, F. E. (1997). *Central auditory processing disorders: New perspectives.* San Diego, CA: Singular Press.

Chervin, R. D., Dillon, J. E., Bassetti, C., Ganoczy, D. A., & Pituch, K. J. (1997). Symptoms of sleep disorders, inattention, and hyperactivity in children. *Sleep, 20,* 1185–1192.

Chmura, J., Krysztofiak, H., Ziemba, A. W., Nazar, K., & Kaciuba-Uscilko, H. (1998). Psychomotor performance during prolonged exercise above and below the blood lactate threshold. *European Journal of Applied Physiology and Occupational Physiology, 77,* 77–80.

Chmura, J., Nazar, K., & Kaciuba-Uscilko, H. (1994). Choice reaction time during graded exercise in relation to blood lactate and plasma catecholamine threshold. *Journal of Sports Medicine, 15,* 172–176.

Chronis, A. M., Chacko, A., Fabiano, G. A., Wymbs, B. T., & Pelham, W. E., Jr. (2004). Enhancements to the behavioral parent training paradigm for families of children with ADHD: Review and future directions. *Clinical Child and Family Psychology Review, 7*, 1–27.

Clarke, A. R., & Barry, R. J. (2004). EEG activity in subtypes of attention-deficit/hyperactivity disorder. *Journal of Neurotherapy, 8*, 43–62.

Clarke, A. R., Barry, R. J., Bond, D., McCarthy, R., & Selikowitz, M. (2002). Effects of stimulant medications on the EEG of children with attention-deficit/hyperactivity disorder. *Psychopharmacology, 164*, 277–284.

Clarke, A. R., Barry, R. J., McCarthy, R., & Selikowitz, M. (2001a). EEG analysis in attention-deficit/hyperactivity disorder: A comparative study of two subtypes. *Psychiatry Research, 81*, 19–29.

Clarke, A. R., Barry, R. J., McCarthy, R., & Selikowitz, M. (2001b). EEG-defined subtypes of children with attention-deficit/hyperactivity disorder. *Clinical Neurophysiology, 112*, 2098–2105.

Clarke, A. R., Barry, R. J., McCarthy, R., Selikowitz, M., Clarke, D. C., & Croft, R. J. (2003). Effects of stimulant medications on children with attention-deficit/hyperactivity disorder and excessive beta activity in their EEG. *Clinical Neurophysiology, 114*, 1729–1737.

Clarke, A. R., Barry, R. J., McCarthy, R., Selikowitz, M., & Croft, R. J. (2002). EEG differences between good and poor responders to methylphenidate in boys with the inattentive type of attention-deficit/hyperactivity disorder. *Clinical Neurophysiology, 113*, 1191–1198.

Claude, D., & Firestone, P. (1995). The development of ADHD boys: A 12-year follow-up. *Canadian Journal of Behavioral Science, 27*, 226–249.

Claycomb, C. D., Ryan, J. J., Miller, L. J., & Schnakenberg-Ott, S. (2004). Relationships among attention deficit hyperactivity disorder, induced labor, and selected physiological and demographic variables. *Journal of Clinical Psychology, 60*, 689–693.

Coburn, K. L., Lauterbach, E. C., Boutros, N. N., Black, K. J., Arciniegas, D. B., & Coffey, C. E. (2006). The value of quantitative electroencephalography in clinical psychiatry: A report by the Committee on Research of the American Neuropsychiatric Association. *Journal of Neuropsychiatry and Clinical Neuroscience, 18*, 460–500.

Colleges for students with learning disabilities and ADD. (2006). Lawrenceville, NJ: Peterson's.

Colquhon, I., & Bunday, S. (1981). A lack of essential fatty acids as a possible cause of hyperactivity in children. *Medical Hypotheses, 7*, 673–679.

Comings, D. E. (2000). Attention-deficit/hyperactivity disorder with Tourette syndrome. In T. E. Brown (Ed.), *Attention-deficit disorders and comorbidities in children, adolescents, and adults* (pp. 363–392). Washington, DC: American Psychiatric Press.

Comings, D. E. (2001). Clinical and molecular genetics of ADHD and Tourette syndrome: Two related polygenic disorders. *Annals of the New York Academy of Sciences, 931,* 50–83.

Comings, D. E., Gade-Andavolu, R., Gonzalez, N., Wu, S., Muhleman, D., Blake, H., et al. (2000a). Comparison of the role of dopamine, serotonin, and noradrenaline genes in ADHD, ODD, and conduct disorder: Multivariate regression analysis of 20 genes. *Clinical Genetics, 57,* 178–196.

Comings, D. E., Gade-Andavolu, R., Gonzalez, N., Wu, S., Muhleman, D., Blake, H., et al. (2000b). Multivariate analysis of associations of 42 genes in ADHD, ODD, and conduct disorder. *Clinical Genetics, 58,* 31–40.

Conners, C. K. (1995). *The Conners' continuous performance test.* North Tonawanda, NY: Multi-Health Systems.

Conners, C. K. (2001). *Conners' Rating Scales—Revised.* North Tonawanda, NY: Multi-Health Systems.

Conners, C. K., Epstein, J. N., March, J. S., Angold, A., Wells, K. C., Klaric, J., et al. (2001). Multimodal treatment of ADHD in the MTA: An alternative outcome analysis. *Journal of the American Academy of Child & Adolescent Psychiatry, 40,* 159–167.

Conners, C. K., Erhardt, D., & Sparrow, E. (1999). *Conners' Adult ADHD Rating Scales.* North Tonawanda, NY: Multi-Health Systems.

Connor, D. F. (2006). Other medications. In R. A. Barkley (Ed.), *Attention-deficit hyperactivity disorder: A handbook for diagnosis and treatment* (pp. 658–677). New York: Guilford Press.

Connor, D. F., Barkley, R. A., & Davis, H. T. (2000). A pilot study of methylphenidate, clonidine, or the combination in ADHD comorbid with aggressive oppositional defiant or conduct disorder. *Clinical Pediatrics, 39,* 15–25.

Cook, J. R., Mausbach, T., Burd, L., Gascon, G. G., Slotnick, H. B., Patterson, B., et al. (1993). A preliminary study of the relationship between central auditory processing and attention deficit disorder. *Journal of Psychiatry & Neuroscience, 18,* 130–137.

Corkum, P. V., & Siegel, L. S. (1993). Is the continuous performance task a valuable research tool for use with children with attention-deficit-hyperactivity disorder? *Journal of Child Psychology and Psychiatry, 34,* 1217–1239.

Corkum, P. V., Tannock, R., & Moldofsky, H. (1998). Sleep disturbances in children with attention-deficit/hyperactivity disorder. *Journal of the American Academy of Child & Adolescent Psychiatry, 37,* 637–646.

Cornish, L. A. (1988). Guanfacine hydrochloride: A centrally acting antihypertensive agent. *Journal of Clinical Pharmacology, 7,* 187–197.

Costello, E. J., Angold, A., Burns, B. J., Stangl, D. K., Tweed, D. L., Erkanli, A., & Worthman, C. M. (1996). The Great Smokey Mountains Study of youth: Functional impairment and serious emotional disturbance. *Archives of General Psychiatry, 53,* 1137–1143.

Costello, E. J., Costello, A. J., & Edelbrock, C. S. (1988). Psychiatric disorders in pediatric primary care. *Archives of General Psychiatry, 45,* 1107–1116.

Cousins, L. S., & Weiss, G. (1993). Parent training and social skills training for children with attention-deficit hyperactivity disorder: How can they be combined for greater effectiveness? *Canadian Journal of Psychiatry, 38,* 449–457.

Craft, L., & Landers, D. M. (1998). The effect of exercise on clinical depression and depression resulting from mental illness: A meta-analysis. *Journal of Sport and Exercise Psychology, 20,* 339–357.

Crawford, M. A. (1992). Essential fatty acids and neurodevelopmental disorder. In N. G. Bazan (Ed.), *Neurobiology of essential fatty acids* (pp. 307–314). New York: Plenum Press.

Cunningham, C. E. (2006). Large-group, community-based family-centered parent training. In R. A. Barkley (Ed.), *Attention-deficit hyperactivity disorder: A handbook for diagnosis and treatment* (pp. 480–498). New York: Guilford Press.

Cunningham, C. E. (2007). A family-centered approach to planning and measuring the outcome of interventions for children with attention-deficit/hyperactivity disorder. *Journal of Pediatric Psychology, 32,* 676–694.

Cunningham, C. E., & Barkley, R. A. (1979). The interactions of hyperactive and normal children with their mothers during free play and structured tasks. *Child Development, 50,* 217–224.

Cunningham, C. E., Bremner, R., & Boyle, M. (1995). Large group community-based parenting programs for families of preschoolers at risk for disruptive behavior disorders: Utilization, cost effectiveness, and outcome. *Journal of Child Psychology and Psychiatry, 36,* 141–159.

David, O. J. (1974). Association between lower level lead concentrations and hyperactivity. *Environmental Health Perspective, 7,* 17–25.

David, O. J., Hoffman, S. P., Clark, J., Grad, G., & Sverd, J. (1983). The relationship of hyperactivity to moderately elevated lead levels. *Archives of Environmental Health, 38,* 341–346.

David, O. J., Hoffman, S. P., Sverd, J., Clark, J., & Voeller, K. (1976). Lead and hyperactivity. Behavioral response to chelation: A pilot study. *American Journal of Psychiatry, 133,* 1155–1158.

Davidson, R. J., & Hugdahl, K. (Eds.). (1995). *Brain asymmetry.* Cambridge, MA: MIT Press.

de la Burde, B., & Choate, M. (1972). Does asymptomatic lead exposure in children have latent sequelae? *Journal of Pediatrics, 81,* 1088–1091.

de la Burde, B., & Choate, M. (1974). Early asymptomatic lead exposure and development at school age. *Journal of Pediatrics, 87,* 638–642.

deBeus, R., Ball, J. D., deBeus, M. E., & Herrington, R. (2003, August). *Attention training with ADHD children: Preliminary findings in a double-blind placebo-controlled study.* Paper presented at the 11th Annual Conference of the International Society for Neuronal Regulation, Houston, TX.

Deinard, A. S., Gilbert, A., Dodds, M., & Egeland, B. (1981). Iron deficiency and behavioral deficits. *Pediatrics, 68,* 828–833.

Deinard, A. S., Murray, M. J., & Egeland, B. (1976). Childhood iron deficiency and impaired attentional development or scholastic performance: Is the evidence sufficient to establish causality? *Pediatrics, 88*, 162–163.

Deming, L., Zhenyun, W., & Daosheng, S. (1991). The relationship of sleep to learning and memory. *International Journal of Mental Health, 20*, 41–47.

Derks, E. M., Hudziak, J. J., Dolan, C. V., Ferdinand, R. F., & Boomsma, D. I. (2006). The relations between DISC–IV *DSM* diagnoses of ADHD and multi-informant CBCL–AP syndrome scores. *Comprehensive Psychiatry, 47*, 116–122.

Derogatis, L. R. (1992). *Symptoms Checklist-90-Revised.* Bloomington, MN: NCS Pearson.

Desmedt, J. E. (1980). P300 is serial tasks: An essential post-decision closure mechanism. In H. H. Kornhuber & L. Deecke (Eds.), *Motivation, motor, and sensory processes of the brain* (pp. 682–686). Amsterdam: Elsevier.

Dinges, D. F., Pack, F., Williams, K., Gillen, K. A., Powell, J. W., Ott, G. E., & Pack, A. I. (1997). Cumulative sleepiness, mood disturbance, and psychomotor vigilance performance decrements during a week of sleep restricted to 4–5 hours per night. *Sleep, 20*, 267–277.

Dougherty, D. D., Bonab, A. A., Spencer, T. J., Rauch, S. L., Madras, B. K., & Fischman, A. J. (1999). Dopamine transporter density in patients with attention deficit hyperactivity disorder. *Lancet, 354*, 2132–2133.

Dragon NaturallySpeaking (Version 9) [Software]. Available from http://www.nuance.com/naturallyspeaking/

Drake, C. L., Roehrs, T. A., Burduvali, E., Bonahoom, A., Rosekind, M., & Roth, T. (2001). Effects of rapid vs. slow accumulation of eight hours of sleep loss. *Psychophysiology, 38*, 979–987.

DuPaul, G. J., Guevremont, D. C., & Barkley, R. A. (1992). Behavioral treatment of attention-deficit hyperactivity disorder in the classroom. *Behavior Modification, 16*, 204–225.

DuPaul, G. J., McGoey, K. E., Eckert, T. L., & VanBrakle, J. (2001). Preschool children with attention deficit/hyperactivity disorder: Impairments in behavioral, social, and school functioning. *Journal of the American Academy of Child & Adolescent Psychiatry, 36*, 1036–1045.

Durmer, J. S., & Dinges, D. F. (2005). Neurocognitive consequences of sleep deprivation. *Seminars in Neurology, 25*, 117–129.

Durston, S. (2003). A review of the biological bases of ADHD: What have we learned from imaging studies? *Mental Retardation and Developmental Disabilities Research Reviews, 9*, 184–195.

Dustman, R. E., Emmerson, R. E., & Shearer, D. E. (1990). Electrophysiology and aging: Slowing, inhibition and aerobic fitness. In M. L. Howe, M. J. Stones, & C. J. Grainerd (Eds.), *Cognitive and behavioral performance factors in atypical aging* (pp. 103–149). New York: Springer-Verlag.

Dwyer, T., Coonan, W., Leitch, D., Hetzel, B. S., & Baghurst, R. A. (1983). An investigation of physical activity on the health of primary school students in South Australia. *International Journal of Epidemiology, 12*, 308–313.

Dye, L., Lluch, A., & Blundell, J. (2000). Macronutrients and performance. *Nutrition, 16*, 1021–1034.

Eakin, L., Minde, K., Hechtman, L., Ochs, E., Krane, E., Bouffard, R., et al. (2004). The marital and family functioning of adults with ADHD and their spouses. *Journal of Attention Disorders, 8*, 1–10.

Egger, J., Carter, C. M., Graham, P. J., Gumley, D., & Soothill, J. F. (1985) Controlled trial of oligoantigenic treatment in the hyperkinetic syndrome. *Lancet, 339*, 540–545.

Egger, J., Stolla, A., & McEwen, L. M. (1992). Controlled trial of hyposensitization in children with food-induced hyperkinetic syndrome. *Lancet, 339*, 1150–1153.

Ehlers, S., & Gillberg, C. (1993). The epidemiology of Asperger syndrome: A total population study. *Journal of Child Psychology and Psychiatry, 34*, 1327–1350.

El-Zein, R. A., Abdel-Rahman, S. Z., Hay, M. J., Lopez, M. S., Bondy, M. L., Morris, D. L., & Legator, M. S. (2005). Cytogenetic effects in children treated with methylphenidate. *Cancer Letters, 230*, 284–291.

Epstein, J. N., Conners, C. K., Hervey, A. S., Toney, S. T., Arnold, L. E., Abikoff, H. B., et al. (2006). Assessing medication effects in the MTA study using neuropsychological measures. *Journal of Child Psychology and Psychiatry, 47*, 446–456.

Ernst, M., Liebenauer, L. L., King, A. C., Fitzgerald, G. A., Cohen, R. M., & Zametkin, A. J. (1994). Reduced brain metabolism in hyperactive girls. *Journal of the American Academy of Child & Adolescent Psychiatry, 33*, 858–868.

Esser, G., Schmidt, M. H., & Woerner, W. (1990). Epidemiology and course of psychiatric disorders in school-age children: Results of a longitudinal study. *Journal of Child Psychology and Psychiatry, 31*, 243–263.

Evans, J. H., Ferre, L., Ford, L. A., & Green, J. L. (1995). Decreasing attention deficit hyperactivity disorder symptoms utilizing an automated classroom reinforcement device. *Psychology in the Schools, 32*, 210–219.

Fallone, G., Acebo, C., Arnedt, J. T., Seifer, R., & Carskadon, M. A. (2001). Effects of acute sleep restriction on behavior, sustained attention, and response inhibition in children. *Perceptual and Motor Skills, 93*, 213–229.

Feagans, L. V., Sanyal, M., Henderson, F., Collier, A., & Applebaum, M. (1987). Relationship of middle ear disease in early childhood to later narrative and attentional skills. *Journal of Pediatrics and Psychology, 12*, 581–594.

Feldman, H., Crumrine, P., Handen, R., Alvin, R., & Teodori, J. (1989). Methylphenidate in children with seizures and attention-deficit disorder. *American Journal of Diseases of Children, 143*, 1081–1086.

Fergusson, D. M., Horwood, L. J., & Lynskey, M. T. (1993). Prevalence and comorbidity of *DSM–III–R* diagnoses in a birth cohort of 15-year-olds. *Journal of the American Academy of Child & Adolescent Psychiatry, 32*, 1127–1134.

Fernstrom, J. D. (1976). The effect of nutritional factors on brain amino acid levels and monoamine synthesis. *Federation Proceedings, 35*, 1151–1156.

Fernstrom, J. D. (1977). Effects of the diet on brain neurotransmitters. *Metabolism*, 26, 207–223.

Fernstrom, J. D. (1981). Effects of the diet on brain function. *Acta Astronautica*, 8, 1035–1042.

Fernstrom, J. D. (1994). Dietary amino acids and brain function. *Journal of the American Dietetic Association*, 94, 71–77.

Fernstrom, J. D., & Wurtman, R. J. (1974). Nutrition and the brain. *Scientific American*, 230(2), 84–91.

Field, T., Diego, M., & Sanders, C. E. (2001). Exercise is positively related to adolescents' relationships and academics. *Adolescence*, 36, 105–110.

Fischer, K., Colombani, P. C., Langhans, W., & Wenk, C. (2001). Cognitive performance and its relationship with postprandial metabolic changes after ingestion of different macronutrients in the morning. *British Journal of Nutrition*, 85, 393–405.

Fischer, K., Colombani, P. C., Langhans, W., & Wenk, C. (2002). Carbohydrate to protein ratio in food and cognitive performance in the morning. *Physiology & Behavior*, 75, 411–423.

Fischer, M., Barkley, R. A., Smallish, L., & Fletcher, K. (2002). Young adult follow-up of hyperactive children: Self-reported psychiatric disorders, comorbidity, and the role of childhood conduct problems and teen CD. *Journal of Abnormal Child Psychology*, 30, 463–475.

Fisher, A., Murray, E., & Bundy, A. (1991). *Sensory integration: Theory and practice*. Philadelphia: F. A. Davis.

Fisher, M. (1997). Persistence of ADHD into adulthood: It depends on whom you ask. *The ADHD Report*, 5, 8–10.

Fisher, S. E., Francks, C., McCracken, J. T., McGough, J. J., Marlow, A. J., MacPhie, I. L., et al. (2002). A genomewide scan for loci involved in attention-deficit/hyperactivity disorder. *American Journal of Human Genetics*, 70, 1183–1196.

Fitzgerald, M., & Kewley, G. (2005). Attention-deficit/hyperactivity disorder and Asperger's disorder? *Journal of the American Academy of Child & Adolescent Psychiatry*, 44, 210.

Foks, M. (2005). Neurofeedback training as an educational intervention in a school setting: How the regulation of arousal states can lead to improved attention and behavior in children with special needs. *Educational and Child Psychology*, 22(3), 67–77.

Foley, H. A., Carlton, C. O., & Howell, R. J. (1996). The relationship of attention deficit hyperactivity disorder and conduct disorder to juvenile delinquency: Legal implications. *Bulletin of the American Academy of Psychiatry and the Law*, 24, 333–345.

Food and Nutrition Board of the National Academy of Sciences. (1989). *Recommended dietary allowances* (10th ed.). Washington, DC: National Academy Press.

Foster-Powell, K., Holt, S. H., & Brand-Miller, J. C. (2002). International table of glycemic index and glycemic load values. *American Journal of Clinical Nutrition*, 76, 5–56.

Fowler, J. S., Volkow, N. D., Ding, Y. S., Wang, G. J., Dewey, S., Fischman, M. S., et al. (1999). Positron emission tomography studies of dopamine-enhancing drugs. *Journal of Clinical Pharmacology, S9*(Suppl.), 13S–16S.

Fox, D. J., Tharp, D. E., & Fox, L. C. (2005). Neurofeedback: An alternative and efficacious treatment for attention deficit hyperactivity disorder. *Applied Psychophysiology and Biofeedback, 30,* 365–373.

Frankel, F., Myatt, R., & Cantwell, D. P. (1995). Training outpatient boys to conform with the social ecology of popular peers: Effects on parent and teacher ratings. *Journal of Clinical Child Psychology, 24,* 300–310.

Frankel, F., Myatt, R., Cantwell, D. P., & Feinberg, D. T. (1997). Parent-assisted transfer of children's social skills training: Effects on children with and without attention-deficit hyperactivity disorder. *Journal of the American Academy of Child & Adolescent Psychiatry, 3,* 1056–1064.

Fuchs, T., Birbaumer, N., Lutzenberger, W., Gruzelier, J. H., & Kaiser, J. (2003). Neurofeedback treatment for attention-deficit/hyperactivity disorder in children: A comparison with methylphenidate. *Applied Psychophysiology and Biofeedback, 28,* 1–12.

Gallucci, F., Bird, H. R., Berardi, C., Gallai, V., Pfanner, P., & Weinberg, A. (1993). Symptoms of ADHD in an Italian school sample: Findings of a pilot study. *Journal of the American Academy of Child & Adolescent Psychiatry, 32,* 1051–1058.

Gammon, G. D., & Brown, T. E. (1993). Fluoxetine and methylphenidate in combination for treatment of attention deficit disorder and comorbid depressive disorder. *Journal of Child and Adolescent Psychopharmacology, 3,* 1–10.

Gascon, G. G., Johnson, R., & Burd, L. (1986). Central auditory processing and attention deficit disorders. *Journal of Child Neurology, 1,* 27–33.

Gentry, L. R., Godersky, J. C., & Thompson, B. (1988). MR imaging of head trauma: Review of the distribution and radiopathologic features of traumatic lesions. *American Journal of Radiology, 150,* 663–672.

Geurts, H. M., Verte, S., Oosterlaan, J., Roeyers, H., & Sergeant, J. A. (2004). How specific are executive functioning deficits in attention deficit hyperactivity disorder and autism? *Journal of Child Psychology and Psychiatry, 45,* 836–854.

Gevins, A., Smith, M. E., McEvoy, L. K., & Yu, D. (1997). High-resolution EEG mapping of cortical activation related to working memory: Effects of task difficulty, type of processing, and practice. *Cerebral Cortex, 7,* 374–385.

Ghaziuddin, M., Weidmer-Mikhail, E., & Ghaziuddin, N. (1998). Comorbidity of Asperger syndrome: A preliminary report. *Journal of Intellectual Disability Research, 42,* 279–283.

Giedd, J. N., Blumenthal, J., Molloy, E., & Castellanos, F. X. (2001). Brain imaging of attention deficit/hyperactivity disorder. *Annals of the New York Academy of Sciences, 931,* 33–49.

Gieseking, C. F., Williams, H. L., & Lubin, A. (1957). The effect of sleep deprivation upon information learning. *American Psychologist, 12,* 406.

Gittelman, R., & Eskinazi, B. (1983). Lead and hyperactivity revisited. *Archives of General Psychiatry, 40,* 827–833.

Goldstein, S. (2005). Coaching as a treatment for ADHD. *Journal of Attention Disorders, 9*, 379–381.

Goldstein, S., & Schwebach, A. J. (2004). The comorbidity of pervasive developmental disorder and attention deficit hyperactivity disorder: Results of a retrospective chart review. *Journal of Autism and Developmental Disorders, 34*, 329–339.

Golub, M. S., Takeuchi, P. T., Keen, C. L., Gershwin, M. E., Hendrickx, A. G., & Lonnerdal, B. (1994). Modulation of behavioral performance of prepubertal monkeys by moderate dietary zinc deprivation. *American Journal of Clinical Nutrition, 60*, 238–243.

Gordon, M. (1983). *The Gordon Diagnostic System.* DeWitt, NY: Gordon Systems.

Gordon, M., Barkley, R. A., & Lovett, B. J. (2006). Tests and observational measures. In R. A. Barkley (Ed.), *Attention-deficit hyperactivity disorder: A handbook for diagnosis and treatment* (pp. 369–388). New York: Guilford Press.

Gordon, M., Thomason, D., Cooper, S., & Ivers, C. L. (1991). Nonmedical treatment of ADHD/hyperactivity: The Attention Training System. *Journal of School Psychology, 29*, 151–159.

Graetz, B. W., Sawyer, M. G., Hazell, P. L., Arney, F., & Baghurst, P. (2001). Validity of *DSM–IV* ADHD subtypes in a nationally representative sample of Australian children and adolescents. *Journal of the American Academy of Child & Adolescent Psychiatry, 40*, 1410–1417.

Granet, D. B., Gomi, C. F., Ventura, R., & Miller-Scholte, A. (2005). The relationship between convergence insufficiency and ADHD. *Strabismus, 13*, 163–168.

Greenberg, L. M. (1994). *Test of Variables of Attention Continuous Performance test manual.* Los Alamitos, CA: Universal Attention Disorders.

Greenberg, L. M., & Kindschi, C. (1996). *TOVA Test of Variables of Attention: Clinical guide.* St. Paul, MN: TOVA Research Foundation

Greenhill, L. L. (2002). Stimulant medication treatment of children with attention deficit hyperactivity disorder. In P. S. Jensen & J. R. Cooper (Eds.), *Attention deficit hyperactivity disorder: State of the science—best practices* (pp. 9-1–9-27). Kingston, NJ: Civic Research Institute.

Greenhill, L. L., Pliszka, D., Dulcan, M. K., Bernet, W., Arnold, V., Beitchman, J., et al. (2002). Practice parameter for the use of stimulant medications in the treatment of children, adolescents, and adults. *Journal of the American Academy of Child & Adolescent Psychiatry, 41*(Suppl. 2), 26–49.

Gresham, F. M., & Elliott, S. N. (1990). *Social skills rating system: Manual.* Circle Pines, MN: American Guidance Service.

Gruber, R., Sadeh, A., & Raviv, A. (2000). Instability of sleep patterns in children with attention-deficit/hyperactivity disorder. *Journal of the American Academy of Child & Adolescent Psychiatry, 39*, 495–501.

Hagerman, R. J., & Falkenstein, A. R. (1987). An association between recurrent otitis media in infancy and hyperactivity. *Clinical Pediatrics, 26*, 253–257.

Hallahan, B., & Garland, M. R. (2004). Essential fatty acids and their role in the treatment of impulsivity disorders. *Prostaglandins, Leukotrienes, and Essential Fatty Acids, 71,* 211–216.

Hallowell, E. M. (1995). Coaching: An adjunct of the treatment of ADHD. *The ADHD Report, 3*(4), 7–9.

Halperin, J. M., Newcorn, J. H., McKay, K. E., Siever, L. J., & Sharma, V. (2003). Growth hormone response to guanfacine in boys with attention deficit hyperactivity disorder: A preliminary study. *Journal of Child and Adolescent Psychopharmacology, 13,* 283–294.

Halverstadt, J. S. (1998). *ADD and romance: Finding fulfillment in love, sex, and relationships.* Dallas, TX: Taylor Press.

Hambidge, M. (2000). Human zinc deficiency. *The Journal of Nutrition, 130*(Suppl. 5), 1344S–1349S.

Harlow, C. W. (1998). Profile of jail inmates, 1996. *Bureau of Justice Statistics Special Report* (Rep. No. NCJ 164620). Washington, DC: U.S. Department of Justice.

Hartsough, C. S., & Lambert, N. M. (1985). Medical factors in hyperactive and normal children: Prenatal, developmental, and health history findings. *American Journal of Orthopsychiatry, 55,* 190–210.

Harvey, W. J., & Reid, G. (2003). Attention-deficit/hyperactivity disorder: A review of research on movement, skill performance, and physical fitness. *Adapted Physical Activity Quarterly, 20,* 1–25.

Hathaway, S. R., & McKinley, J. C. (2001). *The Minnesota Multiphasic Personality Inventory—II.* Minneapolis: University of Minnesota Press.

Hauser, P., Soler, R., Brucker-Davis, F., & Weintraub, B. D. (1997). Thyroid hormones correlate with symptoms of hyperactivity but not inattention in ADHD. *Psychoneuroendocrinology, 22,* 107–114.

Hazell, P. L., & Stuart, J. E. (2003). A randomized controlled trial of clonidine added to psychostimulant medication for hyperactive and aggressive children. *Journal of the American Academy of Child & Adolescent Psychiatry, 42,* 886–894.

Heinrich, H., Gevensleben, H., Freisleder, F. J., Moll, G. H., & Rothenberger, A. (2004). Training of slow cortical potentials in attention-deficit hyperactivity disorder: Evidence for positive behavioral and neuropsychological effects. *Biological Psychiatry, 55,* 772–775.

Hemmer, S. A., Pasternak, J. F., Zecker, S. G., & Trommer, B. L. (2001). Stimulant therapy and seizure risk in children with ADHD. *Pediatric Neurology, 24,* 99–102.

Hermens, D. F. (2006). *An integrated psychophysiological investigation of ADHD.* Unpublished doctoral dissertation, University of Sydney, New South Wales, Australia.

Hermens, D. F., Cooper, N. J., Kohn, M., Clarke, S., & Gordon, E. (2005). Predicting stimulant medication response in ADHD: Evidence from an integrated profile of neuropsychological, psychophysiological, and clinical factors. *Journal of Integrative Neuroscience, 4,* 107–121.

Hermens, D. F., Kohn, M. R., Clarke, S. D., Gordon, E., & Williams, L. M. (2005). Sex differences in adolescent ADHD: Findings from concurrent EEG and EDA. *Clinical Neurophysiology, 116*, 1455–1463.

Hermens, D. F., Williams, L. M., Clarke, S., Kohn, M., Cooper, N., & Gordon, E. (2005). Responses to methylphenidate in adolescent AD/HD: Evidence from concurrently recorded autonomic (EDA) and central (EEG and ERP) measures. *International Journal of Psychophysiology, 58*, 21–33.

Herning, R. I. (1996). Cognitive event-related potentials in populations at risk for substance abuse. *NIDA Research Monographs, 159*, 161–192.

Herskovits, E. H., Megalooikonomou, V., Davatzikos, C., Chen, A., Bryan, R. N., & Gerring, J. P. (1999). Distribution of traumatic brain lesions and attention-deficit/hyperactivity disorder. *Radiology, 213*, 389–394.

Hesslinger, B., van Elst, L. T., Nyberg, E., Dykierek, P., Richter, H., Berner, M., & Ebert, D. (2002). Psychotherapy of attention deficit hyperactivity disorder in adults: A pilot study using a structured skills training program. *European Archives of Psychiatry and Clinical Neuroscience, 252*, 177–184.

Hewitt, J. K., Silberg, J. L., Rutter, M., Simonoff, E., Meyer, J. M., Maes, H., et al. (1997). Genetics and developmental psychopathology: I. Phenotypic assessment in the Virginia Twin Study of Adolescent Behavioral Development. *Journal of Child Psychology and Psychiatry, 28*, 943–963.

Heywood, C., & Beale, I. (2003). EEG biofeedback vs. placebo treatment for attention-deficit/hyperactivity disorder: A pilot study. *Journal of Attention Disorders, 7*, 43–55.

Hikosaka, O., Takikawa, Y., & Kawagoe, R. (2000). Role of the basal ganglia in the control of purposive saccadic eye movements. *Physiological Review, 80*, 953–978.

Hillman, C. H., Snook, E. M., & Jerome, G. J. (2003). Acute cardiovascular exercise and executive control function. *International Journal of Psychophysiology, 48*, 307–314.

Hinshaw, S. P. (2002). Is ADHD an impairing condition in childhood and adolescence? In P. S. Jensen & J. R. Cooper (Eds.), *Attention deficit hyperactivity disorder: State of the science—best practices* (pp. 5-1–5-21). Kingston, NJ: Civic Research Institute.

Hinshaw, S. P., Owens, E. B., Wells, K. C., Kraemer, H. C., Abikoff, H. B., Arnold, L. E., et al. (2000). Family processes and treatment outcome in the MTA: Negative/ineffective parenting practices in relation to multimodal treatment. *Journal of Abnormal Child Psychology, 28*, 555–568.

Hirayama, S., Hamazaki, T., & Terasawa, K. (2004). Effect of docosahexaenoic acid-containing food administration on symptoms of attention-deficit/hyperactivity disorder—A placebo-controlled double-blind study. *European Journal of Clinical Nutrition, 58*, 467–473.

Hirshberg, L. M., Chiu, S., & Frazier, J. A. (2005). Emerging brain-based interventions for children and adolescents: Overview and clinical perspective. *Child and Adolescent Psychiatric Clinics of North America, 14*, 1–19.

Hollingshead, A. B., & Redlich, F. C. (1958). *Social class and mental illness: A community study*. New York: Wiley.

Holtmann, M., Bolte, S., & Poustka, F. (2005). ADHD, Asperger syndrome, and high-functioning autism. *Journal of the American Academy of Child & Adolescent Psychiatry, 44,* 1101.

Hoza, B. (2007). Peer functioning in children with ADHD. *Journal of Pediatric Psychology, 32,* 655–663.

Hoza, B., Gedes, A. C., Mrug, S., Hinshaw, S. P., Bukowski, W. M., Gold, J. A., et al. (2005). Peer assessed outcomes in the multimodal treatment study of children with attention deficit hyperactivity disorder. *Journal of Clinical Child and Adolescent Psychology, 34,* 74–86.

Hughes, J. R., DeLeo, A. J., & Melyn, M. A. (2000). The electroencephalogram in attention deficit-hyperactivity disorder: Emphasis on epileptiform discharges. *Epilepsy & Behavior, 1,* 271–277.

Hunt, R. D., Capper, L., & O'Connell, P. (1990). Clonidine in child and adolescent psychiatry. *Journal of Child and Adolescent Psychopharmacology, 1,* 87–102.

Hunter, L. (2004). The value of school-based mental health services. In K. E. Robinson (Ed.), *Advances in school-based mental health interventions: Best practices and program models* (pp. 1-1–1-10). Kingston, NJ: Civic Research Institute.

Iacono, W. G., Malone, S. M., & McGue, M. (2003). Substance use disorders, externalizing psychopathology, and P300 event-related potential amplitude. *International Journal of Psychophysiology, 48,* 147–178.

Ilsaacs, K. R., Anderson, B. J., Alcantara, A. A., Black, J. E., & Greenough, W. T. (1992). *Journal of Cerebral Blood Flow & Metabolism, 12,* 110–119.

Jacobvitz, D., Sroufe, L. A., Stewart, M., & Leffert, N. (1990). Treatment of attentional and hyperactivity problems in children with sympathomimetic drugs: A comprehensive review. *Journal of the American Academy of Child & Adolescent Psychiatry, 29,* 677–688.

Jensen, A., & Weisz, J. R. (2002). Assessing match and mismatch between practitioner-generated and standardized interview-generated diagnoses for clinic referred children and adolescents. *Journal of Consulting and Clinical Psychology, 70,* 158–168.

Jensen, P. S. (2000). Current concepts and controversies in the diagnosis and treatment of attention deficit hyperactivity disorder. *Current Psychiatry Reports, 2,* 102–109.

Jensen, P. S., Hinshaw, S. P., Kraemer, H. C., Lenora, N., Newcorn, J. H., Abikoff, H. B., et al. (2001). ADHD comorbidity findings from the MTA study: Comparing comorbid subgroups. *Journal of the American Academy of Child & Adolescent Psychiatry, 40,* 147–158.

Jensen, P. S., Hinshaw, S. P., Swanson, J. M., Greenhill, L. L., Conners, C. K., Arnold, L. E., et al. (2001). Findings from the NIMH Multimodal Treatment Study of ADHD (MTA): Implications and applications for primary care providers. *Developmental and Behavioral Pediatrics, 22,* 60–73.

Jensen, P. S., Kettle, L., Roper, M., Sloan, M., Dulcan, M., Hoven, C., et al. (1999). Are stimulants over-prescribed? Treatment of ADHD in 4 U.S. communities. *Journal of the American Academy of Child & Adolescent Psychiatry, 38,* 797–804.

Jensen, P. S., Shervette, R. E., Xenakis, S. N., & Bain, M. W. (1988). Psychosocial and medical histories of stimulant-treated children. *Journal of the American Academy of Child & Adolescent Psychiatry, 27,* 798–801.

Jensen-Doss, A. (2005). Evidence-based diagnosis: Incorporating diagnostic instruments into clinical practice. *Journal of the American Academy of Child & Adolescent Psychiatry, 44,* 947–952.

Jerger, S., Jerger, J., Alford, B. R., & Abrams, S. (1983). Development of speech intelligibility in children with recurrent otitis media. *Ear and Hearing, 4,* 138–145.

Jerome, L. (2000). Central auditory processing disorder and ADHD. *Journal of the American Academy of Child & Adolescent Psychiatry, 39,* 399–400.

Johannes, S., Wieringa, B. M., Nager, W., & Rada, D. (2003). Tourette syndrome and obsessive-compulsive disorder: Event-related potentials show similar mechanisms of frontal inhibition but dissimilar target evaluation processes. *Behavioral Neurology, 14,* 9–14.

Johnstone, S. J., Tardif, H. P., Barry, R. J., & Sands, T. (2001). Nasal bilevel positive airway pressure therapy in children with a sleep-related breathing disorder and attention-deficit hyperactivity disorder: Effects on electrophysiological measures of brain function. *Sleep Medicine, 2,* 407–416.

Jonkman, L. M., Kemner, C., Verbaten, M. N., Koelega, H. S., Camfferman, G., van der Gaag, R. J., et al. (1997). Effects of methylphenidate on event-related potentials and performance of attention-deficit hyperactivity disorder children in auditory and visual selective attention tasks. *Biological Psychiatry, 41,* 690–702.

Kanbayashi, Y., Nakata, Y., Fujii, K., Kita, M., & Wada, K. (1994). ADHD-related behavior among non-referred children: Parents' ratings of DSM–III–R symptoms. *Child Psychiatry and Human Development, 25,* 13–29.

Kaplan, B. J., McNicol, J., Conte, R. A., & Moghadam, H. K. (1989). Dietary replacement in preschool-aged hyperactive boys. *Pediatrics, 83,* 7–17.

Keays, J. J., & Allison, K. R. (1995). The effects of regular moderate to vigorous physical activity on student outcomes: A review. *Canadian Journal of Public Health, 86,* 62–65.

Keith, R. W., & Engineer, P. (1991). Effects of methylphenidate on the auditory processing abilities of children with ADHD. *Journal of Learning Disabilities, 24,* 630–636.

Keller, W. D. (1992). Auditory processing disorder or attention-deficit disorder? In J. Katz, N. Stecker, & D. Henderson (Eds.), *Central auditory processing: A transdisciplinary view* (pp. 107–114). Chicago: Mosby-Yearbook.

Kesaniemi, Y. A., Danforth, Jr., E., Jensen, M. D., Kopelman, P. G., Lefebvre, P., & Reeder, B. A. (2001). Dose-response issues concerning physical activity and health: An evidence-based symposium. *Medical Science, Sports, and Exercise, 33*(Suppl. 6), 351–358.

Kiehl, K. A., Hare, R. D., Liddle, P. F., & McDonald, J. J. (1999). Reduced P300 responses in criminal psychopaths during a visual oddball task. *Biological Psychiatry, 45,* 1498–1507.

Kim, G.-N., Lee, J.-S., Shin, M.-S., Cho, S.-C., & Lee, D.-S. (2002). Regional cerebral perfusion abnormalities in attention deficit/hyperactivity disorder: Statistical parametric mapping analysis. *European Archives of Psychiatry and Clinical Neuroscience, 252,* 219–225.

Kirk, V., Kahn, A., & Brouillette, R. T. (1998). Diagnostic approach to obstructive sleep apnea in children. *Sleep Medicine, 2,* 255–269.

Klein, R. G., & Mannuzza, S. (1991). Long-term outcome of hyperactive children: A review. *Journal of the American Academy of Child & Adolescent Psychiatry, 30,* 383–387.

Klorman, R. (1991). Cognitive event-related potentials in attention deficit disorder. *Journal of Learning Disabilities, 24,* 130–140.

Kotwal, D. B., Burns, W. J., & Montgomery, D. D. (1996). Computer-assisted training for ADHD. *Behavior Modification, 20,* 85–96.

Kozielec, T., & Starobrat-Hermelin, B. (1997). Assessment of magnesium levels in children with attention deficit hyperactivity disorder (ADHD). *Magnesium Research, 10,* 143–146.

Kozielec, T., Starobrat-Hermelin, B., & Kotkowiak, L. (1994). Deficiency of certain trace elements in children with hyperactivity. *Polish Journal of Psychiatry, 28,* 345–353.

Kraus, J. F. (1995). Epidemiological features of brain injury in children: Occurrence, children at risk, causes and manner of injury, severity, and outcomes. In S. H. Broman & M. E. Michel (Eds.), *Traumatic head injury in children* (pp. 22–39). New York: Oxford University Press.

Krause, K. H., Dresel, S. H., Krause, J., Kung, H. F., & Tatsch, K. (2000). Increased striatal dopamine transporter in adult patients with attention deficit hyperactivity disorder: Effects of methylphenidate as measured by single photon emission computed tomography. *Neuroscience Letters, 285,* 107–110.

Kroes, M., Kalff, A. C., Kessels, A. G. H., Steyaert, J., Feron, F., van Someren, A., et al. (2001). Child psychiatric diagnoses in a population of Dutch schoolchildren aged 6 to 8 years. *Journal of the American Academy of Child & Adolescent Psychiatry, 40,* 1401–1409.

Kubitz, K. A., & Mott, A. A. (1996). EEG power spectral densities during and after cycle ergometer exercise. *Research Quarterly for Exercise and Sport, 67,* 91–96.

Kubitz, K. A., & Pothakos, K. (1997). Does aerobic exercise decrease brain activation? *Journal of Sport Exercise Psychology, 19,* 291–301.

Kurzweil 3000 [Software]. Retrieved July 26, 2007. Available from http://www.kurzweiledu.com/kurz3000.aspx

Lahey, B. B., Pelham, W. E., Schaughency, E. A., Atkins, M. S., Murphy, H. A., Hynd, G., et al. (1988). Dimensions and types of attention deficit disorder. *Journal of the American Academy of Child & Adolescent Psychiatry, 27,* 330–335.

Lalonde, J., Turgay, A., & Hudson, J. I. (1998). Attention-deficit hyperactivity disorder subtypes and comorbid disruptive behavior disorders in a child and adolescent mental health clinic. *Canadian Journal of Psychiatry, 43*, 623–628.

Lane, S. J., Miller, L. J., & Hanft, B. E. (2000). Toward a consensus in terminology in sensory integration theory and practice: II. Sensory integration patterns of function and dysfunction. *Sensory Integration Special Interest Section Quarterly, 23*, 1–3.

Laporte, N., Sebire, G., Gillerot, Y., Guerrini, R., & Ghariani, S. (2002). Cognitive epilepsy: ADHD related to focal EEG discharges. *Pediatric Neurology, 27*, 307–311.

Lardon, M. T., & Polich, J. (1996). EEG changes from long-term physical exercise. *Biological Psychology, 44*, 19–30.

LaVaque, T. J., Hammond, D. C., Trudeau, D., Monastra, V. J., Perry, J., & Lehrer, P. (2002). Template for developing guidelines for the evaluation of the clinical effectiveness of psychophysiological interventions. *Applied Psychophysiology and Biofeedback, 27*, 273–281.

Law, S. F., & Schachar, R. J. (1999). Do typical clinical doses of methylphenidate cause tics in children treated for attention-deficit hyperactivity disorder? *Journal of the American Academy of Child & Adolescent Psychiatry, 38*, 944–951.

Lee, D. O., & Ousley, O. Y. (2006). Attention-deficit hyperactivity disorder symptoms in a clinic sample of children and adolescents with pervasive developmental disorders. *Journal of Child and Adolescent Psychopharmacology, 16*, 737–746.

Lee, L., Kepple, J., Wang, Y., Freestone, S., Bakhtiar, R., Wang, Y., & Hossain, M. (2003). Bioavailability of modified-release methylphenidate: Influence of high-fat breakfast when administered intact and when capsule content sprinkled on applesauce. *Biopharmaceutics & Drug Disposition, 24*, 233–243.

Lemkuhl, G., & Thoma, W. (1991). Development in children after severe head injury. In A. Rothenberger (Ed.), *Brain and behavior in child psychiatry* (pp. 267–282). Berlin, Germany: Springer-Verlag.

Leung, P. W. L., Luk, S. L., Ho, T. P., Taylor, E., Mak, F. L., & Bacon-Shone, J. (1996). The diagnosis and prevalence of hyperactivity in Chinese schoolboys. *British Journal of Psychiatry, 168*, 486–496.

Levesque, J., Beauregard, M., & Mensour, B. M. (2006). Effect of neurofeedback training on the neural substrates of selective attention in children with attention-deficit/hyperactivity disorder: A functional magnetic resonance imaging study. *Neuroscience Letters, 394*, 216–221.

Levitan, R. D., Masellis, M., Basile, V. S., Lam, R. W., Jain, U., Kaplan, A. S., et al. (2002). Polymorphism of the serotonin-2A receptor gene (HTR2A) associated with childhood attention deficit hyperactivity disorder (ADHD) in adult women with seasonal affective disorder. *Journal of Affective Disorders, 71*, 229–233.

Levy, F. (1991). The dopamine theory of attention deficit hyperactivity disorder. *Australian and New Zealand Journal of Psychiatry, 25*, 277–283.

Levy, R., Hay, D. A., McStephen, M., Wood, C., & Waldman, J. (1997). Attention deficit hyperactivity disorder: A category or a continuum? Genetic analysis of a large twin study. *Journal of the American Academy of Child & Adolescent Psychiatry, 36,* 737–744.

Lewczyk, C. M., Garland, A. F., Hurlburt, M. S., Gearity, J., & Hough, R. L. (2003). Comparing DISC–IV and clinician diagnoses among youths receiving public mental health services. *Journal of the American Academy of Child & Adolescent Psychiatry, 42,* 349–356.

Lezak, M. (1976). *Neuropsychological assessment.* New York: Oxford University Press.

Li, J., Wang, Y., Qian, Q., Wang, B., & Zhou, R. (2002). Association of 5HT (2A) receptor polymorphism and attention deficit hyperactivity disorder in children. *Zhonghua Yi Xue Za Zhi, 82,* 1173–1176.

Lieberman, H. R., Spring, B. J., & Garfield, G. S. (1986). The behavior effects of food constituents: Strategies used in studies of amino acids, protein, carbohydrate, and caffeine. *Nutrition Reviews, 44*(Suppl.), 61–69.

Linden, M., Habib, T., & Radojevic, V. (1996). A controlled study of the effects of EEG biofeedback on cognition and behavior of children with attention deficit disorders and learning disabilities. *Biofeedback and Self-Regulation, 21,* 35–49.

Loo, S. K. (2003). EEG and neurofeedback findings in ADHD. *The ADHD Report, 11*(3), 1–6.

Loo, S. K., & Barkley, R. A. (2005). Clinical utility of EEG in attention deficit hyperactivity disorder. *Applied Neuropsychology, 12,* 64–76.

Loo, S. K., Hopfer, C., Teale, P. D., & Reite, M. (2004). EEG correlates of methylphendate response in ADHD: Association with cognitive and behavioral measures. *Journal of Clinical Neurophysiology, 21,* 457–464.

Loo, S. K., Teale, P., & Reite, M. (1999). EEG correlates of psychostimulant effects among children with ADHD: A preliminary report. *Biological Psychiatry, 45,* 1657–1660.

Lou, H. C., Henriksen, L., & Bruhn, P. (1984). Focal cerebral hypoperfusion in children with dysphasia and/or attention deficit disorder. *Archives of Neurology, 41,* 825–829.

Lou, H. C., Henriksen, L., & Bruhn, P. (1990). Focal cerebral dysfunction in developmental disabilities. *Lancet, 335,* 8–11.

Lubar, J. F. (1991). Discourse on the development of EEG diagnostics and biofeedback treatment for attention-deficit hyperactivity disorders. *Biofeedback and Self-Regulation, 16,* 201–225.

Lubar, J. F. (2003). Neurofeedback for the management of attention deficit disorders. In M. S. Schwartz & F. Andrasik (Eds.), *Biofeedback: A practitioner's guide* (pp. 409–437). New York: Guilford Press.

Lubar, J. F., Bianchini, K. J., & Calhoun, W. H. (1985). Spectral analysis of EEG differences between children with and without learning disabilities. *Journal of Learning Disabilities, 18,* 403–408.

Lubar, J. F., & Shouse, M. N. (1976). EEG and behavioral changes in a hyperkinetic child concurrent with training of the sensorimotor rhythm (SMR): A preliminary report. *Biofeedback and Self-Regulation, 1,* 293–306.

Lubar, J. F., White, J. N., Swartwood, M. O., & Swartwood, J. N. (1999). Methylphenidate effects on global and complex measures of EEG. *Pediatric Neurology, 21,* 633–637.

Lubar, J. O., & Lubar, J. F. (1984). Electroencephalographic biofeedback of SMR and beta for treatment of attention deficit disorders in a clinical setting. *Biofeedback and Self-Regulation, 9,* 1–23.

Magnie, M. N., Bermon, S., Martin, F., Madany-Lounis, M., Suisse, G., & Muhammad, W. (2000). P300, N400, aerobic fitness, and maximal aerobic exercise. *Psychophysiology, 37,* 369–377.

Mahoney, C. R., Taylor, H. A., Kanarek, R. B., & Samuel, P. (2005). Effect of breakfast composition on cognitive processes in elementary school children. *Physiology & Behavior, 85,* 635–645.

Maidmert, I. D. (2003). The use of antidepressants to treat attention deficit hyperactivity disorder in adults. *Journal of Psychopharmacology, 17,* 332–336.

Mangeot, S. D., Miller, L. J., McIntosh, D. N., McGrath-Clarke, J., Simon, J., Hagerman, R. J., & Goldson, E. (2001). Sensory modulation dysfunction in children with attention-deficit-hyperactivity disorder. *Developmental Medicine & Child Neurology, 43,* 399–406.

Mann, C. A., Lubar, J., Zimmerman, A., Miller, C., & Muenchen, R. (1992). Quantitative analysis of EEG in boys with attention deficit hyperactivity disorder: Controlled study with clinical implications. *Pediatric Neurology, 8,* 30–36.

Mannuzza, S., Klein, R. G., & Addalli, K. A. (1991). Young adult mental status of hyperactive boys and their brothers: A prospective follow-up study. *Journal of the American Academy of Child & Adolescent Psychiatry, 30,* 743–751.

Mannuzza, S., Klein, R., Bessler, A., Malloy, P., & LaPadula, M. (1993). Adult outcomes of hyperactive boys: Educational achievement, occupational rank, and psychiatric status. *Archives of General Psychiatry, 50,* 565–576.

Mannuzza, S., Klein, R., Bessler, A., Malloy, P., & LaPadula, M. (1998). Adult psychiatric status of hyperactive boys grown up. *American Journal of Psychiatry, 155,* 493–498.

Mannuzza, S., Klein, R., Bonagura, N., Palloy, P., Giampino, T. L., & Addalli, K. A. (1991). Hyperactive boys almost grown up: V. Replication of psychiatric status. *Archives of General Psychiatry, 48,* 77–83.

Marcotte, A. C., & Stern, C. (1997). Qualitative analysis of graphomotor output in children with attentional disorder. *Child Neuropsychology, 3,* 147–153.

Marshall, P. (1989). Attention deficit disorder and allergy: A neurochemical model of the relation between the illnesses. *Psychological Bulletin, 106,* 434–446.

Martens, F., & Grant, B. (1980, May–June). A survey of daily physical education in Canada. *Canadian Association of Health, Physical Education, and Recreation (CAHPER) Journal,* 30–38.

Mattes, J. A. (1986). Propranolol for adults with temper outbursts and residual attention deficit disorder. *Journal of Clinical Psychopharmacology, 6,* 299–302.

Maughan, B., Rowe, R., Messer, J., Goodman, R., & Meltzer, H. (2004). Conduct disorder and oppositional defiant disorder in a national sample: Developmental epidemiology. *Journal of Child Psychology and Psychiatry, 45,* 609–621.

Max, J. E., Lindgren, S. D., Knutson, C., Pearson, C. S., Ihrig, D., & Welborn, A. (1998). Child and adolescent traumatic brain injury: Correlates of disruptive behavior disorders. *Brain Injury, 12,* 41–52.

Max, J. E., Smith, W. L., & Sata, Y. (1997). Traumatic brain injury in children and adolescents: Psychiatric disorders in the second three months. *Journal of the American Academy of Child & Adolescent Psychiatry, 36,* 94–102.

McCann, B. S., & Roy-Byrne, P. R. (2004). Screening and diagnostic utility of self-report attention deficit hyperactivity disorder scales in adults. *Comprehensive Psychiatry, 45,* 175–183.

McCann, B. S., Scheele, L., Ward, N., & Roy-Byrne, P. (2000). Discriminant validity of the Wender Utah Rating Scale for attention-deficit/hyperactivity disorder in adults. *Journal of Neuropsychiatry and Clinical Neurosciences, 12,* 240–245.

McCarney, S. B. (2004). *Attention Deficit Disorders Evaluation Scales.* Columbia, MO: Hawthorne Educational Services.

McDermott, C. M., LaHoste, G., Chen, C., Musto, A., Bazan, N. G., & Magee, J. C. (2003). Sleep deprivation causes behavioral, synaptic, and membrane excitability alterations in hippocampal neurons. *The Journal of Neuroscience, 23,* 9687–9695.

McGee, R. A., Clark, S. E., & Symons, D. K. (2000). Does the Conners' Continuous Performance Test aid in ADHD diagnosis? *Journal of Abnormal Child Psychology, 28,* 415–424.

McGee, R. A., Feehan, M., Williams, S., Partridge, F., Silva, P. A., & Kelly, J. (1990). DSM–III disorders in a large sample of adolescents. *Journal of the American Academy of Child & Adolescent Psychiatry, 29,* 611–619.

McIntosh, D. E., Mulkins, R. S., & Dean, R. S. (1995). Utilization of maternal perinatal risk indicators in the differential diagnosis of ADHD and UADD children. *International Journal of Neuroscience, 81,* 35–46.

McIntosh, D. N., Miller, L. J., Shyu, V., & Dunn, W. (1999). Overview of the Short Sensory Profile (SSP). In W. Dunn (Ed.), *The Sensory Profile: Examiner's manual* (pp. 59–73). San Antonio, TX: Psychological Corporation.

McIntosh, D. N., Miller, L. J., Shyu, V., & Hagerman, R. (1999). Sensory-modulation disruption, electrodermal responses, and functional behaviors. *Developmental Medicine & Child Neurology, 41,* 608–615.

Michelson, D., Faries, D., Wernicke, J., Kelsey, D., Kendrick, K., Sallee, F. R., et al. (2001). Atomoxetine in the treatment of children and adolescents with attention-deficit/hyperactivity disorder: A randomized, placebo-controlled, dose-response study. *Pediatrics, 108*(5), 1–9.

Mick, E., Biederman, J., & Faraone, S. V. (1996). Is season of birth a risk factor for attention-deficit hyperactivity disorder? *Journal of the American Academy of Child & Adolescent Psychiatry, 35,* 1470–1476.

Milberger, S., Biederman, J., Faraone, S. V., Guite, J., & Tsuang, M. T. (1997). Pregnancy, delivery, and infancy complications and attention deficit hyperactivity disorder: Issues of gene–environment interaction. *Biological Psychiatry, 41,* 65–75.

Minde, K., Webb, G., & Sykes, D. (1968). Studies on the hyperactive child: VI. Prenatal and paranatal factors associated with hyperactivity. *Developmental Medicine & Child Neurology, 10,* 355–363.

Mitchell, E. A., Aman, M. G., Turbott, S. H., & Manku, M. (1987). Clinical characteristics and serum essential fatty acid levels in hyperactive children. *Clinical Pediatrics, 26,* 406–411.

Molina, B., & Pelham, W. (2003). Childhood predictors of adolescent substance use in a longitudinal study of children with ADHD. *Journal of Abnormal Psychology, 112,* 497–507.

Monastra, V. J. (2000, October). *From IDEAs to action: The IEP as a primary intervention in the treatment of AD/HD.* Paper presented at the 12th Annual International Conference of Children and Adults With Attention Deficit/Hyperactivity Disorder, Chicago.

Monastra, V. J. (2004). Clinical applications of EEG biofeedback. In M. S. Schwartz & F. Andrasik (Eds.), *Biofeedback: A practitioner's guide* (pp. 438–463). New York: Guilford Press.

Monastra, V. J. (2005a). Electroencephalographic biofeedback (neurotherapy) as a treatment for attention deficit hyperactivity disorder: Rationale and empirical foundation. *Child and Adolescent Psychiatric Clinics of North America, 14,* 55–82.

Monastra, V. J. (2005b). Overcoming the barriers to effective treatment for attention-deficit hyperactivity disorder: A neuroeducational approach. *International Journal of Psychophysiology, 58,* 71–80.

Monastra, V. J. (2005c). *Parenting children with ADHD: 10 lessons that medicine cannot teach.* Washington, DC: American Psychological Association.

Monastra, V. J. (2005d). *Working with children with ADHD* [Motion picture]. (Available from the American Psychological Association, 750 First Street, NE, Washington, DC 20002-4242)

Monastra, V. J. (2006). *The Clinical History Questionnaire.* Endicott, NY: Author.

Monastra, V. J. (2007). *Conducting parenting classes in clinical practice: A demonstration of the neuroeducational parent training program* [Motion picture]. (Available from V. J. Monastra, 94 Marshall Drive, Endicott, NY 13760)

Monastra, V. J., & Carlson-Gotz, D. (2006). *Teaching social skills in school settings.* Workshop presented at the annual meeting of the New York State Association of School Psychologists, Syracuse, NY.

Monastra, V. J., Lubar, J. F., & Linden, M. (2001). The development of a quantitative electroencephalographic scanning process for attention deficit-hyperactivity disorder: Reliability and validity studies. *Neuropsychology, 15,* 136–144.

Monastra, V. J., Lubar, J. F., Linden, M., VanDeusen, P., Green, G., Wing, W., et al. (1999). Assessing attention deficit hyperactivity disorder via quantitative electroencephalography: An initial validation study. *Neuropsychology, 13,* 424–433.

Monastra, V. J., Lynn, S., Linden, M., Lubar, J. F., Gruzelier, J., & LaVaque, T. J. (2005). Electroencephalographic biofeedback in the treatment of attention-deficit/hyperactivity disorder. *Applied Psychophysiology and Biofeedback, 30,* 95–114.

Monastra, V. J., & Monastra, D. M. (2004, April). *EEG biofeedback treatment for ADHD: An analysis of behavioral, neuropsychological, and electrophysiological response over a three-year follow-up period.* Paper presented at the annual conference of the Association for Applied Psychophysiology and Biofeedback, Colorado Springs, CO.

Monastra, V. J., Monastra, D. M., & George, D. M. (2002). The effects of stimulant therapy, EEG biofeedback, and parenting style on the primary symptoms of attention-deficit/hyperactivity disorder. *Journal of Applied Psychophysiology and Biofeedback, 27,* 231–249.

Moore, D. R., Hutchings, M. E., & Meyer, S. E. (1991). Binaural masking level differences in children with a history of otitis media. *Audiology, 30,* 91–101.

Moschovakis, A. K., Scudder, C. A., & Highstein, S. M. (1996). The microscopic anatomy and physiology of the mammalian saccadic system. *Progress in Neurobiology, 50,* 133–254.

Mulligan, S. (1996). An analysis of score patterns of children with attention disorders on the sensory integration and praxis tests. *The American Journal of Occupational Therapy, 50,* 647–654.

Multimodal Treatment Study of Children With ADHD Cooperative Group. (1999). A 14-month randomized clinical trial of treatment strategies for attention-deficit/hyperactivity disorder: Multimodal Treatment Study of Children With ADHD. *Archives of General Psychiatry, 56,* 1073–1086.

Multimodal Treatment Study of Children With ADHD Cooperative Group. (2004). National Institute of Mental Health Multimodal Treatment Study of ADHD follow-up: 24-month outcomes of treatment strategies for attention-deficit/hyperactivity disorder. *Pediatrics, 113,* 754–761.

Munoz, D. P., Armstrong, I. T., Hampton, K. A., & Moore, K. D. (2003). Altered control of visual fixation and saccadic eye movements in attention-deficit hyperactivity disorder. *Journal of Neurophysiology, 90,* 503–514.

Munoz, D. P., Dorris, M. C., Pare, M., & Everling, S. (2000). On your mark, get set: Brainstem circuitry underlying saccadic initiation. *Canadian Journal of Physiology and Pharmacology, 78,* 934–944.

Murphy, K. R. (2006). Psychological counseling of adults with ADHD. In R. A. Barkley (Ed.), *Attention-deficit hyperactivity disorder: A handbook for diagnosis and treatment* (pp. 692–703). New York: Guilford Press.

Murphy, K. R., & Barkley, R. A. (1996). Attention deficit hyperactivity disorder in adults. Comorbidities and adaptive impairments. *Comprehensive Psychiatry, 37,* 393–401.

Murphy, K. R., Barkley, R. A., & Bush, T. (2002). Young adults with ADHD: Subtype differences in comorbidity, educational, and clinical history. *Journal of Nervous and Mental Disease, 190,* 147–157.

Murphy, K. R., & Gordon, M. (2006). Assessment of adults with ADHD. In R. A. Barkley (Ed.), *Attention-deficit hyperactivity disorder: A handbook for diagnosis and treatment* (pp. 425–450). New York: Guilford Press.

Musiek, F. E., Gollegly, K., Lamb, L., & Lamb, P. (1990). Selected issues in screening for central auditory processing dysfunction. *Seminars in Hearing, 11,* 372–384.

Mutrie, N., & Biddle, S. (1995). The effects of exercise on mental health in nonclinical populations. In S. Biddle (Ed.), *European perspectives on exercise and sport psychology* (pp. 50–70). Champaign, IL: Human Kinetics.

Nadeau, K. (1996). *Adventures in fast forward: Life, love, and work for the ADD adult.* New York: Brunner/Mazel.

Nakamura, Y., Nishimoto, K., Akamutu, M., Takahashi, M., & Maruyama, A. (1999). The effect of jogging on P300 event-related potentials. *Electroencephalography and Clinical Neurophysiology, 39,* 71–74.

National Institutes of Health. (1998). *NIH consensus statement on the diagnosis and treatment of attention-deficit/hyperactivity disorder.* Bethesda, MD: Author.

National Toxicology Program. (1995). NTP toxicology and carcinogenesis studies of methylphenidate hydrochloride (CAS No. 298-59-9) in F344/N rats and B6C3F1 mice (feed studies). *NTP Technical Reports Series, 439,* 1–299.

Needleman, H. L., Gunnoe, C., Leviton, A., Reed, R., Peresie, H., Maher, C., et al. (1979). Deficits in psychologic and classroom performance of children with elevated dentine lead levels. *New England Journal of Medicine, 300,* 689–695.

Needleman, H. L., Schell, A., Bellinger, D. C., Leviton, L., & Alfred, E. D. (1990). The long-term effects of exposure to low doses of lead in childhood: An 11-year follow-up report. *New England Journal of Medicine, 322,* 83–88.

Nichols, P. L., & Chen, T. C. (1981). *Minimal brain dysfunction: A prospective study.* Hillsdale, NJ: Erlbaum.

Niedermeyer, E., & Naidu, S. B. (1998). Attention deficit disorder and frontal motor disconnection. *Clinical Electroencephalography, 28,* 130–136.

Nigg, J. T. (2000). On inhibition/disinhibition in developmental psychopathology: Views from cognitive and personality psychology and a working inhibition taxonomy. *Psychological Bulletin, 126,* 220–246.

Noterdaeme, M., Amorosa, H., Mildenberger, K., Sitter, S., & Minow, F. (2001). Evaluation of attention problems in children with autism and children with a specific language disorder. *European Child & Adolescent Psychiatry, 10,* 58–66.

Novartis Pharmaceuticals. (2002a). *Focalin product monograph.* East Hanover, NJ: Author.

Novartis Pharmaceuticals. (2002b). *Ritalin product monograph.* East Hanover, NJ: Author.

Offord, D. R., Boyle, M. H., Szatmari, P., Rae-Grant, N. I., Links, P. S., Cadman, D. T., et al. (1987). Ontario Child Health Study: II. Six-month prevalence of disorder and rates of service utilization. *Archives of General Psychiatry, 44,* 832–836.

Ogdie, M. N., MacPhie, I. L., Minassian, L., Yang, M., Fisher, S. E., Franks, C., et al. (2003). A genomewide scan for attention-deficit/hyperactivity disorder in an extended sample: Suggestive linkage on 17p11. *American Journal of Human Genetics, 72,* 1268–1279.

Oski, F. A., Honig, A. S., Helu, B., & Howanitz, P. (1983). Effect of iron therapy on behavior performance in nonanemic, iron-deficient infants. *Pediatrics, 71,* 877–880.

Ozonoff, S., & Strayer, D. L. (1997). Inhibitory function in nonretarded children with autism. *Journal of Autism and Developmental Disorders, 27,* 59–77.

Palumbo, D., Spencer, T., Lynch, J., Co-Chien, H., & Faraone, S. V. (2004). Emergence of tics in children with ADHD: Impact of once-daily OROS ethylphenidate therapy. *Journal of Child and Adolescent Psychopharmacology, 14,* 185–194.

Pastor, P. N., & Reuben, C. A. (2002). Attention deficit disorder and learning disability: United States, 1997–98. *National Center for Health Statistics: Vital and Health Statistics, 10*(206), 1–12.

Pelham, W. E. (2002). Psychosocial interventions for ADHD. In P. S. Jensen & J. R. Cooper (Eds.), *Attention deficit hyperactivity disorder: State of the science—best practices* (pp. 12-1–12-36). Kingston, NJ: Civic Research Institute.

Pelham, W. E., & Hoza, B. (1996). Intensive treatment: A summer treatment program for children with ADHD. In E. D. Hibbs & P. S. Jensen (Eds.), *Psychosocial treatments for child and adolescent disorders: Empirically based strategies for clinical practice* (pp. 311–340). Washington, DC: American Psychological Association.

Pennington, B. F., & Ozonoff, S. (1996). Executive functions and developmental psychopathology. *Journal of Child Psychology and Psychiatry, 37,* 51–87.

Pennington, J. A., & Douglass, J. S. (2004). *Bowes & Church's food values of portions commonly used* (18th ed.). Hagerstown, MD: Lippincott Williams & Wilkins.

Peterson, B. S., Pine, D. S., Cohen, P., & Brook, J. S. (2001). Prospective, longitudinal study of tic, obsessive-compulsive, and attention-deficit/hyperactivity disorders in an epidemiological sample. *Journal of the American Academy of Child & Adolescent Psychiatry, 40,* 685–695.

Pfiffner, L. J., Barkley, R. A., & DuPaul, G. J. (2006). Treatment of ADHD in school settings. In R. A. Barkley (Ed.), *Attention deficit hyperactivity disorder: A handbook for clinical practice* (pp. 547–589). New York: Guilford Press.

Pfiffner, L. J., & McBurnett, K. (1997). Social skills training with parent generalization: Treatment effects for children with attention deficit disorder. *Journal of Consulting and Clinical Psychology, 65,* 749–757.

Physicians' desk reference. (61st ed.). (2007). Montvale, NJ: Thomson Healthcare.

Pillsbury, H. C., Grose, J. H., Coleman, W. L., Conners, C. K., & Hall, J. W. (1995). Binaural function in children with attention-deficit hyperactivity disorder. *Archives of Otolaryngology and Head and Neck Surgery, 121,* 1345–1350.

Pitcher, T. M., Piek, J. P., & Hay, D. A. (2003). Fine and gross motor ability in boys with attention deficit hyperactivity disorder. *Developmental Medicine & Child Neurology, 45,* 525–535.

Pleak, R. R., Birmaher, B., Gavrilescu, A., Abichandani, C., & Williams, D. T. (1988). Mania and neuropsychiatric excitation following carbamazepine. *Journal of the American Academy of Child & Adolescent Psychiatry, 27,* 500–503.

Pliszka, S. R. (2000). Patterns of psychiatric comorbidity with attention-deficit/ hyperactivity disorder. *Child and Adolescent Psychiatric Clinics of North America, 9,* 525–540.

Pliszka, S. R. (2005). The neuropsychopharmacology of attention deficit/hyperactivity disorder. *Biological Psychiatry, 57,* 1385–1390.

Pliszka, S. R., Carlson, C. L., & Swanson, J. M. (1999). *ADHD with comorbid disorders: Clinical assessment and management.* New York: Guilford Press.

Pliszka, S. R., Liotti, M., & Woldorf, M. G. (2000). Inhibitory control in children with attention-deficit/hyperactivity disorder: Event-related potentials identify the processing component and timing of an impaired right frontal response inhibition mechanism. *Biological Psychiatry, 48,* 238–248.

Polich, J., & Herbst, K. L. (2000). P300 as a clinical assay: Rationale, evaluation, and findings. *International Journal of Psychophysiology, 38,* 3–19.

Polich, J., & Kok, A. (1995). Cognitive and biological determinants of P300: An integrative review. *Biological Psychology, 41,* 103–146.

Pollitt, E. (1995). Does breakfast make a difference in school? *Journal of the American Dietetic Association, 95,* 1134–1139.

Pollitt, E., & Mathews, R. (1998). Breakfast and cognition: An integrative summary. *American Journal of Clinical Nutrition, 67*(Suppl. 4), 804–813.

Pollock, I., & Warner, J. O. (1990). Effect of artificial food colors on childhood behavior. *Archives of Disease in Childhood, 65,* 74–77.

Posner, M. I., & Petersen, S. E. (1990). The attention system of the human brain. *Annual Review of Neuroscience, 13,* 25–42.

Prichep, L. S., & John, E. R. (1992). QEEG profiles of psychiatric disorders. *Brain Tomography, 4,* 249–257.

Prince, J. B., Wilens, T. E., Biederman, J., Spencer, T. J., & Wozniak, J. R. (1996). Clonidine for sleep disturbances associated with attention-deficit hyperactivity disorder: A systematic review of 62 cases. *Journal of the American Academy of Child & Adolescent Psychiatry, 35,* 599–605.

Prince, J. B., Wilens, T. E., Spencer, T. J., & Biederman, J. (2006). Pharmacotherapy of ADHD in adults. In R. A. Barkley (Ed.), *Attention-deficit hyperactivity disorder: A handbook for diagnosis and treatment* (pp. 704–736). New York: Guilford Press.

Prochaska, J. O., DiClemente, C. C., & Norcross, J. C. (1992). In search of how people change. Applications to addictive behaviors. *American Psychologist, 47,* 1102–1114.

Rapp, D. J. (1978). Does diet affect hypersensitivity? *Journal of Learning Disabilities, 11,* 56–62.

Rapport, M. D., Carlson, G. A., Kelly, K. L., & Pataki, C. (1993). Methylphenidate and desipramine in hospitalized children: I. Separate and combined effects on cognitive function. *Journal of the American Academy of Child & Adolescent Psychiatry, 32,* 333–342.

Rapport, M. D., & Gordon, M. (1987). *The Attention Training System (ATS).* DeWitt, NY: Gordon Systems.

Rapport, M. D., Loo, S., Isaacs, P., Goya, S., Denney, C., & Scanlan, S. (1996). Methylphenidate and attentional training: Comparative effects on behavior and neurocognitive performance in twin girls with attention-deficit/hyperactivity disorder. *Behavior Modification, 20,* 428–450.

Rasmussen, P., & Gillberg, C. (2001). Natural outcome of ADHD with developmental coordination disorder at age 22 years: A controlled, longitudinal, community-based study. *Journal of the American Academy of Child & Adolescent Psychiatry, 39,* 1424–1431.

Ratey, N. A. (2002). Life coaching for adult ADHD. In S. Goldstein & A. Teeter Ellison (Eds.), *Clinician's guide to adult ADHD: Assessment and intervention* (pp. 261–279). San Diego, CA: Academic Press.

Read & Write [Software]. Retrieved July 26, 2007. Available from http://www.texthelp.com/page.asp?pg_id=10002

ReadPlease! [Software]. Retrieved July 26, 2007. Available from http://www.readplease.com/

Reich, W. (1997). *Diagnostic Interview for Children and Adolescents: Revised DSM–IV version.* Toronto, Ontario, Canada: Multi-Health Systems.

Reitan, R. M., & Wolfson, D. (1985). *The Halstead–Reitan Neuropsychological Test Battery.* Tucson, AZ: Neuropsychology Press.

Reynolds, C., & Kamphaus, R. (1994). *Behavioral Assessment System for Children.* Circle Pines, MN: American Guidance Service.

Riccio, C. A., & French, C. L. (2004). The status of empirical support for treatments of attention deficits. *The Clinical Neuropsychologist, 18,* 528–558.

Riccio, C. A., Hynd, G. W., Cohen, M. J., Hall, J., & Molt, L. (1994). Comorbidity of central auditory processing disorder and attention-deficit hyperactivity disorder. *Journal of the American Academy of Child & Adolescent Psychiatry, 33,* 949–857.

Riccio, C. A., & Reynolds, C. R. (2001). Continuous performance tests are sensitive to ADHD in adults but lack specificity: A review and critique for differential diagnosis. *Annals of the New York Academy of Sciences, 931,* 113–139.

Riccio, C. A., Reynolds, C. R., Lowe, P., & Moore, J. J. (2002). The continuous performance test: A window on the neural substrates for attention? *Archives of Clinical Neuropsychology, 17,* 235–272.

Riccio, C. A., Waldrop, J. J. M., Reynolds, C. R., & Lowe, P. (2001). Effects of stimulants on the continuous performance test (CPT): Implications for CPT use and interpretation. *The Journal of Neuropsychiatry and Clinical Neurosciences, 13,* 326–335.

Richardson, A. J., & Puri, B. K. (2002). A randomized double-blind, placebo-controlled study of the effects of supplementation with highly unsaturated fatty acids on ADHD-related symptoms in children with specific learning difficulties. *Progress in Neuro-Psychopharmacology & Biological Psychiatry, 26,* 233–239.

Robbins, C. A. (2005). ADHD couple and family relationships: Enhancing communication and understanding through imago relationship therapy. *Journal of Clinical Psychology, 61,* 565–577.

Roberts, J. E., Burchinal, M. R., Collier, A. M., Ramey, C. T., Koch, M. A., & Henderson, F. W. (1989). Otitis media in early childhood and cognitive, academic, and classroom performance of the school-aged child. *Pediatrics, 83,* 477–485.

Robin, A. L. (2006). Training families with adolescents with ADHD. In R. A. Barkley (Ed.), *Attention deficit hyperactivity disorder: A handbook for diagnosis and treatment* (pp. 499–546). New York: Guilford Press.

Robin, A. L., & Foster, S. L. (1989). *Negotiating parent–adolescent conflict: Behavioral–family systems approach.* New York: Guilford Press.

Robin, A. L., & Payson, E. (2002). The impact of ADHD on marriage. *The ADHD Report, 10*(3), 9–11.

Robinson, K. E. (2004). *Advances in school-based mental health interventions: Best practices and program models.* Kingston, NJ: Civic Research Institute.

Rogers, J. M., Taubenack, M. W., Daston, G. P., Sulik, K. K., Zucker, R. M., Elstein, K. H., et al. (1995). Zinc deficiency causes optosis but not cell cycle alterations in organogenesis stage rat embryos: Effect of varying duration of deficiency. *Teratology, 52,* 149–159.

Rohde, L. A., Biederman, J., Busnello, E. A., Zimmermann, H., Schmitz, M., Martins, S., et al. (1999). ADHD in a school sample of Brazilian adolescents: A study of prevalence, comorbid conditions, and impairments. *Journal of the American Academy of Child & Adolescent Psychiatry, 38,* 716–722.

Romano, E., Tremblay, R. E., Vitaro, F., Zoccolillo, M., & Pagini, L. (2001). Prevalence of psychiatric diagnoses and the role of perceived impairment: Findings from an adolescent community sample. *Journal of Child Psychology and Psychiatry, 42,* 451–462.

Ross, D. M., & Ross, S. A. (1982). *Hyperactivity: Research, theory, and action.* New York: Wiley.

Rossiter, R. T., & LaVaque, T. J. (1995). A comparison of EEG biofeedback and psychostimulants in treating attention-deficit/hyperactivity disorders. *Journal of Neurotherapy, 1,* 48–59.

Rostain, A. L., & Ramsay, J. R. (2006). A combined treatment approach for adults with ADHD—Results of an open study of 43 patients. *Journal of Attention Disorders, 10,* 150–159.

Rovet, J., & Alvarez, M. (1996). Thyroid hormone and attention in school-age children with congential hypothyroidism. *Journal of Child Psychology and Psychiatry, 37,* 579–585.

Rowe, K. S., & Rowe, K. J. (1994). Synthetic food coloring and behavior: A dose–response effect in a double-blind, placebo-controlled, repeated-measures study. *Journal of Pediatrics, 125,* 691–698.

Roy-Bryne, P., Scheele, L., Brinkley, J., Ward, N., Wiatrak, C., Russo, J., et al. (1997). Adult attention-deficit hyperactivity disorder: Assessment guidelines based on clinical presentation to a specialty clinic. *Comprehensive Psychiatry, 38,* 133–140.

Russell, J. (1997). *Autism as an executive disorder.* Oxford, England: Oxford University Press.

Rutter, M. (1989). Isle of Wight revisited: Twenty-five years of child psychiatric epidemiology. *Journal of the American Academy of Child & Adolescent Psychiatry, 28,* 633–653.

Safren, S. A. (2006). Cognitive–behavioral approaches to ADHD treatment in adulthood. *Journal of Clinical Psychiatry, 67*(Suppl. 8), 46–50.

Safren, S. A., Otto, M. W., Sprich, S., Winett, C. L., Wilens, T. E., & Biederman, J. (2005). Cognitive–behavioral therapy for ADHD in medication-treated adults with continued symptoms. *Behavior Research and Therapy, 43,* 831–842.

Sanders, M. R. (1999). Triple P-Positive Parenting Program: Towards an empirically validated multi-level parenting and family support strategy for the prevention of behavior and emotional problems in children. *Clinical Child and Family Psychology Review, 2,* 71–78.

Sanford, J. A. (1994). *IVA manual.* Richmond, VA: BrainTrain.

Sanford, J. A., & Browne, R. J. (1988). *Captain's Log.* Richmond, VA: BrainTrain.

Satterfield, J. H., Schell, A. M., Backs, R. W., & Hidaka, K. C. (1984). A cross-sectional and longitudinal study of age effects of electrophysiological measures in hyperactive and normal children. *Biological Psychiatry, 19,* 973–990.

Schall, J. D. (1997). Visuomotor areas of the frontal lobe. *Cerebral Cortex, 12,* 527–638.

Schall, U., Schon, A., Zerbin, D., Eggers, C., & Oades, R. D. (1996). Event-related potentials during an auditory discrimination with prepulse inhibition in patients with schizophrenia, obsessive-compulsive disorder and healthy subjects. *International Journal of Neuroscience, 84,* 15–33.

Schmidt, M. H., Mocks, P., Lay, B., Eisert, H. G., Fojkar, R., Fritz-Sigmund, D., et al. (1997). Does oligoantigenic diet influence hyperactive/conduct-disordered children? A controlled trial. *European Child & Adolescent Psychiatry, 6,* 88–95.

Scott, J. P. R., McNaughton, L. R., & Polman, R. C. J. (2006). Effects of sleep deprivation and exercise on cognitive, motor performance and mood. *Physiology & Behavior, 87,* 396–408.

Seifert, J., Scheurpflug, P., Zillessen, K. E., Fallgatter, A., & Warnke, A. (2003). Electrophysiological investigation of the effectiveness of methylphenidate in children with and without ADHD. *Journal of Neural Transmission, 110,* 821–829.

Seiga-Riz, A. M., Popkin, B. M., & Carson, T. (1998). Trends in breakfast consumption for children in the United States from 1965–1991. *American Journal of Clinical Nutrition, 67,* 748–756.

Semrud-Clikeman, M., Filipek, P. A., Biederman, J., & Steingard, R. (1994). Attention-deficit hyperactivity disorder: Magnetic resonance imaging morphometric analysis of the corpus callosum. *Journal of the American Academy of Child & Adolescent Psychiatry, 33,* 875–881.

Semrud-Clikeman, M., Nielsen, K. H., Clinton, A., Sylvester, L., Parle, N., & Connor, R. T. (1999). An intervention approach for children with teacher and parent-identified attention difficulties. *Journal of Learning Disabilities, 32,* 581–590.

Semrud-Clikeman, M., & Wical, B. (1999). Components of attention in children with complex partial seizures with and without ADHD. *Epilepsia, 40,* 211–215.

Sergeant, J. (2005). Modeling attention-deficit/hyperactivity disorder: A critical appraisal of the cognitive–energetic model. *Biological Psychiatry, 57,* 1248–1255.

Sever, Y., Ashkenazi, A., Tyano, S., & Weizman, A. (1997). Iron treatment in children with attention deficit hyperactivity disorder: A preliminary report. *Biological Psychiatry, 35,* 178–180.

Shaffer, D., Fisher, P., Lucas, C., Dulcan, M., & Schwab-Stone, M. (2000). NIMH Diagnostic Interview Schedule for Children, Version IV (NIMH DISC–IV): Description, differences from previous versions, and reliability of some common diagnoses. *Journal of the American Academy of Child & Adolescent Psychiatry, 39,* 28–38.

Shapiro, A. K., & Shapiro, E. (1981). Do stimulants provoke, cause, or exacerbate tics and Tourette syndrome? *Comprehensive Psychiatry, 22,* 265–273.

Shelton, T. L., Barkley, R. A., Crosswait, C., Moorehouse, M., Fletcher, K., Barrett, S., et al. (2000). Multimodal psychoeducational intervention for preschool children with disruptive behavior: Two-year posttreatment follow-up. *Journal of Abnormal Child Psychology, 28,* 253–266.

Shire Pharmaceuticals. (2002). *Adderall XR data on file.* Florence, KY: Author.

Sieg, K. G., Gaffney, G. R., Preston, D. F., & Hellings, J. A. (1995). SPECT brain imaging abnormalities in attention deficit/hyperactivity disorder. *Clinical Nuclear Medicine, 20,* 55–60.

Siever, D. (2003). Applying audio-visual entrainment technology for attention and learning: Part III. *Biofeedback, 31,* 24–29.

Silberg, J., Rutter, M., Meyer, J., Maes, H., Hewitt, J., Simonoff, E., et al. (1996). Genetic and environmental influences on the covariation between hyperactivity and conduct disturbance in juvenile twins. *Journal of Child Psychology and Psychiatry, 37,* 803–816.

Silva, P. A., Chalmers, D., & Stewart, I. (1986). Some audiological, psychological, educational, and behavioral characteristics of children with bilateral otitis media with effusion: A longitudinal study. *Journal of Learning Disabilities, 19,* 165–169.

Silva, P. A., Kirkland, C., Simpson, A., Stewart, I. A., & Williams, S. M. (1982). Some developmental and behavioral problems associated with bilateral otitis media. *Journal of Learning Disabilities, 15,* 417–421.

Silva, R. R., Munoz, D. M., & Alpert, M. (1996). Carbamazepine use in children and adolescents with features of attention-deficit hyperactivity disorder: A meta-analysis. *Journal of the American Academy of Child & Adolescent Psychiatry, 35,* 352–358.

Silver, L. B. (2000). Attention-deficit/hyperactivity disorder in adult life. *Child and Adolescent Psychiatric Clinics of North America, 9,* 511–523.

Simonoff, E. S., Pickles, A., Hewitt, J. K., Silberg, J. L., Rutter, M., Loeber, R., et al. (1995). Multiple raters of disruptive child behavior: Using a genetic strategy to examine shared views and bias. *Behavior Genetics, 25,* 311–326.

Sinclair, G. (1983, March). A daily physical education pilot project. *Canadian Association of Health, Physical Education, and Recreation (CAHPER) Journal,* 22–26.

Slate, S. E., Meyer, T. L., Burns, W. J., & Montgomery, D. D. (1998). Computerized cognitive training for severely emotionally disturbed children with ADHD. *Behavior Modification, 22,* 415–437.

Sleator, E. K., & Pelham, W. E. (1986). *Attention deficit disorder.* Norwalk, CT: Appleton-Century-Crofts.

Smalley, S. L., McGough, J. J., Del'Homme, M., NewDelman, J., Gordon, E., Kim, T., et al. (2000). Familial clustering of symptoms and disruptive behaviors in multiplex families with attention-deficit/hyperactivity disorder. *Journal of the American Academy of Child & Adolescent Psychiatry, 39,* 1135–1143.

Smith, M. E., McEvoy, L. K., & Gevins, A. (1999). Neurophysiological indices of strategy development and skill acquisition. *Brain Research & Cognitive Brain Research, 7,* 389–404.

Smith, M. E., McEvoy, L. K., & Gevins, A. (2002). The impact of moderate sleep loss on neurophysiologic signals during working memory task performance. *Sleep, 25,* 784–794.

Sohlberg, M. M., & Mateer, C. A. (1989). *Attention process training.* Puyallup, WA: Association for Neuropsychological Research and Development.

Solanto, M. J. (1998). Neuropsychopharmacological mechanisms of stimulant drug action in attention-deficit hyperactivity disorder: A review and integration. *Behavioral Brain Research, 94,* 127–152.

Song, D. H., Shin, D. W., Jon, D. I., & Ha, E. H. (2005). Effects of methylphenidate on quantitative EEG of boys with attention-deficit hyperactivity disorder in continuous performance test. *Yonsei Medical Journal, 46,* 34–41.

Span, S. A., Earleywine, M., & Strybel, T. Z. (2002). Confirming the factor structure of attention deficit hyperactivity disorder symptoms in adult, nonclinical samples. *Journal of Psychopathology and Behavioral Assessment, 24,* 129–136.

Spencer, T. J. (2006). Antidepressant and specific norepinephrine reuptake inhibitor treatments. In R. A. Barkley (Ed.), *Attention-deficit hyperactivity disorder: A handbook for diagnosis and treatment* (pp. 648–657). New York: Guilford Press.

Spencer, T. J., Biederman, J., Faraone, S., Mick, E., Coffey, B., Geller, D., et al. (2001). Impact of tic disorders on ADHD outcome across the life cycle: Findings from a large group of adults with and without ADHD. *American Journal of Psychiatry, 158*, 611–617.

Spencer, T. J., Biederman, J., & Wilens, T. E. (1998). Growth deficits in children with attention-deficit/hyperactivity disorder. *Pediatrics, 102*, 501–506.

Spencer, T. J., Biederman, J., & Wilens, T. E. (1999). Attention-deficit/hyperactivity disorder and comorbidity. *Pediatric Clinics of North America, 46*, 915–927.

Spencer, T. J., Biederman, J., Wilens, T. J., & Faraone, S. V. (1998). Adults with attention-deficit/hyperactivity disorder: A controversial diagnosis. *Journal of Clinical Psychiatry, 59*(Suppl. 7), 59–68.

Spencer, T. J., Biederman, J., Wilens, T. E., & Faraone, S. V. (2002). Overview and neurobiology of attention-deficit/hyperactivity disorder. *Journal of Clinical Psychiatry, 63*(Suppl. 12), 3–9.

Spencer, T. J., Biederman, J., Wilens, T., Harding, M., O'Donnell, D., & Griffin, S. (1996). Pharmacotherapy of attention-deficit hyperactivity disorder across the life cycle. *Journal of the American Academy of Child & Adolescent Psychiatry, 35*, 1460–1469.

Spring, B., Maller, O., Wurtman, J., Digman, L., & Cozolino, L. (1982). Effects of protein and carbohydrate meals on mood and performance: Interactions with sex and age. *Journal of Psychiatric Research, 17*, 155–167.

Starobrat-Hermelin, B., & Kozielec, T. (1997). The effects of magnesium physiological supplementation on hyperactivity in children with attention deficit hyperactivity disorder (ADHD): Positive response to magnesium oral loading test. *Magnesium Research, 10*, 143–148.

Sterman, M. B. (1996). Physiological origins and functional correlates of EEG rhythmic activities: Implications for self-regulation. *Biofeedback and Self-Regulation, 21*, 3–33.

Stevens, L. J., Zentall, S. S., Abate, M. L., Kuczek, T., & Burges, J. R. (1996). Omega-3 fatty acids in boys with behavior, learning, and health problems. *Physiology & Behavior, 59*, 915–920.

Stevens, L. J., Zentall, S. S., Deck, J. L., Abate, M. L., Lipp, S. R., & Burgess, J. R. (1995). Essential fatty acid metabolism in boys with attention-deficit hyperactivity disorder, *American Journal of Clinical Nutrition, 62*, 761–768.

Stewart, M. A., Thach, B. T., & Friedin, M. R. (1970). Accidental poisoning and the hyperactive child syndrome. *Diseases of the Nervous System, 31*, 403–407.

Strong Interest Inventory [Instrument]. (2006). Available from http://www.cpp.com/products/strong/index.asp

Stroop, J. R. (1935). Studies of interference in serial verbal reactions. *Journal of Experimental Psychology, 18*, 643–662.

Suffin, S. C., & Emory, W. H. (1995). Neurometric subgroups in attentional and affective disorders and their association with pharmacotherapeutic outcome. *Clinical Electroencephalography, 26*, 76–83.

Surman, C. B., Randall, E. T., & Biederman, J. (2006). Association between attention-deficit/hyperactivity disorder and bulimia nervosa: Analysis of 4 case-control studies. *Journal of Clinical Psychiatry, 67,* 351–354.

Swanson, J. M. (1993). Effect of stimulant medication on hyperactive children: A review of reviews. *Exceptional Child, 60,* 154–162.

Swanson, J. M., & Castellanos, F. X. (2002). Biological bases of ADHD—Neuroanatomy, genetics, and pathophysiology. In P. S. Jensen & J. R. Cooper (Eds.), *Attention deficit hyperactivity disorder: State of the science—best practices* (pp. 7-1–7-20). Kingston, NJ: Civic Research Institute.

Swanson, J. M., Kraemer, H. C., Hinshaw, S. P., Arnold, L. E., Conners, C. K., Abikoff, H. B., et al. (2001). Clinical relevance of the primary findings of the MTA: Success rates based on severity of ADHD and ODD symptoms at the end of treatment. *Journal of the American Academy of Child & Adolescent Psychiatry, 40,* 168–179.

Swanson, J. M., Lerner, M., March, J., & Gresham, F. M. (1999). Assessment and intervention for attention-deficit/hyperactivity disorder in the schools: Lessons from the MTA study. *Pediatric Clinics of North America, 46,* 993–1099.

Swanson, J. M., McBurnett, K., Christian, D., & Wigal, T. (1995). Stimulant medication and treatment of children with ADHD. In T. H. Ollendick & R. J. Prinz (Eds.), *Advances in clinical child psychology* (Vol. 17, pp. 265–322). New York: Plenum Press.

Swanson, J. M., Sandman, C. A., Deutsch, C., & Baren, M. (1983). Methylphenidate hydrochloride given with or before breakfast: I. Behavioral, cognitive, and electrophysiologic effects. *Pediatrics, 72,* 49–55.

Swartwood, M. O., Swartwood, J. N., Lubar, J. F., Timmerman, D. L., Zimmerman, A. W., & Muenchen, R. A. (1998). Methylphenidate effects on EEG, behavior, and performance in boys with ADHD. *Pediatric Neurology, 18,* 244–250.

Swedo, S. E., Leonard, H. L., Garvey, M., Mittleman, B., Allen, A. J., Perimutter, S., et al. (1998). Pediatric autoimmune neuropsychiatric disorders associated with streptococcal infections: Clinical description of the first 50 cases. *American Journal of Psychiatry, 155,* 264–271.

Szatmari, P., Offord, D. R., & Boyle, M. H. (1989a). Correlates, associated impairments, and patterns of service utilization of children with attention deficit disorders: Findings from the Ontario Child Health Study. *Journal of Child Psychology and Psychiatry, 30,* 205–217.

Szatmari, P., Offord, D. R., & Boyle, M. H. (1989b). Ontario Child Health Study: Prevalence of attention deficit disorder with hyperactivity. *Journal of Child Psychology and Psychiatry, 30,* 219–230.

Taylor, F. B., & Russo, J. (2001). Comparing guanfacine and dextroamphetamine for the treatment of adult attention-deficit hyperactivity disorder. *Journal of Clinical Psychopharmacology, 21,* 223–228.

Terman, L. M., & Merrill, M. A. (1960). *Stanford–Binet Intelligence Scale: Manual for the third revision, Form L-M.* Boston: Houghton Mifflin.

Thomas, M., Sing, H., Belenky, G., Holcomb, H., Mayberry, H., Dannals, R., et al. (2000). Neural basis of alertness and cognitive performance impairments during sleepiness: I. Effects of 24 h of sleep deprivation on waking human regional brain activity. *Journal of Sleep Research, 9,* 335–352.

Thomson, J. B., Seidenstrang, R., Kerns, K. A., Sohlberg, M. M., & Mateer, C. A. (1994). *Pay attention!* Puyallup, WA: Association for Neuropsychological Research and Development.

Tillery, K. L., Katz, J., & Keller, W. D. (2000). Effects of methylphenidate (Ritalin) on auditory performance in children with attention and auditory processing disorders. *Journal of Speech, Language, and Hearing Research, 43,* 893–901.

Tomporowski, P., & Ellis, R. (1986). Effects of exercise on cognitive processes: A review. *Psychological Bulletin, 99,* 338–346.

Toomim, H., & Toomim, M. (1999). Clinical observations with brain blood flow biofeedback—the "thinking cap." *Journal of Neurotherapy, 3,* 73.

Toren, P., Eldar, S., Sela, B. A., Wolmer, L., Weitz, R., Inbar, D., et al. (1996). Zinc deficiency in attention-deficit hyperactivity disorder. *Biological Psychiatry, 40,* 1308–1310.

Tourette's Syndrome Study Group. (2002). Treatment of ADHD in children with tics: A randomized controlled trial. *Neurology, 58,* 527–536.

Triolo, S. J., & Murphy, K. R. (1996). *Attention Deficit Scales for Adults (ADSA): Manual for scoring and interpretation.* New York: Brunner/Mazel.

Trommer, B. L., Hoeppner, J. B., Rosenberg, R. S., Armstrong, K. J., & Rothstein, J. A. (1988). Sleep disturbances in children with attention deficit disorder. *Annals of Neurology, 24,* 325–332.

Tryphonas, H., & Trites, R. (1979). Food allergy in children with hyperactivity, learning disabilities, and/or minimal brain dysfunction. *Annals of Allergy, 42,* 22–27.

Tutty, S., Gephart, H., & Wurzbacher, K. (2003). Enhancing behavioral and social skill functioning in children newly diagnosed with attention-deficit hyperactivity disorder in a pediatric setting. *Journal of Developmental and Behavioral Pediatrics, 24,* 51–57.

Uauy, R., Hoffman, P., Peirano, D. G., Birch, E. E., & Birch, E. E. (2001). Essential fatty acids in visual and brain development. *Lipids, 36,* 885–895.

U.S. Department of Health and Human Services. (2000). *Healthy People 2010* (2nd ed.). Washington, DC: U.S. Government Printing Office.

Vaisman, N., Voet, H., Akivis, A., & Vakil, E. (1996). Effect of breakfast timing on the cognitive functions of elementary school students. *Archives of Pediatrics and Adolescent Medicine, 150,* 1089–1092.

van der Stelt, O., van der Molen, M., Boudewijn-Gunning, W., & Kok, A. (2001). Neuroelectrical signs of selective attention to color in boys with attention-deficit hyperactivity disorder. *Cognition Brain Research, 12,* 245–264.

Van Dongen, H. P. A., Maislin, G., Mullington, J. M., & Dinges, D. F. (2003). The cumulative cost of additional wakefulness: Dose-response effects on neurobehavioral functions and sleep physiology from chronic sleep restriction and total sleep deprivation. *Sleep, 26,* 117–126.

Verbaten, M. N., Overtoom, C. C., Koelega, H. S., Swaab-Barneveld, H., van der Gaag, R. J., Guitelaar, J., et al. (1994). Methylphenidate influences on both early and late ERP waves of ADHD children in a continuous performance test. *Journal of Abnormal Child Psychology, 22,* 561–578.

Verhulst, F. C., & Koot, H. M. (1992). *Child psychiatric epidemiology: Concepts, methods, and findings.* Newbury Park, CA: Sage.

Verhulst, F. C., van der Ende, J., Ferdinand, R. F., & Kasius, M. C. (1997). The prevalence of *DSM–III–R* diagnoses in a national sample of Dutch adolescents. *Archives of General Psychiatry, 54,* 329–336.

Voigt, R. G., Liorente, A. M., Jensen, C. L., Fraley, J. K., Beretta, M. C., & Heird, W. E. C. (2001). A randomized, double-blind, placebo-controlled trial of docosahexanoic acid supplementation in children with attention-deficit/hyperactivity disorder. *Journal of Pediatrics, 139,* 189–196.

Volkow, N. D., Ding, Y. S., Fowler, J. S., Wang, G. J., Logan, J., Gatley, J. S., et al. (1995). Is methylphenidate like cocaine? Studies on their pharmacokinetics and distribution in the human brain. *Archives of General Psychiatry, 52,* 456–463.

Volkow, N. D., Wang, G. J., Fowler, J. S., Gatley, S. J., Logan, J., Ding, Y. S., et al. (1998). Dopamine transporters occupancies in the human brain induced by therapeutic doses of oral methylphenidate. *American Journal of Psychiatry, 155,* 1325–1331.

Volkow, N. D., Wang, G. J., Fowler, J. S., Logan, J., Gerasimov, M., Maynard, L., et al. (2001). Therapeutic doses of oral methylphenidate significantly increase extracellular dopamine in the human brain. *Journal of Neuroscience, 21,* RC121.

Ward, M. F., Wender, P. H., & Reimberr, F. W. (1993). The Wender Utah Rating Scale: An aid in the retrospective diagnosis of children with attention deficit hyperactivity disorder. *American Journal of Psychiatry, 150,* 885–890.

Waxmonsky, J. (2003). Assessment and treatment of attention deficit hyperactivity disorder in children with comorbid psychiatric illness. *Current Opinion in Pediatrics, 15,* 476–482.

Weber, P., & Lutschg, J. (2002). Methylphenidate treatment. *Pediatric Neurology, 26,* 261–266.

Wechsler, D. (2004). *Wechsler Individual Achievement Test manual.* San Antonio, TX: Psychological Corporation.

Weinstock, A., Giglio, P., Kerr, S. L., Duffner, P. K., & Cohen, M. E. (2003). Hyperkinetic seizures in children. *Journal of Child Neurology, 18,* 517–524.

Weiss, G., Hechtman, L. T., Milroy, T., & Perlman, T. (1985). Psychiatric status of hyperactives as adults: A controlled prospective 15-year follow-up of 63 hyperactive children. *Journal of the American Academy of Child & Adolescent Psychiatry, 24,* 211–220.

Weiss, L. (1997). *Attention deficit disorder in adults: Practical help and understanding.* New York: Cooper Square Press.

Weiss, M., & Hechtman, L. (1993). *Hyperactive children grown up* (2nd ed.). New York: Guilford Press.

Weiss, R. E., Stein, M. A., & Refetoff, S. (1997). Behavioral effects of liothyronine (L-T3) in children with ADHD in the presence and absence of resistance to thyroid hormone. *Thyroid, 7*, 389–393.

Wells, A. (1990). Panic disorder in association with relaxation-induced anxiety: An attentional training approach to treatment. *Behavior Therapy, 21*, 273–280.

Welner, Z., Welner, A., Stewart, M., Palkes, H., & Wish, E. (1977). A controlled study of siblings of hyperactive children. *Journal of Nervous and Mental Disease, 165*, 110–117.

Welsh, M. C., & Pennington, B. F. (1998). Assessing frontal lobe function in children: Views from developmental psychology. *Developmental Neuropsychology, 4*, 199–230.

Wender, P. H. (1985). Wender Adult Questionnaire—Childhood Characteristics Scale (AQCC). *Psychopharmacological Bulletin, 21*, 927–928.

Wender, P. H., Wolf, L. E., & Wasserstein, J. (2001). Adults with ADHD: An overview. *Annals of the New York Academy of Sciences, 931*, 1–16.

Wentz, E., Lacey, J. H., Waller, G., Rastam, M., Turk, J., & Gillberg, C. (2005). Childhood onset neuropsychiatric disorders in adult eating disorder patients: A pilot study. *European Child & Adolescent Psychiatry, 14*, 431–437.

Wesnes, K. A., Pincock, C., Richardson, D., Helm, G., & Hails, S. (2003). Breakfast reduces declines in attention and memory over the morning in school children. *Appetite, 41*, 329–331.

Wilens, T. E. (2003). Drug therapy for adults with attention-deficit hyperactivity disorder. *Drugs, 63*, 2395–2411.

Wilens, T. E., Biederman, J., Brown, S., Tanguay, S., Monuteaux, M. C., Blake, C., et al. (2002). Psychiatric comorbidity and functioning in clinically referred preschool children and school-age youth with ADHD. *Journal of the American Academy of Child & Adolescent Psychiatry, 41*, 262–268.

Wilens, T. E., & Dodson, W. (2004). A clinical perspective of attention-deficit/hyperactivity disorder into adulthood. *Journal of Clinical Psychiatry, 65*, 1301–1313.

Wilens, T. E., McBurnett, K., Stein, M., Lerner, M., Spencer, T., & Wolraich, M. (2005). ADHD treatment with once-daily OROS methylphenidate: Final results from a long-term open-label study. *Journal of the American Academy of Child & Adolescent Psychiatry, 44*, 1015–1023.

Wilens, T. E., Spencer, T. J., & Biederman, J. (2002). A review of the pharmacotherapy of adults with attention-deficit/hyperactivity disorder. *Journal of Attention Disorders, 5*, 189–202.

Willcutt, E. G., Pennington, B. F., & DeFries, J. C. (2000). Twin study of the etiology of comorbidity between reading disability and attention-deficit/hyperactivity disorder. *American Journal of Medical Genetics, 96*, 293–301.

Williams, H. L., Gieseking, C. F., & Lubin, A. (1966). Some effects of sleep loss on memory. *Perceptual & Motor Skills, 23*, 1287–1293.

Wimmer, F., Hoffmann, R. F., Bonato, R. A., & Moffitt, A. R. (1992). The effects of sleep deprivation on divergent thinking and attention processes. *Journal of Sleep Research, 160*, 223–230.

Winsberg, B. G., Javitt, D. C., & Silipo, G. S. (1997). Electrophysiological indices of information processing in methylphenidate responders. *Biological Psychiatry, 42*, 434–445.

Woodward, L. J., Fergusson, D. M., & Horwood, L. J. (2000). Driving outcomes of young people with attentional difficulties in adolescence. *Journal of the American Academy of Child & Adolescent Psychiatry, 39*, 627–634.

World Health Organization. (1994). *International Classification of Diseases* (10th ed.). Geneva, Switzerland: Author.

Worsley, A., Coonan, W., & Worsley, A. (1987). The first body owner's programme: An integrated school-based physical and nutrition education programme. *Health Promotion, 2*, 39–49.

Wu, J. C., Gillin, J. C., Buchsbaum, M. S., Hershey, T., Hazlett, E., Sicotte, N., & Bunney, W. E., Jr. (1991). The effect of sleep deprivation on cerebral glucose metabolic rate in normal humans assessed with positron emission tomography. *Sleep, 14*, 155–162.

Wurtman, R. J., Wurtman, J. J., Regan, M. M., McDermott, J. M., Tsay, R. H., & Breu, J. J. (2003). Effects of normal meals rich in carbohydrates or proteins on plasma tryptophan and tyrosine ratios. *American Journal of Clinical Nutrition, 77*, 128–132.

Wurtz, R. H., & Goldberg, M. E. (1989). *The neurobiology of saccadic eye movements.* Amsterdam: Elsevier.

Yates, B. J. (1992). Vestibular influences on the sympathetic nervous system. *Brain Research Reviews, 17*, 51–59.

Youdim, M. B. H., Green, A. R., Bloomfield, M. R., Mitchell, B. D., Heal, D. J., & Grahame-Smith, D. G. (1980). The effects of iron deficiency on brain biogenic monoamine biochemistry and function in rats. *Neuropharmacology, 19*, 259–267.

Zagar, R., Arbit, J., Hughes, J. R., Busell, R. E., & Busch, K. (1989). Developmental and disruptive behavior disorders among delinquents. *Journal of the American Academy of Child & Adolescent Psychiatry, 28*, 437–440.

Zametkin, A. J., Nordahl, T. E., Gross, M., King, A. C., Semple, W. E., Rumsey, J., et al. (1990). Cerebral glucose metabolism in adults with hyperactivity of childhood onset. *New England Journal of Medicine, 323*, 1361–1366.

AUTHOR INDEX

Connor, D. F., 123, 124, 125, 126, 127
Conte, R. A., 55
Cook, J. R., 27
Cooke, R. W. I., 53
Coonan, W., 110
Cooper, N. J., 43, 133
Cooper, S., 148
Corkum, P. V., 57
Cornish, L. A., 125
Costello, A. J., 3, 12
Costello, E. J., 3, 4–5, 7, 12, 51
Cousins, L. S., 198
Cozolino, L., 101
Craft, L., 110
Crawford, G., 132
Crawford, M. A., 60
Croft, R. J., 6, 132
Crosby, R., 12
Crumrine, P., 62
Cunningham, C. E., 183, 184

Daosheng, S., 108
Davenport, T. L., 43
David, O. J., 54
Davidson, R. J., 20
Davis, H. T., 123
Dean, R. S., 52
deBeus, M. E., 158
deBeus, R., 158
DeFries, J. C., 36
Deinard, A. S., 59
de la Burde, B., 54
DeLeo, A. J., 61
Dement, W. C., 108
Deming, L., 108
Derks, E. M., 14
Derogatis, L. R., 222
Desmedt, J. F., 75
DiClemente, C. C., 185
Diego, M., 110
Dietrich, M., 12
Digman, L., 101
Dillon, J. E., 57
di Michele, F., 6, 20, 36, 44, 73, 118, 149
Dinges, D. F., 107, 108
Dodds, M., 59
Dodson, W., 3
Dolan, C. V., 14
Dorris, M. C., 63
Dougherty, D. D., 42
Douglass, J. S., 104, 105n
Drake, C. L., 108

Dresel, S. H., 42
Duffner, P. K., 62
Dulcan, M., 70
Dunn, W., 28
DuPaul, G. J., 31, 148, 161, 183
Durmer, J. S., 107, 108
Durston, S., 40
Dustman, R. E., 114
Dwyer, T., 110
Dye, L., 55, 100

Eakin, L., 221
Earleywine, M., 216
Eckert, T. L., 183
Edelbrock, C. S., 3, 12, 14, 15, 136, 183
Edwards, G., 198
Egeland, B., 59
Egger, H. L., 4–5, 51
Egger, J., 55
Eggers, C., 75
Ehlers, S., 26
Elbert, T., 75
Ellington, R. J., 62
Elliott, S. N., 140
Ellis, R., 110
El-Zein, R. A., 121, 122
Emmerson, R. E., 114
Emory, W. H., 44
Engineer, P., 27
Epstein, J. N., 131
Erhardt, D., 72, 213
Erkanli, A., 4–5, 51
Ernst, M., 150
Eskinazi, B., 54
Esser, G., 12
Evans, J. H., 148
Everling, S., 63

Fabiano, G. A., 184
Falkenstein, A. R., 53
Fallgatter, A., 133
Fallone, G., 57
Faraone, S. V., 20, 22, 37, 53, 121, 217
Farley, S. E., 183
Feagans, L. V., 64
Fein, G., 75
Feinberg, D. T., 197
Feldman, H., 62
Ferdinand, R. F., 12, 14
Fergusson, D. M., 12, 31
Fernstrom, J. D., 56, 98
Ferre, L., 148

Field, T., 110
Filipek, P. A., 40
Firestone, P., 13, 14, 15
Fischer, K., 101, 102
Fischer, M., 14, 15, 22, 211
Fisher, A., 28
Fisher, M., 212
Fisher, P., 70
Fisher, S. E., 38
Fitzgerald, M., 26
Fjallberg, M., 57
Fletcher, K., 14, 15, 22, 198, 211
Foks, M., 149, 153
Foley, H. A., 31
Food and Nutrition Board of the National
    Academy of Sciences, 104, 122, 187,
    201, 203, 229, 232, 238
Ford, L., 148
Foster, S. L., 184
Foster-Powell, K., 55
Fowler, J. S., 120
Fox, D. J., 147
Fox, L. J., 147
Frankel, F., 138, 197, 198, 210
Frazier, J. A., 7, 143, 148
Friedin, M. R., 31–32
Freisleder, F. J., 158
French, C. L., 147, 219
Fristad, M., 61
Fuchs, T., 154
Fujii, K., 12

Gaffney, G. R., 150
Gallucci, F., 12
Gammon, G. D., 128
Ganoczy, D. A., 57
Garfield, G. S., 56, 98
Garland, A. F., 14
Garland, M. R., 60
Gascon, G. G., 27
Gavrilescu, A., 127
Gearity, J., 14
Gentry, L. R., 62
George, D. M., 6, 13, 68, 132, 150, 162, 183,
    197, 219
Gephart, H., 198
Gevensleben, H., 158
Gevins, A., 108
Ghariani, S., 62
Ghaziuddin, M., 26
Ghaziuddin, N., 26
Giedd, J. N., 36, 40

Gieseking, C. F., 108,
Giglio, P., 62
Gilbert, A., 59
Gillberg, C., 26, 211
Gillerot, Y., 62
Gittelman, R., 54
Gleser, G., 54
Godersky, J. C., 62
Goldberg, M. E., 63
Golden, C. J., 36
Goldstein, S., 26, 223
Gollegly, K., 64
Golub, M. S., 58
Gomi, C. F., 63
Goodman, R., 15
Gordon, E., 43, 133, 212
Gordon, M., 71, 131, 147, 148, 214
Grad, G., 54
Graetz, B. W., 12
Graham, P. J., 55
Granet, D. B., 63
Grant, B., 110
Green, B., 54
Green, J. L., 148
Greenberg, L. M., 71, 131, 154
Greenhill, L. L., 117, 119, 120, 121, 157
Greenough, W. T., 114
Gresham, F. M., 72, 140
Grose, J. H., 64
Gruber, R., 57
Gruzelier, J. H., 154
Guerrini, R., 62
Guerts, H. M., 25
Guevremont, D. C., 31, 148
Gumley, D, 55
Gunsett, G., 29

Ha, E. H., 132
Habib, T., 150
Hagerman, R., 28
Hagerman, R. J., 53
Hails, S., 55, 101
Hall, J., 25, 64
Hallahan, B., 60
Hallowell, E. M., 223
Halperin, J. M., 125
Halverstadt, J. S., 221
Hamazaki, T., 60
Hambidge, M., 58
Hampton, K. A., 63
Handen, R., 62
Hanft, B. E., 28

Hare, R. D., 75
Harlow, C. W., 31
Harris, M. J., 132
Hartsough, C. S., 31, 52–53
Harvey, W. J., 144
Hathaway, S. R., 136
Hauser, P., 61
Hay, D. A., 28, 36
Hazell, P. L., 12, 128
Hechtman, L., 3, 14, 15, 31, 211
Hehr, B., 59
Heinrich, H., 158
Hellings, J. A., 150
Helm, G., 55, 101
Hemmer, S. A., 62
Henderson, F., 64
Henriksen, L., 149
Herbst, K. L., 75
Hermens, D. F., 6, 43, 44, 132, 133
Herning, R. I., 75
Herrerias, C., 51
Herrington, R., 158
Herskovits, E. H., 62, 63
Hessling, B., 223
Hetzel, B. S., 110
Hewitt, J. K., 14
Heywood, C., 157
Hidaka, K. C., 44, 132
Highstein, S. M., 63
Hikosa, O., 63
Hillman, C. H., 110, 114
Hinshaw, S. P., 5, 7, 14, 15, 19, 25, 30, 121, 140, 173, 183, 185, 197
Hirayama, S., 60
Hirshberg, L. M., 7, 143, 148, 157
Hoeppner, J. B., 57
Hoffman, P., 60
Hoffman, R. F., 108
Hoffman, S. P., 54
Hollingshead, A. B., 31
Hollon, S. D., 148, 157
Holmes, C. S., 12
Holt, S. H., 55
Holtmann, M., 25, 26
Homer, C. J., 51
Honig, A. S., 59
Hopfer, C., 132
Hopkins, M. R., 51
Horwood, L. J., 12, 31
Hough, R. L., 14
Howanitz, P., 59
Howell, C. T., 13–14

Howell, R. J., 31
Hoza, B., 7, 30, 138, 184, 197, 198
Hudson, J. I., 15
Hudziak, J. J., 14
Hugdahl, K., 20
Hughes, J. R., 61
Hunt, R. D., 125, 128
Hunter, L., 161
Hurlburt, M. S., 14
Hutchings, M. E., 64
Hynd, G. W., 25

Iacono, W. G., 75
Individuals With Disabilities Education Act (IDEA), 163
Isaacs, K. R., 114
Ivers, C. L., 148

Jacobvitz, D., 117
Jakim, S., 29
Javitt, D. C., 44
Jensen, A., 14
Jensen, P. S., 5, 7, 14, 15, 19, 31, 33, 51, 121, 133, 140, 173, 197
Jensen-Doss, A., 14
Jerger, J., 64
Jerger, S., 64
Jerome, G. J., 110
Jerome, L., 27
Johannes, S., 75
John, E. R., 44
Johnson, R., 27
Johnstone, S. J., 43, 57, 58, 75, 132
Jon, D. I., 132
Jonkman, L. M., 44

Kaciuba-Uscilko, H., 111
Kahn, A., 57
Kaiser, J., 154
Kamphaus, R., 154
Kanarek, R. B., 55, 101
Kanbayashi, Y., 12
Kaplan, B. J., 55
Kasius, M. C., 12
Katz, J., 27
Kawagoe, R., 63
Keays, J. J., 110
Keenan, K., 37
Keith, R. W., 27
Keller, W. D., 27
Kelly, K. L., 128
Kerns, K. A., 147

Maughan, B., 15
Max, J. E., 62, 63
McBurnett, K., 7, 121, 197, 198
McCann, B. S., 213
McCarney, S. B., 72, 155, 228
McCarthy, R., 6, 43, 44, 73, 132
McConaughy, S. H., 13–14
McDermott, C. M., 108
McDermott, W., 4, 61
McDonald, J. J., 75
McEvoy, L. K., 108
McEwen, L. M., 55
McGee, R. A., 12, 72
McGoey, K. E., 183
McGue, M., 75
McIntosh, D. N., 28, 52
McKay, K. E., 125
McKinley, J. C., 136
McNaughton, L. R., 57
McNicol, J., 55
McStephen, M., 36
Melyn, M. A., 61
Mendelson, M., 222–223
Mensour, B. M., 149
Merkin, H., 43
Merrill, M. A., 143, 144
Messer, J., 15
Metcalfe, D., 54
Metevia, L., 198
Meltzer, H., 15
Meyer, T. L., 143
Meyers, S. E., 64
Michelson, D., 38, 217
Mick, E., 22, 53
Milberger, S., 52, 53
Mildenberger, K., 25
Miller, C., 43
Miller, L. J., 28, 52
Miller-Scholte, A., 63
Milroy, T., 3
Minde, K., 53
Minow, F., 25
Mitchell, E. A., 60
Moffitt, A. R., 108
Moghadam, H. K., 55
Mohammadi, M.-R., 58
Moldofsky, H., 57
Molina, B., 22
Moll, G. H., 158
Molloy, E., 36
Molt, L., 25

Monastra, D. M., 6, 13, 68, 132, 150, 155, 162, 183, 197, 219
Monastra, V. J., 5, 6, 7, 13, 18, 20, 26, 33, 36, 38, 42, 43, 44, 45, 47, 50, 51, 68, 71, 72, 73, 75, 76, 80, 118, 122, 124, 125, 130, 132, 132–133, 133, 133n, 134, 136, 138n, 140, 142n, 143, 147, 148, 149, 150, 151, 153, 154, 155, 156, 158, 162, 166, 167, 176, 178, 183, 184, 185–186, 186, 197, 198, 210, 216, 219
Montgomery, D. D., 143, 148
Moore, D. R., 64
Moore, J. J., 71
Moore, K. D., 63
Moschovkis, A. K., 63
Mott, A. A., 114
MTA Cooperative Group. *See* Multimodal Study of Children With ADHD Cooperative Group
MTA Study. *See* Multimodal Treatment Study of Children with ADHD Cooperative Group
Muenchen, R., 43
Mulkins, R. S., 52
Mulligan, S., 29
Mullington, J. M., 108
Multimodal Treatment Study of Children With ADHD Cooperative Group (MTA), 5, 14, 15, 51, 121, 129, 133, 140, 162, 198
Munoz, D. M., 126
Munoz, D. P., 63
Murphy, K. R., 12, 31, 70, 212, 213, 214, 216, 221, 223
Murray, E., 28
Murray, M. J., 59
Musiek, F. E., 25, 64
Mutrie, N., 110
Myatt, R., 138, 197

Nadeau, K., 221
Nager, W., 75
Naidu, S. B., 36
Nakamura, Y., 110
Nakata, Y., 12
National Institute of Health (NIH), 162, 167
National Toxicology Program, 121
Nazar, K., 111
Needleman, H. L., 54

Newcom, J. H., 125
Nichols, P. L., 53
Niedermeyer, E., 36
Nigam, V. R., 3, 12
Nigg, J. T., 36, 44
Nishimoto, K., 110
Norcross, J. C., 185
Noterdaeme, M., 25
Novartis Pharmaceuticals, 120
Nugent, S. M., 12

Oader, R. D., 75
O'Connell, P., 128
O'Connor, S. J., 75
Offord, D. R., 12, 15
Ogdie, M. N., 38
Oosterlaan, J., 25
Orgill, A. A., 132
Oski, F. A., 59
Ousley, O. Y., 26
Ozonoff, S., 25, 26

Paavonen, E. J., 57
Pagini, L., 12
Palkes, H., 37
Palumbo, D., 121
Pare, M., 63
Pasternak, J. F., 62
Pastor, P. N., 21
Pataki, C., 128
Payson, E., 221
Pelham, W. E., 7, 22, 121, 138, 140, 144,
    184, 197, 198
Pennington, B. F., 25, 36, 43
Pennington, J. A., 104, 105n
Perlman, T., 3
Perrin, J. M., 51
Petersen, S. R., 36
Peterson, B. S., 23
Pfiffner, L. J., 161, 162, 167, 197, 198
Pfingsten, U., 138
Physicans Desk Reference, 20
Piek, J. P., 28
Pierano, D. G., 60
Pillsbury, H. C., 64
Pincock, C., 55, 101
Pine, D. S., 23
Pinkham, S. M., 58
Pitcher, T. M., 28
Pituch, K. J., 57
Pleak, R. R., 127
Pliszka, S. R., 14, 20, 22, 44, 75

Polich, J., 75, 114
Pollitt, E., 55, 100
Pollock, I., 55
Polman, R. C. J., 57
Popkin, B. M., 57
Posner, M. I., 36
Pothakos, K., 114
Poustka, F., 25
Powls, A., 53
Preston, D. F., 150
Prichep, L., 6, 20, 36, 44, 73, 118, 149
Prince, J. B., 122, 123, 138, 217, 218
Prochaska, J. O., 185
Puri, B. K., 60

Qian, Q., 37

Radojevic, V., 150
Radea, D., 75
Ramsay, J. R., 140, 220
Randall, E. T., 24
Rapaport, H. G., 54
Rapoport, J. L., 36
Rapp, D. J., 54
Rapport, M. D., 128, 147, 148
Rasmussen, P., 211
Ratey, N. A., 143, 223
Raviv, A., 57
Realmuto, G. M., 12
Redlich, F. C., 31
Refetoff, S., 61
Rehabilitation Act, 163, 165
Reich, W., 70
Reid, G., 144
Reitan, R. M., 143
Reite, M., 132
Reuben, C. A., 21
Reynolds, C., 71, 72, 131, 154
Rhoads, L. H., 183
Riccio, C. A., 25, 27, 71, 72, 131, 147, 219
Richardson, A. J., 60
Richardson, D., 55, 101
Robbins, C. A., 221
Roberts, J. E., 64
Robin, A. L., 184, 221
Robinson, K. E., 161
Rockstroh, B., 75
Roeyers, H., 25
Rogers, J. M., 58
Rohde, L. A., 12
Romano, E., 12
Rosekind, M. R., 125

Rosenberg, R. S., 57
Ross, D. M., 12
Ross, S. A., 12
Rossiter, R. T., 150, 153, 154, 219
Rostain, A. L., 140, 220
Rothenberger, A., 158
Rothstein, J. A., 57
Rouse, M., 63
Rovet, J., 61
Rowe, K. S., 55
Rowe, R., 15
Roy-Byrne, P., 212, 213
Russell, J., 25, 26
Russo, J., 218
Rutter, M., 18
Ryan, J. J., 52

Sachs, L. A., 29
Sadeh, A., 57
Safren, S. A., 140, 220
Samuel, P., 55, 101
Sanders, C. E., 110
Sanders, M. R., 184
Sands, T., 57
Sanford, J. A., 71, 131, 143, 147
Sanyal, M., 64
Sargent, J., 55
Sata, Y., 62
Satterfield, J. H., 44, 132
Sawyer, M. G., 12
Schachar, R. J., 121
Schall, J. D., 63
Schall, U., 75
Schele, L., 213
Schell, A., 54
Schell, A. M., 44, 132
Scheuerpflug, P., 133
Schmidt, M. H., 12, 55
Schnakenberg-Ott, S., 52
Schon, A., 75
Schwab-Stone, M., 70
Schwebach, A. J., 26
Scott, J. P. R., 57
Scudder, C. A., 63
Sebire, G., 62
Seidenstrang, R., 147
Seifer, R., 57
Seifert, J., 133
Seiga-Riz, A. M., 57
Selikowitz, M., 6, 43, 44, 73, 132
Semrud-Clikeman, M., 40, 62, 148
Serfontein, G., 43, 132

Sergeant, J., 36, 44
Sergeant, J. A., 25
Sever, Y., 59
Shaffer, D., 70
Shapiro, A. K., 121
Shapiro, E., 121
Sharma, V., 125
Shearer, D. E., 114
Shelton, T. L., 31, 173
Shevrette, R. E., 31
Shin, D. W., 132
Shin, M.-S., 150
Shire Pharmaceuticals, 120, 122
Shouse, M. N., 150
Shyu, V., 28
Sieg, K. G., 150
Siever, D., 158
Siever, L. J., 125
Silberg, J., 36
Silipo, G. S., 44
Silva, P. A., 12, 64
Silva, R. R., 126,127
Silver, L. B., 212
Simonoff, E. S., 3, 14
Simpson, A., 64
Sirevaag, E. J., 75
Sitter, S., 25
Slate, S. E., 143
Sleator, E. K., 144
Smalley, S. L., 37
Smallish, L., 14, 15, 22, 211
Smeltzer, D. J., 29
Smith, M. E., 108
Smith, W. L., 62
Smithies, C., 29
Snook, E. M., 110
Sohlberg, M. M., 147, 147–148
Soininen, M., 57
Solanto, M. J., 120
Soler, R., 61
Song, D. H., 132
Soothill, J. F., 55
Span, S. A., 216
Sparrow, E., 72, 213
Spencer, T., 3, 14, 17, 18, 20, 22, 23, 117,
    121, 122, 123, 124, 125, 138, 217
Spreen, O., 144
Spring, B., 101
Spring, B. J., 56, 98
Sroufe, L. A., 117
Starobrat-Hermelin, T., 59
Steere, J. C., 125

Stein, M. A., 61
Steingard, R., 40
Sterman, M. B., 150
Stern, A. C., 144
Stevens, L. J., 60
Stewart, I. A., 64
Stewart, M., 12, 31–32, 37, 117
Stolla, A., 55
Strayer, D. L., 26
Stroop, J. R., 143, 157
Strybel, T., 216
Stuart, J. E., 128
Sturm, R., 54
Suffin, S. C., 44
Surman, C. B., 24
Sverd, J., 54
Sverdrup, E. K., 62
Swanson, J. M., 5, 7, 12, 14, 19, 37, 40, 72, 117, 120, 121, 126, 140, 173, 197
Swartwood, J. N., 132
Swartwood, M. O., 132
Swedo, S. E., 53
Sykes, D., 53
Symons, D. K., 72
Szanton, V. L., 54
Szatmari, P., 12, 14, 15, 32

Takahashi, M., 110
Takikawa, Y., 63
Tannock, R., 57
Tardif, H. P., 57
Tatsch, K., 42
Taylor, F. P., 218
Taylor, H. A., 55, 101
Teale, P. D., 132
Teodori, J., 62
Terasawa, K., 60
Terman, L. M., 143, 144
Thach, B. T., 31–32
Tharp, D. E., 147
Thoma, W. 62
Thomas, M., 108
Thomason, D., 148
Thompson, B., 62
Thomson, J. B., 147
Tillery, K. L., 27
Tomporowski, P., 110
Toomin, H., 158
Toomin, M., 158
Toren, P., 58
Torronen, J., 57
Tourette's Syndrome Study Group, 123

Tremblay, R. E., 12
Triolo, S. J., 213
Trites, R., 54
Trommer, B. L., 57, 62
Tryphonas, H., 54
Turbott, S. H., 60
Turgay, A., 15
Tutty, S., 198
Tyano, S., 59

Uauy, R., 60
U.S. Department of Health and Human Services, 110
U.S. Department of Health and Human Services Center for Disease Control, 61

Vaisman, N., 55
Vakil, E., 55
VanBrakle, J., 183
van der Ende, J., 12
van der Molen, M., 75
van der Stelt, O., 75
Van Dongen, H. P. A., 108
Vendiniapin, A. B., 75
Ventura, R., 63
Verbaten, M. N., 44
Verhulst, F. C., 12, 14
Verte, S., 25
Vignolo, L. A., 143
Vitaro, F., 12
Voeller, K., 54
Voet, H., 55
Volkow, N. D., 37, 42, 120
Votolato, N., 58

Wada, K., 12
Walco, G., 64
Waldman, J., 36
Waldrop, J. J. M., 131
Wang, B., 37
Wang, Y., 37
Ward, C., 222–223
Ward, N., 213
Warner, J. O., 55
Warnke, A., 133
Wasserstein, J., 212
Waxmonsky, J., 14, 20, 22
Webb, G., 53
Weber, P., 62
Wechsler, D., 145
Weidmer-Mikhail, E., 26
Weinstock, A., 62

Weintraub, B. D., 61
Weiss, G., 3, 198
Weiss, L., 221
Weiss, M., 14, 15, 31, 211
Weiss, R. R., 61
Weisz, J. R., 14
Weizman, A., 59
Wells, A., 147
Welner, A., 37
Welner, Z., 37
Welsh, M. C., 43
Wender, P. H., 212, 213, 216
Wenk, C., 101
Wentz, E., 24
Wesnes, K. A., 55, 56, 101
White, J. N., 132
Wical, B., 62
Wieringa, B. M., 75
Wigal, T., 7, 121
Wilens, T. E., 3, 14, 15, 18, 20, 22, 121, 122,
    138, 217
Wilens, T. J., 3
Willcutt, E. G., 36
Williams, D. T., 127
Williams, H. L., 108
Williams, L. M., 132, 133
Williams, S., 12, 64
Wimmer, F., 108
Winsberg, B. G., 44
Wish, E., 37
Woerner, W., 12
Woldorf, M. G., 75
Wolf, L. E., 212

Wolfson, D., 143
Wolraich, M. L., 12
Wood, C., 36
Wood, L. M., 43
Woodward, L. J., 31
World Health Organization, 9
Worsley, A., 110
Wozniak, J. R., 122
Wu, J. C., 108
Wurtman, J., 101
Wurtman, R. J., 98, 102
Wurtz, R. H., 63
Wurzbacher, K., 198
Wymbs, B. T., 184
Wyngaarden, J. B., 4, 61

Xenakis, S. N., 31

Yates, B. J., 29
Youdim, M. B. H., 59
Yu, D., 108

Zagar, R., 31
Zametkin, A. J., 150
Zecker, S. G., 62
Zentall, S. S., 60
Zerbin, D., 75
Zhenyun, W., 108
Zhou, R., 37
Ziemba, A. W., 111
Zillessen, K. E., 133
Zimmerman, A., 43
Zoccolillo, M., 12

SUBJECT INDEX

and case illustration, 243
for depression, 20
Antihypertensive medications, 80, 118, 124–
126, 133
for ADHD and comorbid anxiety and
anger control problems, 140
for adults with ADHD, 218
in case illustration, 241
and qEEG screening, 133
Antipsychotic medications, 127
Anxiety
as comorbid (case illustration), 240–
243
and exercise, 110
and TCAs, 124
Anxiety disorder
ADHD diagnosis distinguished from, 4,
12, 13
as comorbid, 15, 17–19
in case illustration, 230–233
Anxiety problems, in Clinical History Questionnaire, 85
Apnea, 50, 242
Apologies and Amends (strategy), 189, 190
Ascending reticular activating system
(ARAS), 44, 45
Asperger's Disorder (ASP)
in case illustration, 231, 233
as comorbid, 25, 26
Assessment
for ADHD, 4–5, 5, 32, 67–68
in adults, 212–216, 224
in case illustrations, 228–229, 231–
232, 234–235, 237–238, 241–
243
Clinical History Questionnaire for,
71, 73, 76, 77, 81–95
cost analysis of, 80
functional, 136–145 (see also Functional assessment)
goals of, 68
and multiple domains, 46
and NFT program, 159
of pharmacological treatment, 128,
131
preassessment, 68–70
for school-based intervention, 171
session 1, 70–73
session 2, 73–76
session 3, 76–78
session 4, 78–80
and treatment, 33

and medical conditions mimicking
ADHD, 65–66
for zinc levels, 60
See also Diagnosis; Evaluation; Quanti-
tative electroencephalography
Assistive technology, 165–166, 179–180
for adults with ADHD, 224
in case illustrations, 236, 239, 243
Assistive Technology Resources, 247
Association for Applied Psychophysiology &
Biofeedback
treatment criteria of, 157
Web site of, 159, 246
Atomoxetine, 38, 80, 118, 122, 123, 124,
128, 131, 133, 217, 217–218
ATS (Attention Training System), 147, 148
Attention
and nutrition, 98–106
and sleep, 107–110
Attention Deficit Disorders Evaluation
Scales (ADDES), 72, 155, 231, 234
Attention-deficit/hyperactive disorder
(ADHD)
assessment of, 4–5, 5, 32, 67–80, 212–
216 (see also Assessment; Functional
assessment)
and clinical practice, 9, 32–33, 224–225
(see also Clinical practice)
as common symptomatic consequence
of multiple neurological conditions,
36 39, 46, 117
comorbid disorders with, 10, 14–29, 32
(see also Comorbid psychiatric
disorders)
diagnosis of, 4–5, 32–33, 67, 72, 73, 109
diagnostic criteria (core symptoms),
9–12, 13–14
family patterns of, 35
family situations of children with, 30
functional impairment areas of, 3, 29–
32, 46
among adults with ADHD, 216
and dietary habits, 100
in school settings, 161, 171–172 (see
also School-based interventions)
and social skills programs, 197 (see
also Neuroeducational Life Skills
Program for Children and Teenagers)
and treatment plan, 47
genetic foundation of, 5, 6, 12, 36–44,
45–47, 49, 117–118

as health care providers challenge, 7, 32
in home setting, 183 (*see also* Parents of
  ADHD children)
identification of, 3–4
and nutrition, sleep or exercise, 97 (*see
  also* Exercise; Nutrition; Sleep)
prevalence of, 3, 10, 12
subtypes of
  diagnostic, 10, 12
  neurophysiological, 6
treatment for, 47 (*see also* EEG biofeedback; Treatment)
  of adults, 216–224
  multimodal, 32, 135, 159, 162, 244
  and school-based intervention, 161–
    162, 169–170, 176–180
  treatment-resistant (case illustration),
    234–236
  variability of symptoms in, 39
  See also at ADHD
Attention-deficit/hyperactivity disorder,
  combined type, 12
Attention-deficit/hyperactivity disorder, predominately hyperactive–impulsive
  type, 12
Attention-deficit/hyperactivity disorder, pre-
  dominately inattentive type, 12
Attention Deficit Disorder Association, 245
Attention Deficit Scales for Adults (ADSA),
  213
Attention Index (AI), 228, 231, 235, 237,
  241
Attention magazine, 245
Attention problems, in Clinical History
  Questionnaire, 82–83
Attention Process Training, 147
Attention Research Update, 246
Attention Training, 147
Attention Training System (ATS), 147, 148
Auditory Continuous Performance Test, 76
Australia, ADHD prevalence in, 12
Autistic spectrum disorders, as comorbid, 15,
  25–26

Barkley, Russell (ADHD specialist), 246
Beck Depression Inventory, 222–223
Behavioral assessment, functional, 174–175
Behavioral Assessment System for Children,
  154
Behavioral Intervention Plan, 174
Behavioral rating scales, 72, 73, 76, 128
Behavior Management Training, 184

Benzodiazepines, 127
Beta frequencies, 43, 150, 153–154
Biofeedback providers, 159, 246
  Association for Applied Psychophysiol-
    ogy & Biofeedback, 157, 159, 246
  Biofeedback Certification Institute of
    America, 159, 246
  International Society for
    Neurofeedback & Research, 159,
    246
Biosynthesis, of neurotransmitters, 97, 98–
  99, 103
Bipolar disorders, 19, 19–20. *See also* Mood
  disorders
Birth complications, as mimicking ADHD,
  52–53
Birth history, in Clinical History Question-
  naire, 89–90
Brain
  and DCAM perspective, 44–45
  and etiology of ADHD, 36 (*see also* Eti-
    ology of ADHD)
  in neuroimaging studies of ADHD, 40–
    41, 42–44, 45–46
  reward frequencies and inhibit frequen-
    cies for (NFT), 152–153
  See also EEG biofeedback; Quantitative
    electroencephalography
Brain injury (traumatic), as mimicking
  ADHD, 4, 62–63
Brazil, ADHD prevalence in, 12
Breakfast
  cereal in, 106
  and educational performance, 100–103
Breathing, in NLSP, 203
Bulimia Nervosa, 24–25
Buproprion, 118, 123, 123–124, 140, 217,
  218
Business analogy to college career, 179

Calming activities, 192
Canada, ADHD prevalence in, 12
CAPD. *See* Central auditory processing dis-
  order
Captain's Log, 143, 147, 148
Carbamazepine (Tegretol), 20, 118, 126–127
Catecholamines, 98, 111, 120, 123. *See also*
  Dopamine; Norepinephrine
Causes of ADHD. *See* Etiology of ADHD
Central auditory processing disorder (CAPD)
  as comorbid, 25, 27–28
  as mimicking ADHD, 64

in Healthy Life Chart, 112–113
in NLSP, 201–202
in NPTP, 188, 191
for self-care, 195

Facial expressions, in NLSP, 207
FACT (Functional Assessment Checklist for Teachers), 136, 141–142, 172, 174
in NPTP, 187–188
Family counseling, in case illustration, 236
Family history, in Clinical History Questionnaire, 94–95
Fatty acids, essential (deficiencies of), as mimicking ADHD, 50, 60
504 Accommodation Plan, 73, 78, 155, 159, 162, 167
in case illustration, 236
initiation of, 170
in NPTP, 188
and study, 176, 177, 178
5-HT. See Serotonin
Fluency tasks
in functional assessment, 144
in social-skills game, 210
Fluoxetine, 127, 128, 217
fMRI (functional magnetic resonance imaging), 4, 35, 40–41, 46
Food and Drug Administration (FDA), 122, 218
Functional Assessment, 136–145
for adults with ADHD in workplace, 223
vs. functional behavioral assessment, 174–175
in school-based intervention, 170
for IDEA intervention, 163–164
Functional Assessment Checklist for Teachers (FACT), 136, 141–142, 172, 174
in NPTP, 187–188
Functional behavioral assessment, 174–175
Functional impairment in ADHD, areas of, 3, 29–32, 46
among adults with ADHD, 216
and dietary habits, 100
in school settings, 161, 171–172 (see also School-based interventions)
and social skills programs, 185, 197 (see also Neuroeducational Life Skills Program for Children and Teenagers; Neuroeducational Parent Training Program)
and treatment plan, 47

Functional magnetic resonance imaging (fMRI), 4, 35, 40–41, 46

GDS (Gordon Diagnostic System), 71, 72, 131
Genetic foundation of ADHD, 5, 6, 12, 36–39, 49, 117–118
and neuroimaging studies, 39–44
in clinical practice, 45–47
Germany, ADHD prevalence in, 12
Goals, in NLSP, 209
Goldstein, Sam (ADHD specialist), 246
Gordon Diagnostic System (GDS), 71, 72, 131
Guanfacine, 18–19, 26, 118, 122, 123, 124–125, 125, 131, 218, 232, 233

Hallowell, Ned (ADHD specialist), 246
Health care providers
ADHD as challenge for, 7, 32
See also Clinical practice
Healthy Life Chart, 112–113
Heritability
of ADHD, 12
of anxiety disorders, 18
of learning disorders, 21
of substance use disorders, 22
See also Genetic foundation of ADHD
Hollingshead and Redlich Occupational Scale, 31
Hyperactivity, as diagnostic criterion, 11
Hyperactivity problems, in Clinical History Questionnaire, 82–83

IDEA. See Individuals With Disabilities Education Act
IEP. See Individual Education Plan
Imipramine, 118, 123
Impulse control, in NPTP, 192–193
Impulsivity, as diagnostic criterion, 11
Impulsivity problem, in Clinical History Questionnaire, 82–83
Inattention, as diagnostic criterion, 11
Incarceration rate, of ADHD patients, 31
India, ADHD prevalence in, 12
Individual Education Plan (IEP), 73, 78, 155, 159, 162, 167
in case illustrations, 232, 234, 236
and functional assessment, 174
vs. functional behavioral assessment, 174
initiating of, 170

in NPTP, 188
reinforcement and treatment needed with, 172
and review, 173
and study, 176, 177, 178
teachers provided with, 173
Individuals With Disabilities Education Act (Public Law 94-142)(IDEA), 78 163–166
eligibility under, 170–171
in NPTP, 187
Infancy, in Clinical History Questionnaire, 90
Infectious disease, as mimicking ADHD, 53
Initial treatment plan, 76
Intensive Social Skills Training program, 184
Intermediate Variables of Attention, 131
Intermediate Visual and Auditory Continuous Performance Test (IVA), 71, 72
International Society for Neurofeedback and Research, 159, 246
Intervention. *See* Treatment
Intervention, efficacy of (standards for), 148
Iron, 104, 105
Iron deficiency, as mimicking ADHD, 58–59
Italy, ADHD prevalence in, 12
IVA (Intermediate Visual and Auditory Continuous Performance Test), 71, 72

Japan, ADHD prevalence in, 12

Kurzweil 3000 (computer program), 224

Labeling, parents' reluctance toward, 167
Language and motor coordination problems, in Clinical History Questionnaire 87
Language processing and fluency, functional assessment of, 143–144
Large neutral amino acids (LNAA), 99. *See also* Tryptophan; Tyrosine
Lead exposure, and ADHD symptoms, 53–54
Learning disorders
as comorbid, 15, 21–22, 30
in case illustration, 243
return of after assumed cure (case illustration), 236–240
Learning problems (academic skills), in Clinical History Questionnaire, 86–87

Legislation for educational rights
Individuals With Disabilities Education Act (IDEA), 78, 163–166, 170–171 187
Section 504 of Rehabilitation Act (1973), 78, 163, 166–167, 168–169 170–171 (*see also* Section 504 of Rehabilitation Act)
Legislation for workplace rights, 223
Life skills
acquiring of (NPTP), 187, 188–189
for adults with ADHD, 221
See also Social skills programs
Life Skills Questionnaire (LSQ): Adult Form, 136, 139–140, 224
Life Skills Questionnaire (LSQ): Child–Adolescent Form, 136, 137–138, 187 189, 192
Life skills training, 142, 187
LNAA (large neutral amino acids), 99. *See also* Tryptophan; Tyrosine
Lunch
high-carbohydrate, 100
See also under Protein

Magnesium, 104, 105
Magnesium deficiency, as mimicking ADHD, 50, 59–60
Magnetic resonance imaging (MRI), 40–41
Major Depressive Disorder, as comorbid, 19
Mania, 19. *See also* Mood disorders
Marital history, in Clinical History Questionnaire, 95
Marital therapy, for adults with ADHD, 80, 221–223, 225
in case illustration, 243
Massachusetts Institute of Technology, Department of Nutrition and Food Science of, 98
Meals, and symptoms mimicking ADHD, 55–57
Mediation, on ADHD student's plan, 173
Medical conditions
in ADHD patients, 38–39, 49
treatment for, 78–79
Medical conditions mimicking ADHD, 5, 49–50
birth complications, 52–53
and clinical practice, 50–51, 65–66
and diagnosis, 79
and assessment interview, 70–71

Neuropsychological tests, in medication selection and monitoring, 131–134
Neurotherapy. See EEG biofeedback
Neurotransmitters, 98
    biosynthesis of, 97, 98–99, 103
    and protein, 103
New Zealand, ADHD prevalence in, 12
NFT. See EEG biofeedback
NLSP. See Neuroeducational Life Skills Program for Children and Teenagers
No Child Left Behind Act, 166, 167
Nonpharmacological treatments for ADHD, 147. See also EEG biofeedback; Electronic training devices
Noradrenalin, 37, 38, 39, 41, 44
Norepinephrine (NE), 37, 38, 97, 98, 117–118, 120, 123
Nutrition
    and ADHD, 6, 97
    and anemia, 61
    and attention, 98–106
    in case illustration, 229, 230, 231, 232, 238, 239, 239–240, 241, 242, 244
    and causes of impairment, 4, 5, 97
    counseling on, 80
    deficiencies of vitamins, minerals and essential fatty acids, 50, 58–60, 61
    guidelines for, 115
    in Healthy Life Chart, 112–113
    vs. side effects of stimulants, 122
    teaching parents and patients about, 103–106
    See also Dietary habits
Nutritional supplements, 106

Obesity, 145
Obsessive–Compulsive Disorder, 18
Occupational therapy, and comprehensive plan under IDEA, 165
Oppositional and defiance problems, in Clinical History Questionnaire, 83
Oppositional Defiant Disorder
    in case illustration, 237
    as comorbid, 15, 16–17
Organization
    and adult ADHD (case illustration), 240, 243
    and advance notice of school assignments, 179
    on Functional Assessment Checklist, 141
    in NLSP, 208

in NPTP, 193
Organizers, professional, 246
Outburst game, 210

Parent–Child Nonaggression Pact, 190–191
Parent counseling, 80
    for adults with ADHD, 220–221, 225
    in case illustrations, 236, 243
Parenting Children With ADHD: 10 Lessons that Medicine Cannot Teach (Monastra), 184
Parent-to-Parent networks, 196
Parents of ADHD children, 183–184
    nonaggression policy of, 186, 190–191
    programs for, 184
        benefits of, 155
        and clinical practice, 196
        Neuroeducational Life Skills Program for Children and Teenagers (NLSP), 198
        Neuroeducational Parent Training Program (NPTP), 184, 185–196
        about sleep, 109–110
    and treatment noncompliance, 51
Paroxetine, 26, 217
Patient assessment. See Assessment
Patient compliance. See Compliance, treatment
Pay Attention! (electronic training device), 147–148, 148
Peer relationships
    of ADHD children, 30
    and NPTP, 194–195
Performance coach, 223. See also Coaching
Personality Disorder, ADHD diagnosis distinguished from, 12, 13
    Pervasive Developmental Disorder (PDD), ADHD diagnosis distinguished from, 12, 13, 25, 26
PET (positron emission tomography), 4, 35, 40, 41–42, 46, 108, 149, 150
Pharmacological treatment (pharmacology)
    for ADHD, 79–80, 117–118, 135
    for adults with ADHD, 216–219
    and affective disorder, 138
    anticonvulsants, 118, 126–127
    antidepressants, 18, 118, 123–124, 127 (see also Antidepressant medications)
    antihypertensives, 80, 118, 124–126, 133 (see also Antihypertensive medications)

and assessment, 79
and clinical trial, 79
evaluation of (FBA), 175
and genetic research, 39
and insomnia, 109
in overall treatment plan, 159
patient matching to, 6, 118
and compliance, 133–134
in school-based intervention, 173
in clinical practice, 180–181
in study, 177
selection of medication type and dose, 128–131
neuropsychological test and quantitative electroencephalography in, 131–134
stimulants, 118–123 (*see also* Stimulant medications)
for substance use disorders, 22
Pharmacy records, review of (adults with ADHD), 215
Phenylalanine, 56, 98, 99, 105
Physical therapy, and comprehensive plan under IDEA, 165
Planning, in NLSP, 209
Positron emission tomography (PET), 4, 35, 40, 41–42, 46, 108, 149
Practitioner directories, 246
Preassessment, 68–70
Prenatal history, in Clinical History Questionnaire, 88–89
Prenatal medical conditions, as mimicking ADHD, 50, 52
Problem solving, for adults with ADHD, 222
Problem-Solving Communication Training, 184
Problem-solving skills, teaching of
in NLSP, 207–208
in NPTP, 193–194
Products to Aid in Organization (resource), 247
Professionals concerned with ADHD, 246
Propranolol, 124, 218
Protein, 103–104
at breakfast or lunch, 101–102, 103, 106, 187
in case illustration, 229, 238, 242
in common foods, 105
vs. side effects of stimulants, 122
and sleep, 107, 109
Prozac, 241
Psychoactive substance use, in Clinical History Questionnaire, 93–94

Psychostimulants, 62. *See also at* Stimulant
Psychotic Disorder, ADHD diagnosis distinguished from, 12, 13
P300 (P3) component, 74–75
and pharmacological treatment, 133

Quantitative electroencephalography (qEEG), 4, 35, 42–44, 45, 46, 73 128–129
for adults with ADHD, 213, 216
behavioral data gathered through, 175
in case illustrations, 228, 231, 232, 233, 235, 237, 241, 243
for cortical dysregulation, 43, 73–76, 76, 77–78, 80, 118, 149
for differential diagnosis, 20–21
in medication selection and monitoring, 131–134
test sensitivity of, 213
qEEG Scanning Process, 155

RAS (reticular activating system). 41
ascending (ARAS), 44, 45
Ratey, John (ADHD specialist), 246
ReadPlease! (computer program), 224
Read & Write (computer program), 224, 236
Recommended Dietary Allowances (Food and Nutrition Board of the National Academy of Sciences, 122, 187, 201, 203
in case illustrations, 229, 232, 238
Rehabilitation Act of 1973 (Public Law 93-112), Section 504 of. *See* Section 504
of Rehabilitation Act
Reinforcement
in EEG biofeedback, 153
from electronic training devices, 147
and functional behavioral assessment, 174
by parents, 169, 172, 177, 178
and parent-teacher collaboration, 162
in parent training programs, 184
NPTP, 186, 188–189
in social skills programs, 197, 204
of peer-activity rule, 233
in study of school-based interventions, 177–178
task-avoiding behavior as, 175
See also Motivational strategies
Request for Evaluation, 73, 74

Socialization, functional assessment of, 140, 142
    on Checklist (social skills), 141
Socialization and communication problems, in Clinical History Questionnaire 85–86
Social skills deficits, 140
    ADHD combined with (case illustration), 230–233
Social skills programs or training, 80, 142, 197–198
    Neuroeducational Life Skills Program for Children and Teenagers (NLSP) 198–210
    in school-based interventions, 173
Social Skills Rating System, 140
Special education teacher, and IDEA, 164
SPECT (Single photon emission computed tomography), 4, 35, 40, 41–42, 46 149
Stimulant medications, 118–119
    for ADHD plus learning disorder, 22
    for adults with ADHD, 217
    in case illustrations, 232, 242, 243
    clinical benefits of, 120–121
    in combination, 127–128
    and compliance, 133
    and cortical hypoarousal, 149
    and electrophysiological hypoarousal, 132
    failure to respond to (case illustration), 227–230
    and high schooler's schedule, 178
    neurochemistry of, 120
    and neurotherapy, 154–156
        and reason for requesting, 158
    and qEEG examination, 149
    side effects of, 121–123
    with TCAs, 140
    See also Dextroamphetamine; Dextromethylphenidate; Methylphenidate;
        Mixed amphetamine salts
Stimulant rebound, 122
Stimulant therapy, 62, 80
    and fine motor functions, 144
Strong Interest Inventory, 243
Stroop Task, 157
Stroop Word-Color Test, 143
Student rights
    and Individuals With Disabilities Education Act (IDEA), 78, 163–166 (see also

Individuals With Disabilities Education Act)
    and Section 504 of Rehabilitation Act (1973), 78, 163, 166–167, 168–169
        (see also Section 504 of Rehabilitation Act)
Substance use
    in case illustration, 238, 239
    in Clinical History Questionnaire, 93–94
Substance use disorders
    as comorbid, 15, 22–23
    and P3 component, 75
Support groups, 245
Symptom Checklist—90—R, 222

TCAs. See Tricyclic antidepressants
Teasing, response to, 195
    in NLSP, 206
Telephone screening interview, 68–70
Test of Variables of Attention (TOVA), 71, 72, 131, 154, 155
    Auditory Version of, 73
    in case illustrations, 228, 231, 234, 236, 241, 243
"Test Your food IQ" game, 201
Therapy. See Clinical practice; Treatment
Thermometer as analogy to qEEG, 75
Theta frequencies, 43, 150, 153–154
Thyroid disorders, as mimicking ADHD, 60–61
Tic disorders
    and antihypertensives, 125
    as comorbid, 15, 23–24
Tics, neuromuscular, 121, 123
Time Stands Still (strategy), 188, 190
Token Test, 143
Tourette's Disorder, 23, 23–24
    and P3 component, 75
    See also Tic disorders; Tics, neuromuscular
TOVA (Test of Variables of Attention), 71, 72, 131, 154, 155
    Auditory Version of, 73
    in case illustrations, 228, 231, 234, 236, 241, 243
Transient tic disorder, 23
Traumatic brain injury, as mimicking ADHD, 4, 49, 62
Treatment
    for ADHD, 47
    of adults, 216–224

ABOUT THE AUTHOR

Vincent J. Monastra, PhD, is a clinical psychologist and director of the FPI Attention Disorders Clinic in Endicott, New York. He is also an adjunct associate professor in the Department of Psychology at Binghamton University. During the past 3 decades, he has conducted a series of studies involving more than 10,000 individuals with disorders of attention and behavioral control, resulting in the publication of numerous scientific articles, a book chapter, and the award-winning book *Parenting Children With ADHD: 10 Lessons That Medicine Cannot Teach* (American Psychological Association [APA], 2005). His skills as a master diagnostician and therapist have been recognized and are archived in several educational videotaped programs, including *Working With Children With ADHD* (APA, 2005). His research examining the neurophysiological characteristics of children and teens with ADHD, as well as his treatment studies investigating the role of parenting style, school intervention, nutrition, and electroencephalographic biofeedback in the overall care of patients with ADHD, is internationally recognized and has led to several scientific awards, including the President's Award and the Hans Berger Award, bestowed by the Association for Applied Psychophysiology & Biofeedback for his groundbreaking research. He is listed among the innovative researchers recognized in *Reader's Digest*'s 2004 edition of *Medical Breakthroughs*.